T0215671

Contrast Sensitivity

Proceedings of the Retina Research Foundation Symposia

Volume Five

Proceedings of the Retinal Research Foundation Symposia

Contrast Sensitivity

Proceedings of the Retina Research Foundation Symposia

Volume Five

edited by
Robert Shapley and Dominic Man-Kit Lam

A Bradford Book
The MIT Press
Cambridge, Massachusetts
London, England

Proceedings of the Retina Research Foundation Symposia
Volume Five
Contrast Sensitivity

This book was set in Palatino by Asco Trade Typesetting Ltd.

Library of Congress Cataloging-in-Publication Data

Contrast sensitivity / edited by Robert Shapley, Dominic Man-Kit Lam.
     p.   cm. — (Proceedings of the Retina Research Foundation
  Symposia; v. 5)
  "A Bradford book."
  Includes bibliographical references and index.
   ISBN 978-0-262-19339-9 (hc. : alk. paper) — 978-0-262-51940-3 (pb. : alk.. paper)
   1. Contrast sensitivity (Vision)—Congresses. 2. Visual pathways—Congresses.
3. Retinal ganglion cells—Congresses.   I. Shapley, R. M. II. Lam, Dominic Man-Kit.
III. Series: Retina Research Foundation (U.S.). Symposium. Proceedings of the Retina
Research Foundation Symposium; v. 5.
QP479.R469   1988 vol. 5
[RE79.C65]
599'.01823 s—dc20
[152.14]   93-22432
                                                                              CIP

MIT Press is pleased to keep this title available in print by manufacturing single copies, on demand, via digital printing technology.

Contents

Contributors

A. B. Bonds
Department of Electrical Engineering
Vanderbilt University
Nashville, Tennessee

R. K. Brening
Department of Ophthalmology
University of Washington
Seattle, Washington

David R. Copenhagen
Department of Ophthalmology
University of California, San
Francisco
San Francisco, California

M. Carter Cornwall
Department of Physiology
Boston University
Boston, Massachusetts

Karen K. De Valois
Department of Psychology
University of California, Berkeley
Berkeley, California

Russell L. De Valois
Department of Psychology
University of California, Berkeley
Berkeley, California

Don B. Dixon
Department of Ophthalmology
University of California, San
Francisco
San Francisco, California

Christina Enroth-Cugell
Biomedical Engineering Department
Northwestern University
Evanston, Illinois

Gordon L. Fain
Departments of Ophthalmology and
Physiological Science
University of California, Los Angeles
Los Angeles, California

Robert F. Hess
McGill Vision Research Centre
McGill University
Montreal, Quebec, Canada

Ehud Kaplan
The Laboratory of Biophysics
Rockefeller University
New York, New York

Gordon E. Legge
Minnesota Laboratory for
Low-Vision Research
Department of Psychology
University of Minnesota
Minneapolis, Minnesota

Peter Lennie
Center for Visual Science and
Department of Psychology
University of Rochester
Rochester, New York

Peter R. MacLeish
Department of Ophthalmology
Cornell University Medical College
New York, New York

Scott Mittman
Department of Ophthalmology
University of California, San
Francisco
San Francisco, California

Pratik Mukherjee
The Laboratory of Biophysics
Rockefeller University
New York, New York

Ken-ichi Naka
Departments of Ophthalmology and
Physiology and Biophysics
New York University School of
Medicine
New York, New York

Keith Purpura
Department of Neurology
Cornell University Medical College
New York, New York

D. Regan
Department of Ophthalmology
University of Toronto
Toronto, Canada

J. G. Robson
Physiological Laboratory
Cambridge University
Cambridge, England

R. W. Rodieck
Department of Ophthalmology
University of Washington
Seattle, Washington

Hiroko Sakai
Department of Ophthalmology
New York University School of
Medicine
New York, New York

Robert Shapley
Center for Neural Science
New York University
New York, New York

Malcolm M. Slaughter
Department of Biophysical Sciences
State University of New York, Buffalo
Buffalo, New York

W. Rowland Taylor
Department of Ophthalmology
University of California, San Francisco
San Francisco, California

Ning Tian
Department of Biophysical Sciences
State University of New York, Buffalo
Buffalo, New York

J. B. Troy
Biomedical Engineering Department
Northwestern University
Evanston, Illinois

M. Watanabe
Department of Physiology
Institute for Developmental Research
Aichi, Japan

Preface

This book is about how we see the world in terms of contrast. It is also about persistence and continuity in science. The book grew out of the Fifth Annual Retina Research Foundation Symposium, which took place in The Woodlands, Texas, during March 1992. The theme of that meeting was "Contrast Sensitivity from Receptors to Clinic." The meeting was sponsored by the Retina Research Foundation in collaboration with the Alice R. McPherson Laboratory of Retina Research of the Center for Biotechnology, Baylor College of Medicine and The Woodlands Corporation. The symposium included the annual presentation of the W. H. Helmerich III Award, which was given in 1992 to Christina Enroth-Cugell of Northwestern University. The themes of the meeting and the book are closely associated with past and present research interests of Dr. Enroth-Cugell, so this book is a fitting tribute to her influence on retinal neurophysiology and visual perception. Dr. Enroth-Cugell's chapter is a written version of her Helmerich Award Lecture.

The authors of the chapters in this book have attempted to present the state of research in visual signal processing, the retina and central visual pathways, and the study of contrast sensitivity in humans. The field is surveyed from fundamental processes in receptor outer segments all the way to perceptual processes in humans that use information from visual contrast for reading and form discrimination. Possible clinical implications are discussed in the later chapters of the book. Theoretical implications are discussed continuously throughout the volume.

We wish to thank the Retina Research Foundation for supporting the meeting that provided the impetus for this book. We also wish to thank Teddy Woodyard of Baylor College of Medicine, Center for Biotechnology, who assisted us in all phases of this enterprise. We owe additional thanks to Fiona Stevens of The MIT Press, who has done such a fine job bringing the book to an expectant public.

Finally, we would also like to thank Christina Enroth-Cugell for providing the occasion for such an excellent meeting and the subject for what we hope will be a correspondingly good book.

R. S.
D. M.-K. L.

Introduction

The eye, the retina, and the entire visual pathway are concerned with an organism's interaction with the world of light. It is the main theme of this book that a large fraction of that interaction is determined by contrast in the light signal—where *contrast* is another way of saying *relative change*. The sensitivity to contrast is the subject of the book, and most chapters are about either the functional basis or the functional consequences of visual contrast sensitivity.

What I want to address in this introduction is why there is a close association of the investigation of contrast sensitivity with a systems analysis approach to the visual system, and how the nature of the study of contrast sensitivity has been affected by applying the tools of systems analysis to the visual system. This is not a necessary association, but, as often happens in science, is a consequence of the interests and backgrounds of the scientists who investigated contrast sensitivity and how they were influenced by their contemporaries in other scientific fields. Whether necessary or not, there is a definite correlation between the study of contrast sensitivity and the use of sinusoidal gratings or similar sophisticated visual stimuli. Understanding why there is this correlation reveals a lot about the state of vision research now, as well as its future.

The problem of sensitivity of the visual system to contrast arises naturally when one considers the nature of vision and the illuminated world. Vision has to do with reconstructing the nature of the surfaces of objects around the observer. One could consider visual perception as a long-range sense of touch; we use our eyes to "feel" the surfaces we watch. The textures, colors, and shapes of surfaces tell us the nature of the object we are attempting to perceive. It is important to us to know whether these objects are predators or prey; animal, vegetable, mineral. One should also stress the "long-range" aspect of vision. The sooner the observer perceives the nature of the visual surface, the better the chances of the observer's survival. Therefore, the farther away the object can be perceived correctly, the better. Perception at a distance demands high sensitivity to contrast, as will be discussed later.

The visual systems we study evolved in an environment in which reflecting objects were illuminated by the sun. The average value of solar illumination may vary by a factor of more than a million, but the ratio of the amount of light reflected from an object to the amount of light reflected from a reflecting background behind the object is approximately invariant. Therefore, if neural responses and perception were based on relative change, on something like the ratio of the light from an object to the light from its background, then perception would be stable and would not be affected by the vagaries of sunlight and weather. Another way of looking at the visual environment is as a time-varying stimulus that, as the eyes move, sweeps across positions on the retina and thereby drives retinal neurons and their central visual targets. According to this concept, the visual world may have a wide range of average values of illumination. However, the fractional modulation as the retinal image of an object sweeps across a retinal position will be fixed and invariant with changes in the level of illumination. According to this view, the task of visual neurons is to respond to amounts of fractional modulation around a steady level of illumination—to perturbations around an operating point. The name we give to relative modulation, fractional modulation, relative change, and perturbation is *contrast*.

LIGHT AND DARK ADAPTATION

The neural mechanisms that regulate the contrast sensitivity of the retina when is it exposed to significant changes in illumination are called *light adaptation* and *dark adaptation*. Light adaptation is the most important of the two in the context of this book, because it is the process that keeps contrast sensitivity stable under natural operating conditions: the regulation of the gain and time course of retinal response as mean illumination varies. Dark adaptation can be viewed as the recovery of the retina from overload after it is exposed to a light that is too intense for light adaptation to regulate successfully. It is the slow recovery of dark-adapted retinal sensitivity after very intense illumination. The relation between light and dark adaptation is treated in chapter 1 by Gordon Fain and M. Carter Cornwall.

This is a subject that has interested visual physiologists and psychophysicists for a long time. The functional consequences of light adaptation for vision are mentioned in my chapter in this book with Ehud Kaplan and Keith Purpura (chapter 2), which follows lines of argument that Christina Enroth-Cugell and I advanced in our 1984 review paper on retinal adaptation (Shapley and Enroth-Cugell, 1984). It is also of interest that our recent work indicates that an important site of light adaptation is in cone photoreceptors. This is not a new idea, but it is now supported with novel evidence about response time course. In our 1984 paper, Dr. Enroth-Cugell and I concluded that there had to be hierarchical light adaptation processes because of the existence of parallel and multiple retinal pathways of signal processing. It is clear that the functional importance of light adaptation is the preservation of high levels of contrast sensitivity at high levels of illumination where vision's dependence on contrast is greatest.

While the retinal mechanisms for light adaptation are still somewhat mysterious, there has been a lot of progress recently in the study of the functional organization of the retina. In particular, the study of neurotransmission has yielded some elegant results, which are described and discussed in this book by D. Copenhagen, S. Mittman, W. R. Taylor, and D. B. Dixon (in chapter 3), as well as by M. Slaughter and N. Tian in chapter 4.

CONTRAST SENSITIVITY

Human contrast sensitivity is prodigious and in fact strains the capabilities of electronic display devices including television and computer graphics displays. The optimum human performance for detecting a static black/white border is a contrast threshold of less than 1 percent change in modulation across the border. In tasks involving color or motion detection we may be able to perform even better than in the detection of a static black/white border. Though the visual system can respond over an enormous range of operating points, its response range around any single operating point is limited by the nature of neural signal processing. However, this range limitation is not a severe constraint in vision because the range of contrasts in the natural world is also limited. We can detect very low levels of contrast, yet we are rarely overwhelmed by saturating levels of contrast. The neural mechanisms that produce prodigious contrast sensitivity, yet also protect us from saturation and overload, are *light adaptation*, described above, and cortical contrast gain control, which is discussed in chapter 12 by A. B. Bonds.

Now we are at a point at which we can consider why the physics of light and objects, and the consequent importance of contrast, attracted the interest of scientists who studied the nervous system as a physical communication system. The study of a system driven by small perturbations around an operating point is a well-analyzed area of systems analysis and usually leads to a linear analysis in the small signal regime. The beauty of linear systems analysis is its clarity and simplicity: from a finite, basic set of measurements, one can predict the linear system's response to any stimulus one might imagine (as long as it lies within the linear range of operation). Thus, one can understand a linear system completely. Furthermore, there are lexicons of linear systems with particular structures: serial cascades, parallel channels, negative feedback circuits, or damped oscillators. This means that, if one can fit the behavior of a measured system with an analytic function, one has a reasonable chance of inferring the underlying connectivity or functional sequence that produces the behavior, or at least its functional equivalent, by looking it up in the linear systems dictionary. In the case of the visual system, this linear approach has been used to characterize visual neural networks in the retinas of cats and monkeys, the eyes of horseshoe crabs, and the mammalian visual cortex, not to mention its use to describe of the human observer at threshold.

Many of the pioneers of linear systems analysis as it has been applied to vision are represented in this book: Robert Rodieck, John Robson, Christina Enroth-Cugell, and Karen and Russell De Valois. My own training in the laboratory of Hartline and Ratliff, along with the elegant work of Bruce Knight and colleagues (Knight, Toyoda, and Dodge 1970) directed me to this point of view also, and the influence of those pioneers has pervaded my own thinking, as can be seen in chapter 7, which I wrote with Kaplan and Purpura.

Linear Systems and Receptive Fields

It is useful to consider the relationship, which is close to equivalence, between a linear systems approach to visual signal processing and the classical receptive field approach that Hartline introduced into visual neuroscience following Sherringtonian principles. The receptive field of a visual neuron is that region of visual space that maps onto the neuron. Quantitatively, for linear visual neurons one may describe this spatial summation using the spatial sensitivity distribution. This function, introduced by Rodieck in his analysis of the receptive fields of cat retinal ganglion cells, is the visual, neural analogue of the pointspread function of an optical system. The spatial description or representation of a neuron's receptive field has a direct equivalent in the spatial frequency domain: the spatial frequency sensitivity function or, as it is usually called, the *contrast sensitivity function*. Both qualitatively and quantitatively these two functions—spatial sensitivity and spatial frequency sensitivity— are a paired description, in the two domains of space and spatial frequency, of

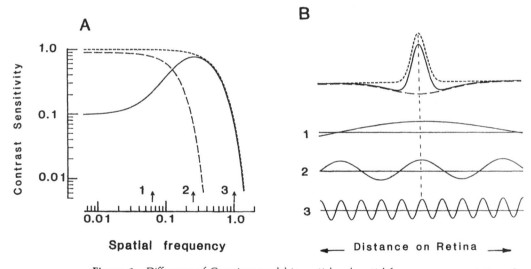

Figure 1 Difference of Gaussians model in spatial and spatial frequency representations. In (A) are shown the contrast sensitivity (spatial frequency response) curves for a center Gaussian (small dashes), for a surround Gaussian (larger dashes), and for a difference of Gaussians model (continuous curve). In (B) the same functions are depicted in a spatial representation. The difference of Gaussians spatial profile is the continuous curve in (B). Contrast sensitivity and spatial frequency are given in relative units here. In neurophysiological experiments, contrast sensitivity is usually defined as the reciprocal of the contrast required to produce a criterion, usually small, response. In the lower part of (B) are shown three sinusoidal grating waveforms that could be used to measure the spatial frequency response of a neuron. The corresponding spatial frequencies are indicated in (A) by the numbered arrows. (Modified from Enroth-Cugell and Robson 1984)

the same physical phenomenon, namely neuronal convergence and spatial summation.

The characteristic features of these two functions, illustrated in figure 1 (modified from the Friedenwald lecture of Enroth-Cugell and Robson 1984), teach us about the functional implications of signal processing in even the simplest linear neurons. For instance, the spatial spread of the spatial sensitivity function is a measure of the amount of neuronal convergence. Correspondingly, the spatial frequency cutoff at high spatial frequency is a measure of the same convergence. For particular mathematical models, there is a direct analytical relationship between spatial spread and spatial frequency cutoff. For example, in the well-known Difference of Gaussians (DOG) model shown in figure 1, the spatial spread and spatial frequency cutoff are reciprocals. Furthermore, both spatial spread and spatial frequency cutoff tell us about the range of resolution of the neuron—to how small an object it can respond and how fine a pattern it can resolve.

In this way we can analyze how the properties of convergence limit our ability to see infinitely far away, because adding signals from many receptors causes limitations on resolution and therefore on the distance range over which details of objects can be discriminated from the uniform background. In this way we can also understand how higher amplification of signal compared to noise and therefore higher contrast sensitivity will elevate the contrast sensitivity function and allow for better resolution. These considerations are the basis for a critical understanding of what limits our ability to recognize targets at a distance, a subject mentioned near the beginning of this essay.

Nonlinear Systems

We have seen that the natural description of linear visual neurons in terms of linear systems leads naturally to the use of sine gratings as spatial stimuli and to the description of spatial summation in terms of responses to sine gratings. However, sinusoidal stimuli are not the only tools of systems analysis, and many interesting neural networks cannot be approximated by linear systems. The famous Y-type cat retinal ganglion cells discovered by Enroth-Cugell and Robson are a good example of visual neurons fed by an essentially nonlinear network. There are many other ways besides linear systems analysis with sine waves to study neural networks and neurons these days, some of which are described in this book. For instance, Panos Marmarells and Ken Naka introduced the use of "white noise analysis" to characterize nonlinear retinal networks based on theories of nonlinear system identification devised by Norbert Wiener. Other techniques along this line include the sum-of-sinusoids approach developed by Jonathan Victor and the maximal-length-shift-register-sequence, or "m-sequence," method crafted by Erich Sutter. These and other nonlinear systems identification approaches are necessary for a complete and accurate study of many naturally occurring neural networks that have nonlinear stages as part of their basic signal-processing paths.

SPATIOTEMPORAL INTERACTIONS

We should realize that spatiotemporal interactions are tremendously important in both linear and nonlinear neural networks, particularly in the visual system. For instance, the understanding of visual motion detection and discrimination depends on a full spatiotemporal analysis. While above I have emphasized spatial systems analysis for the sake of simplicity, the interested reader should be aware that the application of systems techniques to temporal signal processing and temporal filtering is also an important area of vision research. In fact, the winner of the 1992 Helmerich Award from the Retina Research Foundation, Dr. Christina Enroth-Cugell, has throughout her career studied the nature and source of the time course of response of retinal ganglion cells. The determinants of the temporal properties of vision include temporal integration in photoreceptors, temporal filtering in the retina and the lateral geniculate nucleus (LGN), conduction delays between the retina and the LGN and between the LGN and the cerebral cortex, and filtering and time delays in the neural networks within the cortex. These issues are discussed in several chapters in this book. For example, my chapter with Ehud Kaplan and Keith Purpura (chapter 7) is about the change of time course of response with light adaptation and how this implies that cone photoreceptor adaptation may play a large part in regulating contrast sensitivity in the primate retina. The chapter by Kaplan, Pratik, Mukherjee and me (chapter 10) also deals with changes in dynamics, this time in relation to changes of information flow through the lateral geniculate nucleus.

PARALLEL PATHWAYS

One area of the study of visual information processing has emerged from attention to contrast sensitivity, namely *parallel retinocortical channels*. Initially there was a focus on X and Y cat retinal ganglion cells that grew out of the discoveries described in the Enroth-Cugell and Robson (1966) paper. More recently, there has been a lot of interest in the P (parvocellular-projecting) and M (magnocellular-projecting) pathways in primates, and in particular the contrast sensitivity of neurons in the different parallel pathways.

I believe it is important to understand that the distinction between X and Y cells, from which all this work issued, was fundamentally based on the linearity of signal summation within a neural network. The distinction was initially based on whether a ganglion cell's mean discharge rate was increased or invariant with the presentation of a drifting grating pattern. The Y cells were those retinal ganglion cells that fired impulses more rapidly when a pattern was drifting across the retina than when they viewed a blank, evenly illuminated field. The X cells were those cells that kept an even pace of average impulse firing whether the pattern was drifting or the viewing field was blank.

This distinction is a test of the superposition of DC, in other words average, light-evoked neural signals, with time-varying signals. In a sense it is the simplest test of superposition one could imagine. A system that obeys superposition, a linear system, will keep its average output the same independent of the presence, or changes in amplitude, of time-varying signals. This simplest, very elegant test was the forerunner of all the linear/nonlinear systems analysis that was aimed at X and Y cells later. It was a natural test of neural networks if one was thinking of them as physical communication networks. According to my arguments above, therefore, the initial discovery of parallel retinocortical pathways in cat retinal ganglion cells was a natural consequence of considerations of the retina as a processor of contrast and as a physical communication system.

The importance of contrast to the understanding of primate P and M pathways is more subtle. Based on the relative size of the receptive field, relative conduction velocity, and time course of response, several authors have attempted to make a functional analogy between primate P cells and cat X cells and between primate M cells and cat Y cells. In my opinion, this idea is wrong for a number of reasons, which are elaborated in detail elsewhere (for example, in Shapley and Perry 1986). For one thing, it leaves out the big issue of color sensitivity and selectivity. P cells seem designed to be sensitive and selective for color, and in this way they are not like color-blind cat X cells at all.

Furthermore—and this is where this subject connects with contrast—the contrast gain {slope of response vs. contrast curve in the limit of low contrast} is much lower for P cells than for X cells when achromatic patterns are used as stimuli. Recently other researchers and I have found that the lower achromatic contrast gain in P cells is directly related to their color sensitivity. Thus, from the point of view of contrast sensitivity of the neurons, P cells and X cells are designed to be very functionally dissimilar. It is remarkable, however, that the contrast gains of primate M cells and cat X cells are quite similar. This is illustrated by figure 2 (from work by Ehud Kaplan and me), which shows response vs. contrast functions for a cat X ganglion cell, a macaque M cell, and a macaque P cell.

The link between cellular contrast sensitivity and behavioral contrast sensitivity remains problematical. Based mainly on the lesion evidence of Merigan and colleagues, it seems that detection of static achromatic grating patterns depends more on the integrity of the P cell pathway than on that of the M cell pathway, even though individual P cells may be almost a log unit less sensitive to contrast than individual M cells. The explanation offered, for instance by Peter Lennie in chapter 11 this book, is that there must be some way of pooling signals from P cells to enable them to support behavioral contrast sensitivity. Finding such sites of pooling of P-pathway signals would support such an hypothesis. Another possible explanation is that so far the lesion experiments for technical reasons have probed contrast sensitivity in the peripheral visual field, where it is quite poor—so poor that it might be supported by the contrast sensitivity of peripheral P cells. It is a puzzle why the more contrast-sensitive M cells do not contribute to detection in the visual field periphery, since the brain seems to be throwing away information from

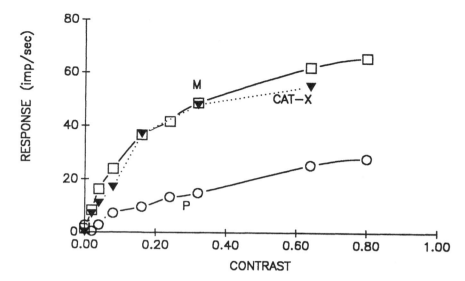

Figure 2 Response vs. contrast for retinal ganglion cells of the cat and monkey. Data from a P cell circles) and from an M cell (squares) from one monkey are plotted as amplitude of response vs. contrast of a drifting optimal grating stimulus. Also shown are data from a cat X cell (filled triangles and dotted line). These data are typical. The experiment was done under midphotopic conditions (approximately 1000 td) with achromatic gratings drifting at around 4 Hz temporal frequency.

M cells it could use for detection. In my view, this is an area in which more research is needed in the future to clarify what seems cloudy today.

The area of parallel processing is heavily represented in this book. Peter Lennie considers the question of P and M pathway function explicitly in chapter 11. In chapter 8 R. W. Rodieck, R. K. Brening, and M. Watanabe deal with the anatomical substrate of parallel processing in the retina. J. B. Troy has written chapter 6 about receptive field models of different classes of retinal ganglion cells in the cat. The idea of parallel channels for information flow is intrinsic to the discussion of labeled lines for color and and pattern in chapter 13 by Karen and Russell DeValois. In chapters 15–17 on the assessment of human visual performance, Gordon Legge, Robert Hess, and D. Martin Regan, respectively, employ the concept of parallel channels in their studies of contrast processing in the human retina and brain.

IMAGE PROCESSING

The success of the systems approach and the use of contrast sensitivity measurements should not distract us from the enormous gaps in our understanding of visual perception and the neural basis for perception. In general, I feel that scientific texts and volumes like this one tend to put too much emphasis on what we understand and have done rather than highlighting what we do not understand now and how we might proceed. This last section of the introduction is an attempted corrective, for this book at least.

One important question that we cannot answer here and now is how the shape of a visual object is represented in the brain. Related to this is the question of how we remember shapes and use these memories to recognize a newly presented object as familiar. Thus far the systems approach has been applied microscopically to single-cell activity. Many attempts to enlarge the scope of systems techniques to neural ensembles are in the early stages of development, and these may help crack the problem of shape. However, there has been psychophysical work in the area of so-called "higher-level" vision that suggests that a simple extension of systems techniques upwards or outwards will not be sufficient. Therefore, there may be a need to find the neural basis for shape primitives—what Julesz calls "textons" or what other might call features—and how these featural elements interact may be crucial for shape representation.

Rather than a version of the visual image that has been filtered through an array of passive linear and nonlinear spatiotemporal filters, the representation of shape in the brain may instead depend on the correlated and patterned activity of feature detectors wired to extract some global aspects of form. The nature of this correlation or of the patterned activity is unclear, and this is where I feel new methods and new ideas are most needed—to understand how image processing is done.

Possibly symmetry, aspect ratio, smoothness, or compactness are global descriptors that emerge from such image processing based on as yet poorly understood interactions between local feature detectors. Then the collection of global descriptors may be just the form representation. Alternatively, there may be an intermediate representation of groups of features as intermediate-level object primitives: the "geons" of Irving Biederman. Another idea is that local features are combined to extract visual surfaces or planes at different apparent depths from the observer and that spatiotemporal image processing is confined within these extracted surfaces or planes. My presentation of these ideas is speculative, without a clear path to a theory. I offer them here not as correct ideas, but as examples of the kind of thinking that may be required for us to progress toward an understanding of perception.

I must finish this introduction by stating, first, that the opinions contained in it are my own, and none of the other authors in the book are responsible for what is written above; and in fact, I am sure some contributors would take issue with some of my controversial points. Second, it was a pleasure to take part in the Retina Research Foundation Symposium in March 1992, which gave birth to this volume. It was a particular pleasure because the symposium honored Christina Enroth-Cugell, who is one of the finest people in vision research. Let me thank Dominic Lam, who had the idea to organize the symposium and to write this book, and who has cooperated in editing this volume. Finally, the authors did a splendid job with their chapters, and I hope that readers will enjoy and study the book because of them.

Robert Shapley

REFERENCES

Enroth-Cugell, C., and Robson, J. G. (1966) The contrast sensitivity of retinal ganglion cells of the cat. J. Physiol. 187: 517–552.

Enroth-Cugell, C., and Robson, J. G. (1984) Functional characteristics and diversity of cat retinal ganglion cells. Investigative Ophthalmology 25, 250–267.

Knight, B. W., Dodge, F. A., and Toyoda, J. I. (1970) A quantitative description of the dynamics of excitation and inhibition in the eye of *Limulus*. J. Gen. Physiol. 56, 421–437.

Shapley, R., and Enroth-Cugell, C. (1984) Visual adaptation and retinal gain controls. In N. Osborne and G. Chader, eds. Progress in Retinal Research, vol. 3, pp. 263–346. London: Pergamon.

Shapley, R., and Perry, V. H. (1986) Cat and monkey retinal ganglion cells and their visual functional roles. Trends in Neurosciences 9, 229–235.

I Retinal Processing of Visual Signals

In this section the machinery of the retina is described and analyzed. The basis for response dependence on contrast is the neural network of the retina, so this section lays the groundwork for the phenomena studied throughout the volume.

Gordon Fain and Carter Cornwall have studied the cellular mechanisms of light and dark adaptation in photoreceptors. Their elegant work revives the concept of the *equivalent background* produced by bleached photopigment. Peter MacLeish provides novel and impressive evidence of functional specialization within single cone photoreceptors of the monkey retina using the powerful new technique of calcium imaging. The chapter by David Copenhagen and his colleagues, Scott Mittman, W. Rowland Taylor, and Don B. Dixon, describes the latest work on the effect of glutamate receptors on retinal neurons and the role they might play in dynamic signal processing. Malcolm Slaughter and Ning Tian describe their research on GABA receptors in the retina and how they might function to control retinal signal processing. The retinal processing section concludes with an analytical essay by Ken Naka and Hiroko Sakai about the possibility of analyzing signal processing in a nervous system that resembles our own.

1 Light and Dark Adaptation in Vertebrate Photoreceptors

Gordon L. Fain and M. Carter Cornwall

The bleaching of pigment molecules by light in a vertebrate photoreceptor activates a cascade of biochemical reactions which ultimately leads to a change in conductance in the outer segment membrane of the rod or cone (see Stryer 1986, 1988). Extensive investigation during the last two decades has shown that the activated form of rhodopsin (meta II or R^*) binds the G-protein transducin, causing the exchange of GTP for GDP on the transducin α subunit (T_α). The activated T_α's then bind to and remove the γ inhibitory subunits of the cyclic GMP phosphodiesterase (PDE). The removal of these subunits greatly increases the hydrolytic rate of the PDE, and the increased hydrolysis of cGMP by the PDE causes the concentration of cGMP in the outer segment to decrease.

The outer segment plasma membranes of rods and cones contain specialized channels permeable to monovalent and divalent cations which are opened by binding to intracellular cGMP (Yau and Baylor 1989; Kaupp 1991). The intracellular concentration of free cGMP in darkness in a rod is normally 5–10 μM (see Pugh and Lamb 1990), and the probability of channel opening in darkness is estimated to be only 0.01–0.02 (Nakatani and Yau 1988a). However, this is sufficient to produce a standing inward current of 30–50 pA flowing into the outer segment, carried predominantly by Na^+ and Ca^{2+}, which maintains the membrane potential of the rod or cone at the rather depolarized value of -30 to -35 mV. The light-induced decrease in cGMP by the PDE reduces the probability of channel opening, the channels close, the circulating current decreases, and the photoreceptor hyperpolarizes.

In addition to triggering this excitatory cascade, light also sets in motion a sequence of events that modulate transduction (Fain and Matthews 1990). We shall refer to these events collectively as *adaptation*. We shall distinguish two forms: the steady-state decrease in sensitivity produced by steady background light, which we shall call *light adaptation* or *background adaptation*; and the decrease and subsequent recovery of sensitivity that occur after exposure to light that is strong enough to bleach a significant percentage (> 1 percent) of the visual pigment, which we shall refer to as *dark adaptation* or *bleaching adaptation*. The distinction between these two forms of adaptation is in some respects arbitrary, since background lights, if they are bright enough, can bleach a significant fraction of the photopigment, and the desensitization produced by bleaches seems similar in many respects to that produced by backgrounds. Nevertheless, it is convenient to discuss these two forms of adaptation separately, since they emerge from two distinct experimental protocols for investigating the modulation of excitation, which have formed the basis of considerable previous investigation.

LIGHT ADAPTATION

When a rod or cone is exposed to steady background illumination, the sensitivity of the photoreceptor decreases (Kleinschmidt and Dowling 1975; Fain 1976). This can be seen in figure 1.1, which shows recordings from a rod of the salamander *Ambystoma tigrinum* that have been made with the suction pipette method (Baylor, Lamb, and Yau 1979a; Schnapf and McBurney 1980). The stimulus marker at the top of the figure shows the duration of presentation of a background light and the timing and intensity of brief flashes superimposed upon the background. In the first trace, marked dark, there was no background, and the response amplitude increased with flash intensity according to the dark-adapted response-intensity function of the receptor. In the two traces below, the background intensities were 0.24 and 1.57 photons $\mu m^{-2} s^{-1}$, and the background light produced a steady decrease in the amplitude of the circulating current. When flashes at the same intensities as for the dark-adapted receptor were superimposed upon the background, additional transient decreases in circulating current were observed.

As the background intensity increased, progressively brighter flashes were needed to produce changes in current of the same amplitude. Thus the *sensitivity*, or change in current per unit light intensity, became smaller as the background was made brighter. For both rods and cones sensitivity has been shown to decline approximately proportionally to background intensity according to the Weber-Fechner Law,

$$S_F/S_F^D = (1 + I_B/I_o)^{-1} \tag{1.1}$$

where S_F is the flash sensitivity, S_F^D is the flash sensitivity in darkness, I_B is the background intensity, and I_o is a constant often referred to as the *dark light* (see figure 1.6B and Fain and Matthews 1990; Pugh and Lamb 1990). I_o is only a few pigment molecules bleached per receptor per second for rods (Bastian and Fain 1979) but is orders of magnitude larger for cones (see for example Matthews, Fain, Murphy, and Lamb 1990).

Figure 1.1 also shows that, in the presence of background light, the whole response-intensity function moves to brighter flash intensities. This can be seen more clearly in figure 1.2, which plots for a different rod from the same species the response-intensity functions for flashes in darkness and in the presence of seven background intensities. The data points give the peak change in photocurrent as a function of flash intensity. As the background is made brighter, the response-intensity curve moves to the right, toward higher flash intensities. In addition, the maximum amplitude of the receptor response to flashes decreases. This is a trivial consequence of the steady response

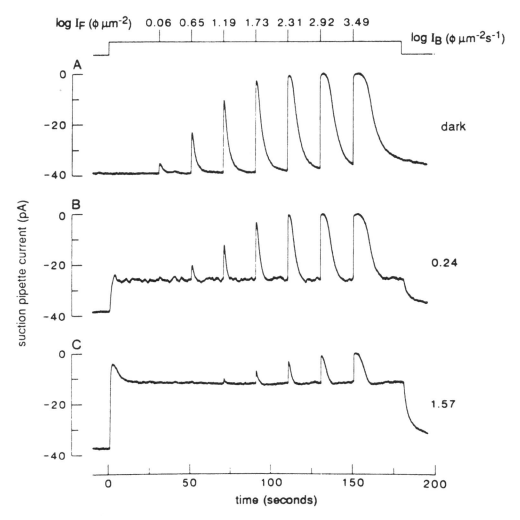

Figure 1.1 Responses of salamander rod to flashes of light of increasing intensity in darkness (A) and in the presence of background illumination of two different intensities (B and C). Currents were recorded using the suction pipette technique (Baylor et al. 1979; Schnapf and McBurney 1980) from a single rod isolated by mechanical disruption from a dark-adapted retina. Methods for recording and optical stimulation are as in Lamb et al. 1986. Flashes were 20 msec long at 500 nm. Flash intensities were the same for (A–C) and are given at the top of the figure adjacent to the stimulus indications in units of photons (ϕ) μm^{-2}. Background intensities (at 500 nm) are given to the right of the traces in units of photons μm^{-2} s^{-1}. (Reprinted with permission from Matthews 1990)

Fain & Cornwall: Light and Dark Adaptation

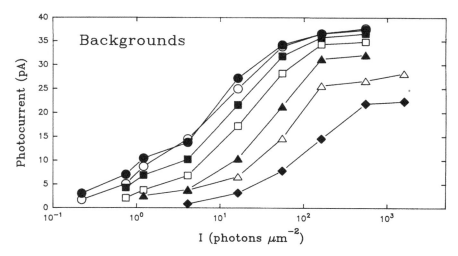

Figure 1.2 Response-intensity curves for salamander rod in darkness and in background light. The ordinate gives the photocurrent response, measured using the suction electrode technique, to brief (20 msec) flashes of 520-nm light. Responses are measured relative to the steady-state current in the presence of background illumination. Symbols indicate peak amplitude of response in darkness (filled circles) and in the presence of continuous 520-nm illumination of the following intensities (in photons $\mu m^{-2} s^{-1}$): 0.042 (open circles), 0.16 (filled squares), 0.52 (open squares), 1.8 (filled triangles), 5.8 (open triangles), and 20 (diamonds). Test and background beams were calibrated as in Cornwall et al. (1990). Light intensities in units of photons μm^{-2} can be converted to Rh* per photoreceptor by multiplying by a collecting area of approximately 20 μm^2 (Lamb et al. 1986).

produced by the background (see figure 1.1), since the brighter the background, the smaller the circulating current available to be decreased by superimposed flashes.

The movement of the response-intensity function is one of the mechanisms responsible for adjusting the operating range of the visual system as the ambient light intensity changes (Walraven et al. 1990). For our purposes, the significance of the results in figures 1.1 and 1.2 is that they show that much of the shifting of the operating range occurs at the first stage of visual processing, within the photoreceptors themselves. Similar results have been obtained from both rods and cones in a variety of species (see Fain and Matthews 1990; Pugh and Lamb 1990), including mammals (Tamura, Nakatani, and Yau 1989, 1991; Matthews, 1990a).

Acceleration of Response Decay

Fuortes and Hodgkin (1964) first suggested for the horseshoe crab *Limulus polyphemus* that changes in photoreceptor sensitivity might be intimately related to changes in response waveform. Background light produces a pronounced quickening of the receptor response, in *Limulus* and in vertebrates, which is probably in large part responsible for the well-known increase in temporal resolution produced by increases in ambient light intensity. Fuortes and Hodgkin proposed that the changes in sensitivity and changes in waveform might be manifestations of the same processes, which compress the time scale of excitation.

For vertebrate photoreceptors, the predominant effect of backgrounds on receptor waveform is to quicken the time course of decay (Baylor and Hodgkin 1974). We illustrate this for salamander rods in figure 1.3 (see also Fain, Lamb, Matthews, and Murphy 1989). In part A we have plotted small-amplitude responses recorded from a rod in darkness and in several background intensities. The responses have been plotted per unit flash intensity—that is, in units of sensitivity. The reason for doing this is to permit comparison of the waveforms of responses produced in different backgrounds by flashes of different intensities. Since small-amplitude receptor responses are nearly linear, dividing by the flash intensity is nearly equivalent to normalizing responses to the same flash intensity of 1 photon per μm^2.

The results in figure 1.3A show that, as the intensity of the background is increased, the peak amplitude of the sensitivity decreases, as we have previously observed. Notice, however, that the change in sensitivity is accompanied by a characteristic alteration in the response waveform. The intial phase of the response is nearly the same, even for fairly large changes in sensitivity. This would suggest that the rates of the initial stages in the enzymatic cascade from rhodopsin bleaching to PDE hydrolysis are unaffected by background light (Torre, Matthews, and Lamb 1986). What is changed is the time course of decay: as the background intensity increases, the responses decay more and more quickly. This can also be seen in part B, for which three of the responses in part A have been normalized to the same peak amplitude to facilitate the comparison of the response waveforms.

Baylor and Hodgkin (1974) first suggested that this acceleration of decay is the basic mechanism responsible for the change in sensitivity during light adaptation. Some process seems to be activated after a delay, which brings the flash response back to the baseline at a rate which becomes faster and faster the brighter the ambient intensity. This accelerating decay "cuts off" the response more and more quickly, so that peak amplitude and thus the sensitivity decrease in background light.

A Role for Ca^{2+} in Light Adaptation

The evidence that changes in time course of decay and photoreceptor sensitivity are intimately related has been greatly strengthened by the discovery that both are regulated by changes in intracellular Ca^{2+} (Matthews, Murphy, Fain, and Lamb 1988; Nakatani and Yau 1988b; Fain et al. 1989; Matthews et al. 1990). About 10–15 percent of the dark current is normally carried by Ca^{2+} (Yau and Baylor 1989), and in the salamander this amounts to about 10^7 Ca^{2+} entering the rod per second. This Ca^{2+} is extruded by a $Na^+/(Ca^{2+}, K^+)$ counter-transport system (Cervetto, Lagnado, Perry, Robinson, and McNaughton 1989), which is present in the outer segment

Backgrounds

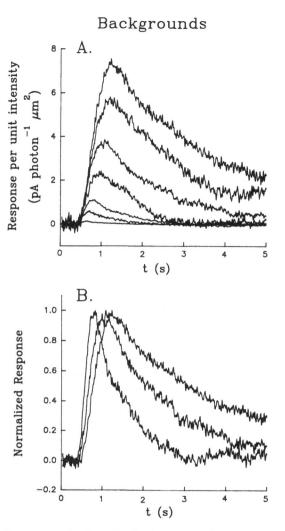

Figure 1.3 Small-amplitude responses of salamander rod in darkness and in background light. (A) Responses to brief (20 msec) 520-nm flashes plotted as sensitivities (response amplitude divided by light intensity) recorded in darkness and in the presence of background illumination. The largest response was recorded in darkness, and sensitivity then decreased systematically as background intensity was increased. Background intensities (520 nm) were as follows (in photons μm^{-2} s^{-1}): 0.042, 0.16, 0.52, 1.8, 5.8, and 20. Flash intensities (from largest sensitivity to smallest) were as follows (in photons μm^{-2}): 0.75, 0.75, 1.21, 1.21, 4.09, 4.09, and 16.3. Peak amplitude of flash responses in these backgrounds at these flash intensities as fractions of the maximum peak amplitude of flash response in the same background (i/i_{max}) were as follows: 0.21, 0.18, 0.19, 0.14, 0.25, 0.16, 0.20. (B) Same responses as in (A) but normalized to a common peak amplitude of 1.0. The response decaying most slowly was recorded in darkness, intermediate response, in 0.16 photons μm^{-2} s^{-1} background, and most rapidly decaying response, in 1.8 photons μm^{-2} s^{-1} background. Flash intensities were 0.75, 1.21, and 4.09 photons μm^{-2}, respectively. The methods used to record and calibrate the light intensities were as in figure 1.2.

membrane (Reid, Friedel, Molday, and Cook 1990). Since light reduces the dark current but has no direct effect on the counter-transporter (Nakatani and Yau 1988a), the concentration of free Ca^{2+} in the outer segment would be expected to decrease during illumination, and this has been demonstrated by direct measurement (McNaughton, Cervetto, and Nunn 1986; Ratto, Payne, Owen, and Tsien 1988).

There is considerable evidence that the intracellular concentration of Ca^{2+} regulates the time course of response decay. This has been shown by retarding the light-induced change in Ca^{2+} either (1) by introducing Ca^{2+} buffers such as BAPTA (Torre et al. 1986) and Quin (Korenbrot and Miller 1986) into the receptor cytosol or (2) by minimizing Ca^{2+} influx and efflux across the plasma membrane (Matthews et al. 1988; Nakatani and Yau 1988b). The effects of these two treatments on the rod photocurrent are illustrated in figure 1.4. Part A shows what happens after BAPTA incorporation. The decay of the response is greatly prolonged, as if buffering Ca^{2+} prevented or greatly slowed the activation of a process normally responsible for bringing the current back to its dark-adapted level.

Part B of figure 1.4 shows the effect of minimizing the influx and efflux of Ca^{2+}. Influx was decreased by reducing the extracellular concentration of Ca^{2+} from 1–2 mM to 1–3 μM. Efflux was simultaneously minimized by replacing Na^+ in the extracellular medium with guanidium$^+$, which permeates the light-sensitive conductance but cannot substitute for Na^+ in $Na^+/(Ca^{2+}, K^+)$ exchange. Similar results have been obtained when Na^+ was substituted with Li^+ (Fain et al. 1989). Li^+ and guanidium$^+$ produce a circulating current that is suppressed by illumination, but the transport of Ca^{2+} out of the rod is greatly inhibited. The effect of minimizing both the influx and efflux of Ca^{2+} on the response waveform is nearly identical to that of BAPTA incorporation.

Treatments that minimize changes in intracellular Ca^{2+} also abolish light adaptation, as illustrated in figure 1.5 (Nakatani and Yau 1988b; Fain et al. 1989). Part A compares responses in a dark-adapted cell to brief flashes in Ringer solution (labeled R) and in a low-Ca^{2+} guanidinium solution like that used for the experiments of figure 1.4B. Once again we see that slowing changes in Ca^{2+} greatly retards the time course of decay. In the other two parts of this figure we show responses of the same rod to prolonged steps of background illumination in Ringer solution (part B) and in the low-Ca^{2+} guanidinium solution (part C). The noisier traces are the actual recorded responses. The smooth curves give the waveforms predicted if the responses to steps were a simple, linear summation of the responses to flashes.

To construct these curves, the responses to the flashes in part A were scaled by the ratio of step and flash intensities and by the integration time of the cell, and they were then integrated over the duration of the step response (see Fain et al. 1989 for details). In Ringer solution, the results of these calculations give a satisfactory fit to the recorded responses at early times, but the responses soon sag below the predictions. This is not too surprising since the onset of

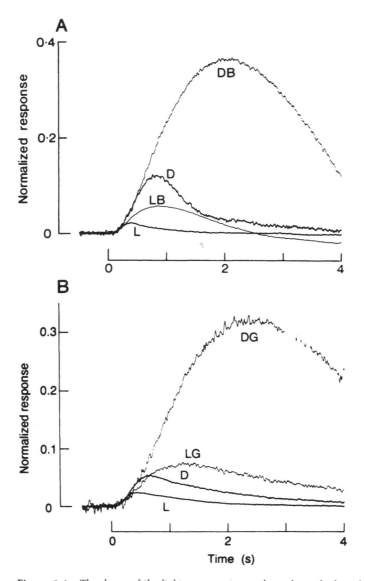

Figure 1.4 The decay of the light response is greatly prolonged when changes in Ca^{2+} are inhibited. Responses are plotted as sensitivities (as in figure 1.3A) and have been normalized to the value of the circulating current. The methods of recording and optical stimulation were as in figure 1.1. (A) Responses to flashes before and after the incorporation of the Ca^{2+} chelator BAPTA from a patch pipette. Trace D, dark-adapted control, trace L, light-adapted control, traces DB and DL are after BAPTA incorporation. The flash intensities (500 nm) were 0.85 (D, DB) and 6.5 (L, LB) photons μm^{-2}, and the background for L and LB was 17 photons μm^{-2} s^{-1} (500 nm).(B) Flash responses in Ringer solution and in low-Ca^{2+}/zero-Na^{+} solution. The $[Ca^{2+}]_0$ was 3 μM, and Na^{+} was replaced with guanidinium^{+}. Traces D and L are dark-adapted and light-adapted responses in Ringer solution, and DG and LG are similar responses in the low-Ca^{2+}/zero-Na^{+} solution. The steady 500-nm background light for L and LG was 2.4 photons μm^{-2} s^{-1}, and the 500-nm flash intensities (in photons μm^{-2}) were D, 1.2; DG, 0.56; L, 4.5; and LG, 2.2. (Reprinted with permission from Fain and Matthews 1990)

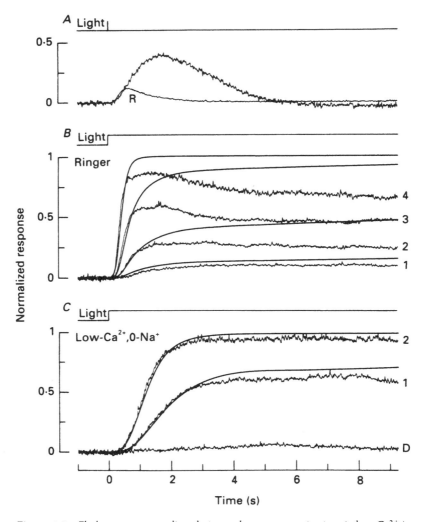

Figure 1.5 Flash responses sum linearly to produce responses to steps in low-Ca^{2+}/zero-Na^+ solution but not in Ringer solution. (A) Flash responses normalized to the value of the circulating current in Ringer solution (R) and in low-Ca^{2+}/zero-Na^+ solution, recorded from the same salamander rod. The methods of recording and light stimulation are as in figure 1.1. The upper trace indicates the timing of a 500-nm, 20-msec flash of intensity 2.8 photons μm^{-2}. (B) Step responses from the same rod as in (A) recorded in Ringer solution (noisy traces), as well as predictions of step responses calculated from linear summation of response to flash in Ringer solution (smooth traces). Responses to flashes were scaled by the ratio of step and flash intensities and by the integration time of the cell, and they were then integrated over the duration of the step response with correction for response compression (see Fain et al. 1989).(C) Same as for (B) but in low-Ca^{2+}/zero-Na^+ solution. The responses are from the same rod as in (A) and (B). Traces at the top of (B) and (C) give the timing of step illuminations at intensities (in photons μm^{-2} s^{-1}) indicated by the numerals to the right of the traces: D, darkness; 1, 2.4; 2, 9.1; 3, 37; and 4, 140. (Reprinted with permission from Fain et al. 1989)

light adaptation produces a time-dependent decrease in the sensitivity of the response, which is reflected by the decrease in the photocurrent. What is surprising is that in low-Ca^{2+} guanidinium solution, the responses agree much more closely. It is as if the photoreceptor in this solution were summing photons with a sensitivity which did not change during the presentation of the background. The results in figure 1.5 are from a rod, but similar results have also been obtained from cones (Nakatani Yau 1988b; Matthews et al. 1990).

The data in figure 1.6 provide another demonstration that light adaptation is suppressed when changes in Ca^{2+} concentration are minimized (Matthews et al. 1990). This time we show results from cones (for a similar experiment with rods, see Matthews et al. 1988). In part A we show the response-intensity functions of several receptors in Ringer solution (filled symbols) and in low-Ca^{2+}, zero-Na^+ solution (open symbols) for steady-state responses to background steps. Each symbol type gives results from a different cell. In Ringer, the slope of the relation for steps of light is quite shallow, much shallower than similar relations for flashes (see figure 1.2). The reason for this is that steps of light are sufficiently prolonged to trigger the time-dependent onset of light adaptation, which produces a sag in the response (see figure 1.5B). This produces a decrease in the steady-state amplitude that becomes increasingly pronounced as the step intensity is increased. A similar effect occurs to some extent even during responses to brief flashes, but it becomes more pronounced the longer the duration of the stimulus.

In low-Ca^{2+}, zero-Na^+ solution the response-intensity curve is much steeper. If exposure to this solution abolished light adaptation, this curve would represent the simple summation of single quantum responses. It would be steeper because there would be no sagging of the response. In support of this notion, we note that a curve of exactly this same shape can be used to fit the response-intensity function for flashes in low-Ca^{2+}, zero-Na^+ solution. It is necessary only to translate the curve along the intensity axis by the value of the integration time of the cell (Matthews et al. 1990).

In part B of figure 1.6 we show measurements of receptor sensitivity as a function of background intensity for the same cells as in part A. In Ringer solution sensitivity declines according to the Weber-Fechner law (equation 1.1), as previously described. In low-Ca^{2+}, zero-Na^+ solution, sensitivity declines much more steeply as the background light is increased. This may seem paradoxical, since we have been arguing that exposure to this solution eliminates light adaptation. Why should the sensitivity change at all?

The reason for the change in sensitivity can be appreciated from the data in part A. As the background light is increased, the steady response of the receptors to light reduces the circulating current and decreases the dynamic range by decreasing the amount of current remaining to be suppressed. If this were the only mechanism responsible for the change of sensitivity in low-Ca^{2+}, zero-Na^+ solution, the decrease of sensitivity should decline as the normalized derivative of the response-intensity function in part A. The exact

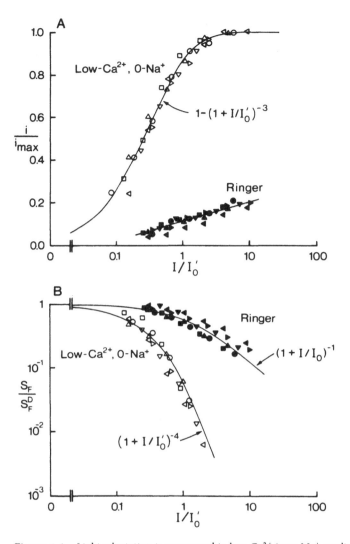

Figure 1.6 Light adaptation is suppressed in low-Ca²⁺/zero-Na⁺ medium. Data points were recorded from salamander cones. Open and filled symbols (e.g., open and filled circles) are from the same cone in low-Ca²⁺/zero-Na⁺ and Ringer solution, respectively. Symbols of different shapes (e.g., circles and squares) are from different receptors. The methods of recording and light stimulation are as in figure 1.1 (see Matthews et al. 1990). (A) Steady response as a function of steady background intensity. Points in Ringer solution have been fitted with a straight line by eye. Points in low-Ca²⁺/zero-Na⁺ solution have been fitted with the equation $i/i_{max} = 1 - (1 + I/I_0')^{-3}$, where i is the photocurrent, i_{max} is the saturating value of the photocurrent, I is the steady background intensity, and I_0' is a constant (see Matthews et al. 1990). (B) Sensitivity as a function of background light for the same receptors as in (A). Sensitivity in the presence of background illumination (S_F) has been plotted as a fraction of sensitivity in darkness (S_F^D). The curve through data in Ringer solution has been fitted with Weber-Fechner law (Eq. 1.1). The curve through data in low-Ca²⁺/zero-Na⁺ solution has been fitted with the normalized derivative of the curve used to fit the response amplitude in (A). (Reprinted with permission from Fain and Matthews 1990)

form of the equations used to fit the data has been described in detail (see Matthews et al. 1990), but it is not important in the present context. What is important is that the normalized derivative of the curve in part A fits the curve. in part B. When changes in Ca^{2+} are minimized, the active process that regulates sensitivity during light adaptation is eliminated. What is left is simply the compression of the response against its maximum value, which causes the sensitivity to decrease merely by reducing the number of channels available to be closed.

The Mechanism of Light Adaptation

Recent experiments have demonstrated that changes in Ca^{2+} concentration may regulate sensitivity by modulating the activity of the enzyme that synthesizes cGMP, guanylyl cyclase. Guanylyl cyclase is regulated by Ca^{2+} (Koch and Stryer 1988). The lower the concentration of Ca^{2+} the greater the stimulation of the cyclase. The effect on cyclase appears to occur within a range of free Ca^{2+} concentrations of 0.05 to 0.5 μM (see Koch and Stryer 1988) that is within the physiological range for the photoreceptor (McNaughton, Cervetto, and Nunn, 1986; Ratto et al. 1988).

The activity of Ca^{2+}-dependent guanylyl cyclase could modulate sensitivity in the following way. Light stimulation produces an activation of phosphodiesterase and a decrease in free cGMP concentration. The decrease in cGMP causes the channels to close and the Ca^{2+} concentration to decrease. If the decrease in Ca^{2+} activated the guanylyl cyclase, then the cyclase would resynthesize cGMP and restore its concentration. As the cGMP concentration recovered, the channels would open back up and the light response would decay. The greater the velocity of the cyclase, the faster the rate of recovery of the photoresponse. If the cyclase rate were increased by a decrease in Ca^{2+} concentration, then the steady decrease in Ca^{2+} produced by background light would produce an acceleration of response decay which would be more and more pronounced the brighter the background. As a result, sensitivity would decrease and the dynamic range of the receptor would shift to higher flash intensities. There is evidence that the rate of the guanylyl cyclase increases when receptors are illuminated (Ames, Walseth, Heyman, Barad, Graeff, and Goldberg 1986; Hodgkin and Nunn 1988). Further evidence for this comes from our own experiments, as we describe below (see Bleached Pigment Excites the Transduction Cascade).

Background light also appears to modulate the rate of the guanylyl phosphodiesterase (PDE). This was first demonstrated convincingly by Kawamura and Murakami (1991), who recorded from rods under conditions in which the contribution of the guanylyl cyclase to the waveform of the light response was minimized. With the cyclase contribution sufficiently small, the response waveform should reflect only time-dependent activation of the PDE. Kawamura and Murakami showed that the light response under these conditions decays much more rapidly in a low (i.e., light-adapted) Ca^{2+} than in high

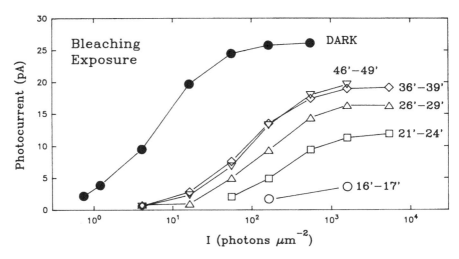

Figure 1.7 Response-intensity curves of salamander rod in darkness and after exposure to bleaching light. The ordinate gives the photocurrent response, measured using the suction electrode technique, to brief (20-msec) flashes of 520-nm light. Responses were measured relative to the steady-state current after bleach. Symbols give the peak amplitude of response in darkness (filled circles) and at various times after exposure for 8 sec to light with an intensity of 2.0×10^7 photons μm^2 s^{-1} at 520 nm (open symbols). The numbers above or to right of curves with open symbols give the approximate time intervals (in minutes after the bleach) during which the response-intensity measurements were made. The methods for recording and light stimulation were as in figure 1.2. Light intensities in units of photons μm^{-2} can be converted to Rh* per photoreceptor by multiplying by a collecting area of approximately 20 μm^2 (Lamb et al. 1986).

Ca^{2+}. They further showed that this effect is dependent on a soluble protein which they called S-modulin.

More recently, Kawamura (1992) has studied light-dependent activation of PDE in vitro. Both the fraction of light-activated PDE and the PDE lifetime are decreased as the Ca^{2+} is lowered. The modulation of the PDE again has an absolute requirement for S-modulin and occurs over a range of Ca^{2+} concentrations which includes the physiological range. Thus as Ca^{2+} concentration decreases in the light, the velocity of the PDE decreases, and the gain of phototransduction is turned down.

Experiments that measure light-activated PDE do not distinguish between direct effects on the PDE itself and indirect effects on one of the stages of transduction which precedes PDE activation. It now seems clear that the principal effect of Ca^{2+} and S-modulin is to modulate the lifetime of activated rhodopsin (R*) (Kawamura, 1993). This seems to work in the following way. In high Ca^{2+}, S-modulin inhibits rhodopsin kinase, the enzyme that phosphorylates rhodopsin and terminates R*. In low Ca^{2+}, the kinase is accelerated, and the lifetime of R* is reduced. As the lifetime of R* is decreased, there is less time for R* to interact with transducin, and fewer PDE molecules are activated.

In summary, there appear to be at least two mechanisms responsible for light adaptation, both mediated by a decrease in Ca^{2+}. On the one hand, lowered Ca^{2+} activates the guanylyl cyclase, which accelerates the rate of resynthesis of cGMP. On the other hand, the decrease in Ca^{2+} leads to a reduction in the lifetime of R^*, which decreases cGMP hydrolysis by the PDE. Both mechanisms would be expected to reduce sensitivity and accelerate the recovery of the light response. Both, acting together, may be entirely responsible for light adaptation, but other Ca^{2+}-dependent or even Ca^{2+}-independent mechanisms may remain to be discovered.

DARK ADAPTATION

Strong bleaching lights also have profound effects on photoreceptor sensitivity. It has long been known that the bleaching of a significant fraction of the visual pigment in a rod depresses sensitivity to a much greater extent than would be expected simply on the basis of the decrease in the probability of photon absorption (for reviews, see Barlow 1964, 1972; Ripps and Pepperberg 1987; Lamb 1990). In the intact rat or human (Dowling 1960; Rushton 1961) or in an eyecup preparation (Dowling and Ripps 1970), sensitivity recovers as rhodopsin is regenerated by the recombination of opsin with 11-*cis* retinal synthesized by the retinal pigment epithelium (RPE). In an isolated photoreceptor (in the absence of the RPE), sensitivity remains depressed after a bleach unless 11-*cis* retinal is added exogenously (Pepperberg, Lurie, Brown, and Dowling 1976; Yoshikami and Nöll 1978; Cornwall, Fein, and MacNichol 1990). In both intact and isolated photoreceptors, sensitivity has a similar, nonlinear dependence on the concentration of rhodopsin (Dowling 1960; Rushton 1961; Ripps and Pepperberg 1987). The significance of this function has been the subject of considerable speculation (see Rushton, 1965; Pepperberg 1984; Lamb 1990), but it remains unclear why sensitivity is so depressed after bleaching and why the recovery of sensitivity depends so closely upon the regeneration of the photopigment.

In an isolated rod of an amphibian, bright bleaching light initially produces complete suppression of the circulating current, which then recovers slowly in darkness (Cornwall et al. 1990). As the circulating current increases, the sensitivity recovers, and both current and sensitivity stabilize after a time that depends upon the intensity of the bleaching illumination. A typical result is given in figure 1.7. In this experiment, the response-intensity function was first measured in darkness (filled circles). The cell was then exposed for 8 seconds to light with an intensity of 2.0×10^7 photons μm^2 s^{-1}. The pigment absorption of this cell was not measured before and after bleaching, so we do not know exactly how much rhodopsin was bleached. Since the rod was isolated from the pigment epithelium, we shall make the simplifying assumption that no regeneration of pigment occurred (however, see Cocozza and Ostroy 1987). We can then calculate that the light produced a stable bleach of approximately 70 percent of the pigment, assuming a photosensitivity for A_2-based pigments of 7.4×10^{-9} μm^2 (Dartnall 1972).

The open circles show response-intensity functions measured at several times after the bleach. The slow recovery of sensitivity presumably reflects the slow time course with which pigment intermediates and the PDE and cyclase rates reach a steady state. After about 45 minutes the sensitivity and maximum amplitude of the response stabilized at levels which are considerably below those for the dark-adapted receptor.

Other experiments have shown that little further recovery occurs, even after several hours (Corson, Cornwall, MacNichol, Jin, Johnson, Derguini, Crouch, and Nakanishi 1990). The effect of bleaching on the response-intensity function superficially resembles the effect of background light (see figure 1.2), but careful comparison indicates that the effects are not precisely the same. In particular, the maximum amplitude of the response (and hence the amplitude of the circulating current) seems to be larger after a bleach than in the presence of a background for a similar decrease in sensitivity, even after taking into consideration the loss in sensitivity due to the loss in quantum catch (Cornwall et al. 1990).

The Response Waveform

Bleaching also alters the time course of the light response (Cornwall et al. 1990; Matthews et al. 1990; Cornwall, Ripps, Chappell, and Jones 1989). In figure 1.8 we compare the response waveforms from the same rod in darkness and after two bleaching exposures. The format of this figure is identical to that of figure 1.3: in part A we show small-amplitude responses plotted as sensitivities, and in part B the peak amplitudes of the responses in A have been normalized. The largest response in A was recorded at the beginning of the experiment, in darkness. A bleaching exposure was then given which bleached 7 percent of the pigment. After waiting 20 minutes for the sensitivity and amplitude of circulating current to stabilize, the response waveform was again recorded, and the sensitivity had fallen by about a factor of two. A second bleaching exposure was then given and was calculated to have bleached 25 percent of the remaining pigment (for a total bleach of 30 percent). After a further 41 minutes, sensitivity stabilized at about one-tenth that of the rod in darkness. The bleaches do not appear to have altered the initial rise time of the response (see also Kahlert, Pepperberg, and Hofmann 1990). As for background light, the principal effect of bleaching was to accelerate the time course of decay.

One way to compare the effects of backgrounds and bleaches is to compare changes in the integration time of the small-amplitude response. The integration time (t_i) is defined as the integral of the response divided by the maximum amplitude (Baylor and Hodgkin 1973). For both rods and cones, t_i decreases with increasing background light (see for example Matthews et al. 1990). This is to be expected, since the acceleration of response decay decreases the integral of the response waveform. Since bleaches also accelerate decay time (see figure 1.8), they might also be expected to decrease t_i.

Bleaches

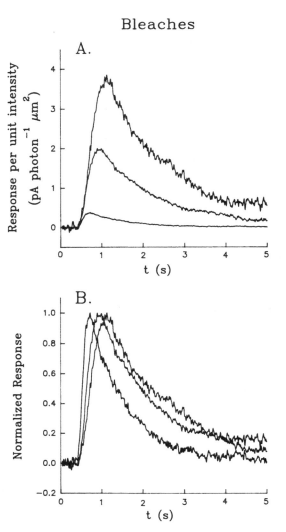

Figure 1.8 Small-amplitude responses of salamander rod in darkness and after exposure to bleaching lights. (A) Responses to brief (20-msec) 520-nm flashes plotted as sensitivities (response amplitude divided by light intensity) recorded in darkness (largest response) and at steady state after exposure to bleaching light with an intensity of 2.0×10^7 photons μm^{-2} s^{-1} at 520 nm for 0.5 s (intermediate response) and for 2.0 s (smallest response). Flash intensities (from the largest response to the smallest) were 1.21, 4.09, and 16.3 photons μm^{-2}. Peak amplitudes of flash responses as a fraction of the maximum peak amplitudes under the same conditions (i/i_{max}) were 0.20, 0.39, and 0.39. (B) Same responses as in (A) but normalized to a common peak amplitude of 1.0. The response decaying most slowly was recorded in darkness; intermediate response, after a 0.5-s bleach; and most rapidly decaying response, after a 2.0-s bleach. Flash intensities were as in (A). The methods for recording and calibrating the light intensities were as in figure 1.2.

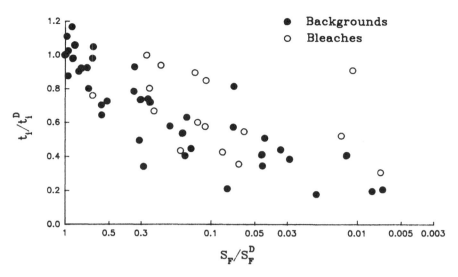

Figure 1.9 Integration time decreases as a similar function of decrease of sensitivity in background light and after bleaches. The integration time of small-amplitude response (t_i) was measured as the integral of the response in pA-s divided by the maximum amplitude in pA (Baylor and Hodgkin 1973). The responses were integrated using the trapezoidal rule in MCAD (MathSoft, Inc., Cambridge, Massachusetts). Values of t_i were normalized for each cell to the integration time in darkness (t_i^D) and plotted as a function of the sensitivity of that cell (S_F) normalized to its value in darkness (S_F^D). Filled symbols are from responses in background light, and open symbols are from responses at steady state after bleaching exposures.

The effect of bleaches and backgrounds on integration time is illustrated for salamander rods in figure 1.9, which plots the ratio of t_i to its value in darkness (t_i^D) against the log of the ratio of the flash sensitivity (S_F) to its value in darkness (S_F^D). The filled symbols are for responses recorded in the presence of background light, and the open symbols are for bleaches. Although there is considerable scatter, the decline in integration time is comparable in both cases.

The data in figures 1.8 and 1.9 indicate that similar processes might be responsible for the changes in response kinetics during light and dark adaptation. However, this inference should be drawn with caution. Several attempts have been made to compare the exact shape of the receptor response in backgrounds and after bleaches, and all have concluded that the waveform is not precisely the same for the same change in sensitivity (Liebovic, Dowling, and Kim 1987; Matthews et al. 1990; Cornwall et al. 1989). However, this comparison is difficult to make quantitatively since there is a large variation in response waveform from receptor to receptor within the same species (and with time, even for a recording from a single cell).

Regeneration with 11-*cis* Retinal

In an isolated photoreceptor the changes in sensitivity and waveform produced by bleaching light (see figures 1.7–1.9) are irreversible unless exoge-

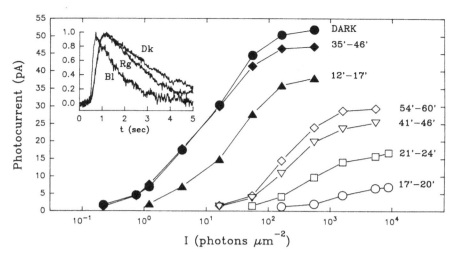

Figure 1.10 Response-intensity curves of salamander rod in darkness, after exposure to bleaching light, and after addition of 11-*cis* retinal. The ordinate gives the photocurrent response, measured using the suction electrode technique, to brief (20-msec) flashes of 520-nm light. The responses were measured relative to steady-state current. Symbols give the peak amplitudes of response in darkness (filled circles), after exposure for 16 sec to light with an intensity of 2.0×10^7 photons μm^{-2} at 520 nm (open symbols), and after the addition of 11-*cis* retinal (filled triangles, diamonds). Numbers to the right of curves give the approximate time intervals in minutes after bleach (for open symbols) or after addition of 11-*cis* retinal (for closed symbols) during which the response-intensity measurements were made. The methods for recording and light stimulation were the same as in figure 1.2. The 11-*cis* retinal was added to liposomes as in Cornwall et al. (1990). Inset: Waveform of small-amplitude responses recorded from the same cell in darkness (Dk), 55 min after bleach (Bl), and 36 min after adding 11-*cis* retinal (Rg). The ordinate gives the response amplitude normalized to the peak amplitude recorded for each response. Flash intensities (in photons μm^{-2} at 520 nm) and peak response amplitudes (in pA) were 0.75 and 4.58 (Dk), 55 and 4.39 (Lt), and 0.75 and 4.35 (Rg).

nous chromophore is added. In the presence of added 11-*cis* retinal the photopigment can regenerate, and both sensitivity and waveform can recover nearly to the dark-adapted state (Pepperberg et al. 1976; Yoshikami and Nöll, 1978; Cornwall et al. 1990) . A typical result is given in figure 1.10. The filled circles give the response-intensity function in the dark-adapted cell at the beginning of the experiment. A light was then given which, in the absence of regeneration, would have produced a stable bleach of 91 percent of the pigment. The open symbols show four response-intensity curves measured at various times after the bleach. After about an hour, sensitivity and circulating current had stabilized at values considerably below those previously recorded in darkness. The 11-*cis* retinal chromophore was then added in liposomes as previously described (Cornwall et al. 1990; Corson et al. 1990). Two additional response-intensity functions were measured at 12 to 17 minutes (▲) and at 35 to 46 minutes (◆) after the addition of the chromophore. The sensitivity and maximum amplitude of the response recovered nearly to their dark-adapted values.

The waveforms of normalized, small-amplitude responses from this same cell are shown in the inset to figure 1.10. The response decaying the most slowly (labeled Dk) is the one from the dark-adapted receptor. The rapidly decaying response (Bl) was recorded about 55 minutes after the bleach, when the sensitivity of the response had stabilized. The third response (Rg), similar to the one recorded in darkness but decaying not quite as slowly, was recorded 36 minutes after adding 11-*cis* retinal. The addition of chromophore produced a significant recovery in the decay time of the response.

THE MECHANISM OF DARK ADAPTATION

Since backgrounds and bleaches produce similar effects on sensitivity and response waveforms, they may act at least in part by a common mechanism. A suggestion of this sort was first made sixty years ago by W. S. Stiles and B. H. Crawford (1932), who proposed that bleaches produce an "equivalent background light," a sort of invisible afterglow which reduces sensitivity just as real background light does. They then showed that the changes in threshold produced by varying the temporal and spatial characteristics of visual targets were similar during light and dark adaptation and could be quantitatively accounted for by postulating an equivalent background of the appropriate magnitude (Crawford 1937, 1947).

The hypothesis of an equivalent background has had a profound effect on our thinking about dark adaptation. As we attempt to translate this notion to the level of the photoreceptor, it is important to keep in mind that Stiles and Crawford measured thresholds, psychophysically from human observers, whereas the measurements we have been describing are from single rods and cones. For dim backgrounds and small bleaches, the threshold as measured psychophysically may not be determined by the sensitivity of single receptors, but rather by a summation pool somewhere in the retina or the central nervous system (see Rushton 1965; Powers and Green 1990). For bright backgrounds and large bleaches, the behavioral threshold is more likely to be determined by the photoreceptors themselves. Fortunately, the notion of an equivalent background also seems to be useful under these conditions (Blakemore and Rushton 1965), and these are also the conditions under which direct measurements can be made from the photoreceptors. It is therefore worth considering whether the equivalent background hypothesis might explain the effects of bleaches on single rods and cones.

In its strongest form, the equivalent background hypothesis states that every aspect of the photoreceptor response is affected identically after bleaches and in the presence of backgrounds. As we have already seen, this seems unlikely to be true. The circulating current is usually somewhat larger after a bleach than in the presence of a background for the same change in sensitivity (Cornwall et al. 1990). The waveform of the receptor response is often somewhat different in the two cases (Liebovic et al. 1987; Matthews et al. 1990; Cornwall et al. 1989). The spread of the sensitivity change up and down the outer segment is also different for a spatially restricted bleach or background (Cornwall et al. 1990). Nonetheless, backgrounds and bleaches produce generally similar effects: the decay time shortens, the circulating current decreases, and the sensitivity declines.

Given these similarities and differences, we are inclined to adopt as a working hypothesis a weaker form of the equivalent background hypothesis. We propose that bleached pigment in some way stimulates the transduction cascade: in an isolated rod, bleaching produces a sustained activation of the PDE and cyclase and a sustained decrease in the concentration of Ca^{2+}, which is relieved by the addition of exogenous 11-*cis* retinal and regeneration of the photopigment. We propose that at least some of the effects of bleaches on the responses of rods and cones are produced by this sustained excitation, which acts like an equivalent background. We shall not attempt at this stage to explain the differences between the effects of backgrounds and bleaches (Cornwall et al. 1990), but we anticipate that explanations will emerge as our understanding of the mechanism of adaptation becomes more complete.

Bleached Pigment Excites the Transduction Casacade

If the bleaching of pigment produces an equivalent background excitation of the photoreceptor, bleaching should cause a sustained activation of the transduction cascade. We have recently verified this hypothesis by showing that the bleaching of pigment in an isolated salamander rod produces a sustained activation of the PDE and cyclase (Cornwall and Fain 1992 and in preparation). Using methods devised by Hodgkin and Nunn (1988), we examined the effects of backgrounds and bleaching on the velocities of the PDE and cyclase by suddenly exposing the rods either to Li^+ Ringer solution or to Ringer containing IBMX. Sudden exposure of a rod to Li^+ Ringer should cause the concentration of Ca^{2+} in the outer segment to rise suddenly, since Li^+ is unable to substitute for Na^+ in the countertransport of $Na^+/(Ca^{2+}, K^+)$. The rise in Ca^{2+} should greatly reduce the velocity of the cyclase (Koch and Stryer 1988). In the absence of cGMP synthesis, the basal level of PDE activity will cause hydrolysis of cGMP until none is left and the channels all close. The greater the velocity of the PDE, the faster the time constant with which the current decreases. Cyclase velocity, on the other hand, can be estimated from the maximal rate of current increase after sudden exposure to 0.5 mM IBMX. IBMX should inhibit most of the PDE, and the current should increase as the cyclase synthesizes cGMP.

We find that steady background illumination produces an increase in both PDE and cyclase velocities, with both increasing monotonically over 2 to 3 log units of background intensity. Our results with backgrounds are similar to those previously published by Hodgkin and Nunn (1988) and by Cobbs (1991). We also find that bleaching a substantial fraction of the visual pigment (>5 percent) in an isolated rod produces an increase in PDE and cyclase velocities and, the bigger the bleach, the larger the increase in velocity. In isolated rods the changes in PDE and cyclase velocities are essentially irreversible, even after 1 to 2 hours. If exogenous 11-*cis* retinal is added to liposomes, both cyclase and PDE rates return to approximately their dark-adapted values as the photoreceptors recover sensitivity and circulating current (see figure 1.10).

These experiments show that bleached pigment activates the transduction cascade much as background light does. By comparing changes ln PDE rates for bleaches and backgrounds, we have estimated that the overall efficiency of excitation by bleached pigment is of the order of $10^{-6}-10^{-7}$ that of R*. Our experiments do not distinguish whether bleached pigment excites the PDE directly or whether excitation occurs via transducin.

The Equivalent Background Is Not Produced by Recycling through R*

When rhodopsin is excited by light, the pigment passes through a series of intermediates to metarhodopsin II (or R*), which interacts with transducin and triggers visual excitation. R* then decays to metarhodopsin III and to opsin. When 70 to 90 percent of the pigment of an isolated salamander rod is bleached, sensitivity stabilizes after 45 to 60 minutes (see figures 1.7 and 1.10), and the cyclase and PDE rates are greatly accelerated (Cornwall and Fain 1992 and in preparation). Since most of the meta II will have decayed, it is of some interest to know which form of the pigment is responsible for stimulating the PDE and cyclase.

It seems to us that there are at least three possibilities. Excitation might be produced by a small amount of meta II remaining in the rod. This meta II would probably be phosphorylated by the reactions that turn off R* (see Stryer 1986, 1988), but the phosphorylation may be reversible and the dephosphorylation of meta II might recycle the pigment through an active form, much like R* itself (Lisman 1985; Lamb 1990). A second possibility, similar to the first, is that meta III or some other intermediate recycles back to meta II and eventually to R* (Lamb 1981). Finally, meta II, meta III, or some other intermediate, perhaps even opsin itself, might directly excite the transduction cascade without recycling through R* (Rushton 1965; Corson et al. 1990).

The first two possibilities seem unlikely to us. If the equivalent background were produced by recycling through R*, it should be possible to see single-photon events much like those recorded in background light. In steady light, the circulating current of a rod is noisy since photon events occur randomly. This can be seen figure 1.11, which shows 60-second duration records of the steady-state baseline current from a salamander rod in darkness and in backgrounds of three different intensitites. In darkness, the baseline current shows little noise since the rate of spontaneous events is low. In a dim background ($I_B = 0.55$), the frequency of events is much higher and the amplitude of the single-photon response is large because the sensitivity of the cell is high. In a brighter background ($I_B = 3.7$), the number of events increases further, but their amplitude decreases as the sensitivity of the rod declines. As the background is made even brighter ($I_B = 37$), the sensitivity becomes so small that the noise becomes barely detectable, and the current trace is nearly as quiet as that recorded from the cell in darkness. A similar phenomenon has been

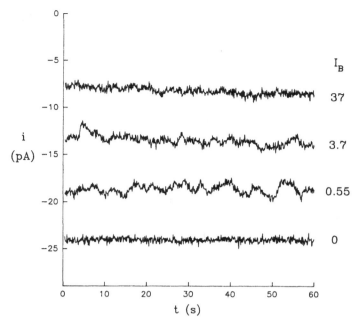

Figure 1.11 The steady-state baseline current recorded from an isolated salamander rod using the suction pipette method in darkness and in background light of three different intensities. All traces are from the same cell. The ordinate gives the value of the circulating current in pA. The absolute values of the currents were estimated from the peak amplitude of the response of the cell to saturating flashes. The intensity of the background light (I_B) is given to the right of each of the traces in units of photons $\mu m^{-2} s^{-1}$.

described for rods of the toad *Bufo marinus* (see figure 1 of Baylor, Lamb, and Yau 1979b).

If the equivalent background excitation were produced by recycling through R^* very similar background noise should be recorded from rods at steady state after bleaches. We have looked for this noise and have never been able to observe it. For isolated rods subjected to bleaching light, the baseline current at steady state is similar to that of a dark-adapted rod, regardless of the size of the bleach. Even for photoreceptors subjected to bleaches of 7 to 14 percent of the pigment, which produce stable decreases in sensitivity of only 2 to 5 fold, there is no detectable photon noise at steady state in darkness after the bleach. Our measurements suggest that, no matter how the equivalent background is generated, the number of light-sensitive channels closed by a single bleached pigment molecule is at least 5 to 10 times smaller than that produced by R^*.

Increased noise has been observed in toad rods after small bleaches of 1 percent or so of the pigment (Lamb 1980, 1986), and similar events have been seen in primate rods (Schnapf, Kraft, Nunn, and Baylor 1987) and in those of the salamander (M. C. Cornwall, unpublished observations). The significance of these events is unclear. It is possible that they contribute to the desensitization of the retina as a whole, perhaps by summation in an "adaptation pool" in some proximal cell such as a bipolar or ganglion cell (Lamb 1980, 1986). If so, these effects seem to occur only over a rather restricted range of light exposures. We have been unable to obtain evidence that increased noise plays a significant role in the decreases in sensitivity and changes in waveform recorded from rods after larger bleaches, and we think it unlikely that noise makes an important contribution to the normal course of recovery of visual sensitivity after exposure to bright light.

The Equivalent Background May Be Produced by Opsin Itself

If the equivalent background excitation is not produced by pigment recycling through R*, it must be produced by some other form of bleached pigment directly exciting transducin or PDE. We think this is likely to be opsin itself, as was first suggested by Horace Barlow (1964) and by William Rushton (1965). There are several indications that this might be so. Dowling (1960) showed many years ago that the extent of desensitization produced by bleaching has the same dependence on rhodopsin concentration as on vitamin A depletion. The simplest explanation of this finding is that the intermediate producing the desensitization in both cases is opsin (but see Engbretson and Witkovsky 1978). Another indication that opsin is the desensitizing intermediate is the result of studies by Brin and Ripps (1977), who showed that treatment of skate retina with hydroxylamine greatly speeds the kinetics of meta II and meta III decay and would be expected to produce a large change in the steady-state concentrations of these intermediates; however, there is little effect of hydroxylamine on photoreceptor sensitivity after a bleach. If neither meta II nor meta III is responsible for desensitization, only opsin would remain as a likely alternative.

These experiments are suggestive, but more compelling evidence that opsin is the substance responsible for the equivalent background desensitization comes from recent results with analogues of 11-*cis* retinal (figure 1.12). Corson and colleagues (1990) have shown that two 11-*cis*-locked analogues (11-*cis*-locked-retinal and 11-*cis*-locked-13-*cis*-retinal) are able to remove most of the desensitization produced by bleaching. These compounds bind to opsin and form a Schiff base linkage with the protein, but the pigment so formed is not bleachable and is incapable of triggering transduction. Nevertheless, the equivalent background excitation is largely quieted, and the sensitivity and waveform of the receptor response return nearly to those recorded in darkness.

Similar effects have been now been shown to be produced by other analogues, for example β-ionone and 9-*cis* C17 aldehyde, which do not even form a Schiff base linkage with opsin (Jin, Crouch, Corson, Katz, MacNichol and Cornwall, 1993). The remarkable thing about these analogues is that it is possible to add them (in liposomes), produce resensitization and recovery of receptor waveform, and then wash the analogues out and regain the desensitization and accelerated responses characteristic of the bleached cell. The ana-

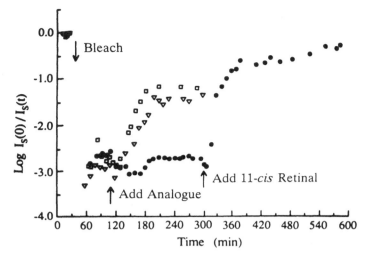

Figure 1.12 The time course of a change in sensitivity after bleaching and addition of 11-*cis* retinal or one its analogs. Each symbol represents data from a different cell. The ordinate gives the $\log_{10}$ of the ratio of the semisaturation constant in darkness ($I_S(0)$) to the semisaturation constant measured at the time indicated along the abscissa ($I_S(t)$). This quantity is generally within 0.1 to 0.2 log units of $\log_{10}(S_F/S_F^p)$. At the first arrow, 520 nm light of 6.6×10^7 photons $\mu m^{-2} s^{-1}$ was given for 5 min to produce a stable bleach of approximately 93 percent of the pigment. At the second arrow, an analog was added to the liposomes (for the used methods, see Corson et al. 1990). The analogs were all-*trans* retinal (circles), 11-*cis*-locked retinal (triangles), and 11-*cis*-locked-13-*cis* retinal (squares). At the third arrow, 11-*cis* retinal was added to the cells represented by circles only. (Reprinted with permission from Corson et al. 1990)

logue can be added and washed out several times for the same cell, and sensitivity increases and decreases each time. It is difficult to see how this could occur unless the form of the pigment producing the desensitization was devoid of chromophore.

DARK ADAPTATION, NIGHT BLINDNESS AND RETINITIS PIGMENTOSA

In Figure 1.13 we summarize the mechanisms that we believe are responsible for adaptation in vertebrate photoreceptors. We believe that light adaptation is produced by a decrease in concentration of Ca^{2+}, which acts at least in part by activating the guanylate cyclase. In addition, the decrease in the concentration of Ca^{2+} probably also alters the lifetime of R*, by altering the activity of the rhodopsin kinase (Kawamura, 1993). Bleaching exposures also decrease sensitivity, at least in part by generating an equivalent background, which we suppose cause desensitization by a mechanism similar to that occurring in real backgrounds. We believe that the equivalent background is produced by opsin, which directly activates either transducin or the PDE.

Whatever the mechanism, the overall gain of excitation produced by opsin is of the order of $10^{-6}-10^{-7}$ that produced by light, since the desensitization

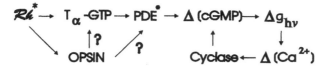

Figure 1.13 A scheme indicating proposed mechanisms for sensitivity regulation during light and dark adaptation in vertebrate photoreceptors. See text.

produced by 10^8 bleached pigment molecules is approximately the same as that produced by $10-100$ R^*'s. Furthermore, a single activated opsin molecule must produce a change in the light-sensitive conductance at least 5 to 10 times smaller than a single R^* in order to account for the much smaller noise seen after bleaches than in the presence of backgrounds for the same change in sensitivity. We presume that the equivalent background produces a steady decrease in the concentration of Ca^{2+} just as real background light does, leading to a steady increase in the cyclase rate and the speeding up and desensitization of the light response (Matthews, Fain and Cornwall 1993).

The scheme in figure 1.13 poses the question of how opsin activates T_{α} or PDE. Although direct activation of the transduction cascade by opsin has not previously been demonstrated (see, for example, Robinson, Cohen, Shukovsky, and Oprian 1992), our experiments (Cornwall and Fain 1992 and in preparation) suggest that the gain of activation by opsin might be as low as one cGMP hydrolyzed per opsin per second, too low to be observed in vitro. The activation of transducin has recently been shown for a mutant form of opsin, for which lysine 296 (which normally forms the Schiff base linkage with 11-*cis* retinal) has been replaced by a glycine residue (Robinson et al. 1992). The activation is observed in the absence of chromophore and in complete darkness. If this mutant form can activate, it is natural to suppose that native opsin can do so as well, without chromophore and in complete darkness, though perhaps with an efficiency too low to be detected biochemically.

We view the slow recovery of sensitivity after a bleach as a kind of unavoidable mistake. Many a cave man must have come to grief as a result of it. One can only suppose that the pronounced loss of sensitivity produced by bleaching is the inevitable result of the high concentration of bleached opsin in the photoreceptor. Perhaps nature knows no way of designing the opsin molecule that completely eliminates the equivalent background. Instead of dismay at the imperfection of our visual system, we should rather express amazement that a molecule that is capable of signaling responses to single photons with chromophore still produces activation without chromophore, but with a gain six orders of magnitude or more smaller.

The scheme in figure 1.13 also offers an explanation of night blindness. If sensitivity decreases during vitamin A deprivation according to the same function of rhodopsin concentration as during dark adaptation (Dowling 1960), then the explanation of decrease in sensitivity may be the same. It is usually thought that night blindness is caused by a lack of vitamin A. In a certain sense, of course, this is true. However, if the decrease in sensitivity is much larger than one would expect merely from the decrease in quantum catch, then it seems to us more accurate to say that the problem is not too little vitamin A, but rather too much opsin. Opsin deprived of its chromophore may produce background excitation much like that produced after bleaching, and the resulting desensitization may be mostly responsible for the increase in threshold. It would be of considerable interest to record from photoreceptors from vitamin A-deprived animals to see if their responses resemble those recorded after bleaching exposure.

Prolonged vitamin A deprivation eventually produces widespread degeneration of the photoreceptors (Dowling and Wald 1960). It is often supposed that this occurs because of some instability in the photoreceptor membranes, which is caused by the absence of 11-*cis* retinal. Our results suggest a different explanation (Fain and Lisman, 1993). We think it conceivable that continuous low-level activation of the transduction cascade by opsin causes the degeneration. This would explain why continuous exposure to light at levels far below those that cause thermal damage can also produce photoreceptor degeneration (Noell, Walker, Kang, and Berman 1966; Noell and Albrecht 1971).

Our observations may also help us understand the origin of some forms of retinitis pigmentosa (Fain and Lisman, 1993). It is now known that a significant percentage of cases of retinitis pigmentosa are caused by mutations in the gene for rhodopsin (Dryja et al. 1990; Sung et al. 1991). One example of such a mutation that produces retinitis pigmentosa is the substitution of lysine at position 296 of the opsin molecule (Xeen, Inglehearn, Lester, Bashir, Jay, Bird, and Battacharya 1991). Robinson and colleagues (1992) have shown that mutations at position 296 can produce continuous activation of the transduction cascade, and other rhodopsin mutations may produce similar effects. Continuous activation by the mutant form of the pigment would be expected to depress sensitivity, much as opsin does after bleaching or vitamin A deprivation. We would predict that, for these patients, sensitivity would be more depressed than could be accounted for by decrease in pigment concentration (see for example Perlman and Auerbach 1981). We do not know why continuous activation should lead to degeneration. An explanation may perhaps emerge from a clearer understanding of the mechanisms responsible for sensitivity modulation in the photoreceptors.

ACKNOWLEDGMENT

We are grateful to John Lisman, of Brandeis University, Boston for his critical comments on an earlier version of this manuscript.

REFERENCES

Ames A, III, Walseth TF, Heyman RA, Barad M, Graeff RM, Goldberg ND (1986) Light-induced increases in cGMP metabolic flux correspond with electrical responses of photoreceptors. J Biol Chem 261:13034–13042.

Barlow HB (1964) Dark-adaptation: a new hypothesis. Vision Res 4:47–58.

Barlow HB (1972) Dark and light adaptation: psychophysics. In: Handbook of Sensory Physiology, Vol VII/4 (Jameson D, Hurvich LM, eds), pp 1—28. Berlin: Springer-Verlag.

Bastian BL, Fain GL (1979) Light adaptation in toad rods: requirement for an internal messenger which is not calcium. J Physiol 297:493—520.

Baylor DA, Hodgkin AL (1973) Detection and resolution of visual stimuli by turtle photoreceptors. J Physiol 234:163—198.

Baylor DA, Hodgkin AL (1974) Changes in time scale and sensitivity in turtle photoreceptors. J Physiol 242:729—758.

Baylor DA, Lamb TD (1982) Local effects of bleaching in retinal rods of the toad. J Physiol 328:49—71.

Baylor DA, Lamb TD, Yau K-W (1979a) The membrane current of single rod outer segments. J Physiol 288:589—611.

Baylor DA, Lamb TD, Yau K-W (1979b) Responses of retinal rods to single photons. J Physiol 288:613—634.

Blakemore CB, Rushton WAH (196S) Dark adaptation and increment threshold in a rod monochromat. J Physiol 181:612—628.

Brin KP, Ripps H (1977) Rhodopsin photoproducts and rod sensitivity in the skate retina. J Gen Physiol 69:97—120.

Cervetto L, Lagnado L, Perry RJ, Robinson DW, McNaughton PA (1989) Extrusion of calcium from rod outer segments is driven by both sodium and potassium gradients. Nature 337:740—743.

Cobbs WH (1991) Light and dark active phosphodiesterase regulation in salamander rods. J Gen Physiol 98:575—614.

Cocozza JD, Ostroy SE (1987) Factors affecting the regeneration of rhodopsin in the isolated amphibian retina. Vision Res 27:1085—1091.

Cornwall MC, Fain GL (1992) Bleaching of rhodopsin in isolated rods causes a sustained activation of PDE and cyclase which is reversed by pigment regeneration. Invest Ophthalmol Vis Sci ARVO Suppl 33:1103.

Cornwall MC, Fein A, MacNichol EF Jr (1990) Cellular mechanisms that underlie bleaching and background adaptation. J Gen Physiol 96:345—372.

Cornwall MC, Ripps H, Chappell R, Jones G (1989) Membrane current responses of skate photoreceptors. J Gen Physiol 94:633—647.

Corson DW, Cornwall MC, MacNichol EF, Jin J, Johnson R, Derguini F, Crouch RK, Nakanishi K (1990) Sensitization of bleached rod photoreceptors by 11-cis-locked analogues of retinal. Proc Natl Acad Sci USA 87:6823—6827.

Crawford BH (1937) The change of visual sensitivity with time. Proc Roy Soc B 123:68—69.

Crawford BH (1947) Visual adaptation in relation to brief conditioning stimuli. Proc Roy Soc B 134:283—302.

Dartnall HJA (1972) Photosensitivity. In: Handbook of Sensory Physiology, Vol VII/l (Dartnall HJA, ed), pp 122—145. Berlin: Springer-Verlag.

Dowling JE (1960) The chemistry of visual adaptation in the rat. Nature 188:114—118.

Dowling JE, Ripps H (1970) Visual adaptation in the retina of the skate. J Gen Physiol 56:491—520.

Dowling JE, Wald G (1960) The biological function of vitamin A acid. Proc Natl Acad Sci USA 46:587—608.

Dryja TP, McGee TL, Reichel E, Hahn LB, Cowley GS, Yandel DW, Sandberg MA, Berson EL (1990). A point mutation of the rhodopsin gene in one form of retinitis pigmentosa. Nature 343:364–366.

Engbretson GA, Witkovsky P (1978) Rod sensitivity and visual pigment concentration in *Xenopus*. J Gen Physiol 72:801–819.

Fain GL (1976) Sensitivity of toad rods: dependence on wavelength and background. J Physiol 261:71–101.

Fain GL, Lisman JE (1993) Photoreceptor degeneration in vitamin A deprivation and retinitis pigmentosa: the equivalent light hypothesis. Exp Eye Res, in press.

Fain GL, Matthews HR (1990) Calcium and the mechanism of light adaptation in vertebrate photoreceptors. Trends Neurosci 13:378–384.

Fain GL, Lamb TD, Matthews HR, Murphy RLW (1989) Cytoplasmic calcium concentration as the messenger for light adaptation in salamander rods. J Physiol 416:215–243.

Fuortes MGF, Hodgkin AL (1964) Changes in time scale and sensitivity in the ommatidia of *Limulus*. J Physiol 172:239–263.

Hodgkin AL, Nunn BJ (1988) Control of light-sensitive current in salamander rods. J Physiol 403:439–471.

Jin, J., Crouch, RK, Corson, DW, Katz, BM, MacNichol, EF, Cornwall, MC (1993). Non-covalent occupancy of the retinal binding pochet of opsin diminishes bleaching adaptation of retinal cones. Neuron, in press.

Kahlert M, Pepperberg DR, Hofmann KP (1990) Effect of bleached rhodopsin on signal amplification in rod visual receptors. Nature 345:537–539.

Kaupp UB (1991) The cyclic nucleotide-gated channels of vertebrate photoreceptors and olfactory epithelium. Trends Neurosci 14:150–157.

Kawamura S (1993) Rhodopsin phosphorylation as a mechanism of cyclic GMP phosphodiesterase regulation by S-modulin. Nature 362:855–857.

Kawamura S, Murakami M (1991) Calcium-dependent regulation of cyclic GMP phosphodiesterase by a protein from frog retinal rods. Nature 349:420–423.

Kowamura S, Murakami M (1991) Calcium-dependent regulation of cyclic GMP phosphodiesterase by a protein from frog retinal rods. Nature 349:420–423.

Keen TJ, Inglehearn CF, Lester DH, Bashir R, Jay M, Bird AC, Bhattacharya SS (1991) Autosomal dominant retinitis pigmentosa: four new mutations in rhodopsin, one of them in the retinal attachment site. Genomics 11:199–205.

Kleinschmidt J, Dowling JE (1975) Intracellular recordings from gecko photoreceptors during light and dark adaptation. J Gen Physiol 66:617–648.

Koch K-W, Stryer L (1988) Highly cooperative feedback control of retinal rod guanylate cyclase by calcium ions. Nature 334:64–66.

Korenbrot JI, Miller DL (1986) Cytoplasmic free calcium concentration in dark-adapted retinal rod outer segments. Vision Res 29:939–948.

Lamb TD (1980) Spontaneous quantal events induced in toad rods by pigment bleaching. Nature 287:349–351.

Lamb TD (1981) The involvement of rod photoreceptors in dark adaptation. Vision Res 21:1773–1782.

Lamb TD (1990) Dark adaptation: a re-examination. In: Night Vision, chp 5 (Hess RF, Sharpe LT, Nordby K, eds), pp 177–222, 499–503. Cambridge: Cambridge University Press.

Lamb TD, Matthews HR, Torre V (1986) Incorporation of calcium buffer into salamander retinal rods: a rejection of the calcium hypothesis of phototransduction. J Physiol 372:315–349.

Lamb TD, McNaughton PA, Yau K-W (1981) Spatial spread of activation and background desensitization in rod outer segments. J Physiol 319:463–496.

Leibovic KN, Dowling JE, Kim YY (1987) Background and bleaching equivalence in steady-state adaptation of vertebrate rods. J Neurosci 7:1056–1063.

Lisman J (1985) The role of metarhodopsin in the generation of spontaneous quantum bumps in ultraviolet receptors of *Limulus* median eye. J Gen Physiol 85:171–187.

Matthews HR (1990a) Evidence implicating cytoplasmic calcium concentration as the messenger for light adaptation in rod photoreceptros isolated from guinea-pig retina. J Physiol 425:48P.

Matthews HR (1990b) Messengers of transduction and adaptation in vertebrate photoreceptors. In: Light and Life in the Sea, Ch 11 (Herring PJ, Campbell AK, Whitfield M, Maddock L, eds), pp 185–198. Cambridge: Cambridge University Press.

Matthews HR, Fain GL, Cornwall, MC (1993) Role of Ca^{2+} in bleaching adaptation in cones isolated from the salamander retina. J Physiol 467:354P.

Matthews HR, Fain GL, Murphy RLW, Lamb TD (1990) Light adaptation in cone photo-receptors of the salamander: a role for cytoplasmic calcium. J Physiol 420:447–469.

Matthews HR, Murphy RLW, Fain GL, Lamb TD (1988) Photoreceptor light adaptation is mediated by cytoplasmic calcium concentration. Nature 334:67–69

McNaughton PA, Cervetto L, Nunn BJ (1986) Measurement of the intracellular calcium concentration in salamander rods. Nature 322:261–263.

Nakatani K, Yau K-W (1988a) Calcium and magnesium fluxes across the plasma membrane of the toad rod outer segment. J Physiol 395:695–729.

Nakatani K, Yau X-W (1988b) Calcium and light adaptation in retinal rods and cones. Nature 334:69–71.

Noell WK, Albrecht R (1971) Irreversible effects of visible light on the retina: role of vitamin A. Science 172:76–79.

Noell WK, Walker VS, Kang BS, Berman S (1966) Retinal damage by light in rats. Invest Ophthalmol Vision Sci 5:450–473.

Pepperberg DR (1984) Rhodopsin and visual adaptation: analysis of photoreceptor thresholds in the isolated skate retina. Vision Res 24:357–366.

Pepperberg DR, Lurie M, Brown PK, Dowling JE (1976) Visual adaptation: effects of externally applied retinal on the light-adapted, isolated skate retina. Science 191:394–396.

Perlman I, Auerbach E (1981) The relationship between visual sensitivity and rhodopsin density in retinitis pigmentosa. Invest Ophthalmol Vision Sci 20:758–765.

Powers MK, Green DG (1990) Physiological mechanisms of visual adaptation at low light levels. In: Night Vision, Chp 3 (Hess Rf, Sharpe LI, Nordby K, eds), pp 125–145, 493–497. Cambridge: Cambridge Univ Press.

Pugh EN, Lamb TD (1990) Cyclic GMP amd calcium: the internal messengers of excitation and adaptation in vertebrate photoreceptors. Vision Res 30:1923–1948.

Ratto GM, Payne R, Owen WG, Tsien RY (1988) The concentration of cytosolic free Ca^{2+} in vertebrate rod outer segments measured with fura-2. J Neurosci 8:3240–3246.

Reid D, Friedel U, Molday RF, Cook NJ (1990) Identification of the sodium-calcium exchanger as the major ricin-binding glycoprotein of bovine rod outer segments and its localization to the plasma membrane. Biochemistry 29:1601–1607.

Ripps H, Pepperberg DR (1987) Photoreceptor processes in visual adaptation. Neurosci Res, Suppl 6, S87–S106.

Robinson PR, Cohen GB, Zhukovsky EA, Oprian DD (1992) Constitutive activation of rhodopsin by mutation of LYS^{296}. Neuron 9:719–725.

Rushton WAH (1961) Rhodopsin measurement and dark adaptation in a subject deficient in cone vision. J Physiol 156:193–205.

Rushton WAH (1965) The Ferrier Lecture, 1962. Visual adaptation. Proc R Soc B 162:20–46.

Schnapf JL, Kraft TW, Nunn BJ, Baylor DA (1987) Spectral sensitivity and dark adaptation in primate photoreceptors. Invest Ophthalmol Vis Sci, ARVO Suppl, 28:50.

Schnapf JL, McBurney RN (1980) Light-induced changes in membrane current in cone outer segments of tiger salamander and turtle. Nature 287:239–241.

Stiles WS, Crawford BH (1932) Equivalent adaptation levels in localized retinal areas. In: Report of a Joint Discussion on Vision, June 3, 1932, Imperial College of Science, pp 194–211. London: Physical Society.

Stryer L (1986) Cyclic GMP cascade of vision. Ann Rev Neurosci 9:87–119.

Stryer L (1988) Molecular basis of visual excitation. Cold Spring Harbor Symp Quant Biol 53:283–294.

Sung C-H, Davenport CM, Hennessey JC, Maumenee IH, Jacobson SG, Heckenlively JR, Nowakowski R, Fishman G, Gouras R, Nathans J (1991) Rhodopsin mutations in autosomal dominant retinitis pigmentosa. Proc Natl Acad Sci USA 88:6481–6485.

Tamura T, Nakatani K, Yau K-W (1989) Light adaptation in cat retinal rods. Science 245:755–757.

Tamura T, Nakatani K, Yau K-W (1991) Calcium feedback and sensitivity regulation in primate rods. J Gen Physiol 98:95–130.

Torre V, Matthews HR, Lamb TD (1986) Role of calcium in regulating the cyclic GMP cascade of phototransduction in retinal rods. Proc Natl Acad Sci USA 83:7109–7113.

Walraven J, Enroth-Cugell C, Hood DC, MacLeod DIA, Schnapf JL (1990) The control of visual sensitivity: Receptoral and post receptoral processes. In: Visual Perception: The Neurophysiological Foundations (Spillmann L & Werner JS eds), pp 53–101. New York: Academic Press.

Yau K-W, Baylor DA (1989) Cyclic GMP-activated conductance of retinal photoreceptor cells. Ann Rev Neurosci 12:289–327

Yoshikami S, Noll GN (1978) Isolated retinas synthesize visual pigments from retinol congeners delivered by liposomes. Science 200:1393–1395.

Fura-2 Imaging of Calcium in Monkey Solitary Cones

Peter R. MacLeish

Intracellular recording from photoreceptors from a variety of vertebrates has shown the presence of voltage-gated calcium channels, probably used in calcium-dependent synaptic transmission (Trifonov 1968; Kaneko and Shimazaki 1976; Schwartz 1986), and a number of calcium-activated channels whose activity is expected to modify the time course of the signals generated by light (Bader et al. 1982; Atwell et al. 1982; Barnes and Hille 1989; Maricq and Korenbrot 1988, Yagi and MacLeish 1989; Thorenson and Burkhardt 1991). In the electrophysiological experiments, the total membrane current was recorded and the precise location of the conductance mechanisms was not investigated in any great detail. In the present report I have combined electrical recording with optical imaging in monkey cones with a view to obtaining a better idea of the spatial organization of calcium entry and of changes in cytoplasmic free calcium.

DISSOCIATION

Monkey cones were isolated from retinae following treatment with papain (Lam 1972; MacLeish et al. 1984). Enucleation was carried out under deep surgical anaesthesia just prior to the euthanasia of animals that were used in studies of cortical function. Isolated cones were identified by their characteristic morphology and by staining them with a cone-specific mouse monoclonal antibody that was isolated in our laboratory. Figure 2.1 consists of two photomicrographs of the same fixed monkey cone after 1 day in culture. It shows the differential interference contrast image to the left and the fluorescence image to the right following labeling with our cone-specific antibody. As is typical, the outer segment is missing and the cell body has rounded up. A thin fiber connects the cell body to an enlarged terminal. Cells could be maintained in culture for up to 2 weeks in a variety of media. The most commonly used was L-15 growth medium supplemented with 200 to 500 μg/ml of bovine serum albumin, 16 mM of glucose, and 10 μg/ml of gentamicin. Whereas the cells survived for weeks, the electrical recordings deteriorated around the fourth day, primarily because of the difficulty of maintaining stable high-resistance seals.

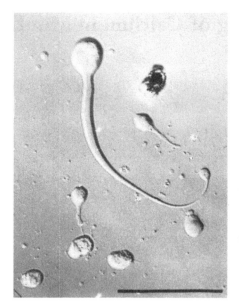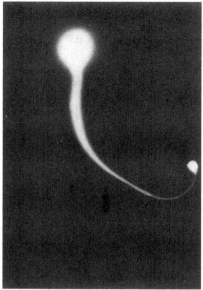

Figure 2.1 Photomicrographs of fixed monkey retinal cells. (Left) DIC image of a group of cells after 1 day in culture. A long fiber connects the rounded cell body of a cone to the terminal enlargement; outer segment is missing. (Right) fluorescence image showing specificity of labeling with a cone-specific antibody. Secondary antibody was conjugated to fluorescein. Calibration bar: 50 μm.

FURA-2 FILLING AND RECORDING

To monitor changes in intracellular free calcium, single wavelength measurements were made of fura-2 fluorescence. Cells were filled with fura-2 by treating them with fura-2 AM for half an hour in a calcium-free medium. Following rinsing, the preparation was illuminated with 380 nm light while recording at 510 nm (Grynkiewicz et al. 1986). All retinal cells were brilliantly fluorescent, indicating effective filling with fura-2. The light intensity was recorded with a cooled CCD camera (Photometrics, Ltd., Tucson, Az.), and images were created and analyzed using a computer system (Lasser-Ross et al. 1991). Typically a 300×200 pixel array with 4×4 binning was imaged at 20 frames per second. Membrane potential was controlled with patch pipettes in the whole-cell configuration of the patch-clamp technique (Hamill et al. 1981). The bathing medium contained (in mM) NaCl 139, KCl 3, HEPES 1, $MgCl_2$ 1, phenol red 0.02, glucose 16. The pH was adjusted to 7.2 to 7.4 with NaOH. The pipette solution contained (in mM) KCl 136, $MgCl_2$ 5, ATP (Na_2) 1, HEPES 10, and EGTA 0.05. The pH was adjusted to 7.5 with approximately 10 mM NaOH.

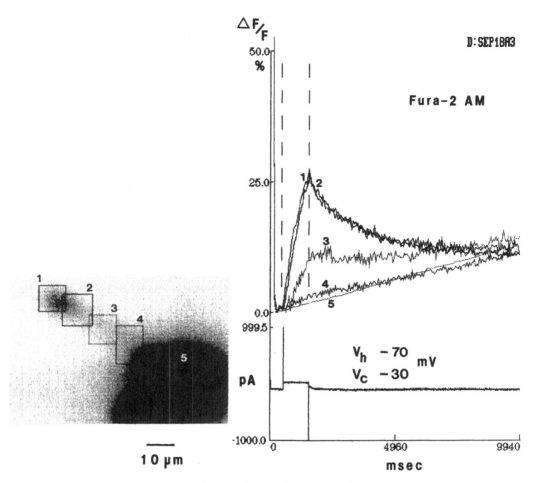

Figure 2.2 Fractional changes of fura-2 fluorescence. The traces show the fractional change in fluorescence as a function of time within the corresponding numbered box covering different parts of the cone cell shown in the left image. The cell body is on the lower right and the fiber extends upward to the left and ends within box 1. The cell voltage was clamped at -70 mV (V_h) and stepped to -30 mV (V_c) for the period shown in the current (bottom, right) trace. The fractional change varied almost linearly during the voltage step and began to decline immediately after the voltage was returned to -70 mV. The largest and fastest changes occurred at or near the terminal.

FLUORESCENCE CHANGES DUE TO LARGE DEPOLARIZATION

For our study of cones, voltage was clamped to various levels while recording the fluorescent light with the CCD camera system. Figure 2.2 shows the response to a depolarizing step to -30 mV (V_c), a voltage at which the calcium channels are activated, from a holding potential of -70 mV (V_h), a voltage at which the calcium channels are inactive, and illustrates a number of features that were consistently found in our recordings. Rises in calcium are signaled by upward deflections and are taken as such when they are time locked with the potential changes, as is seen in this figure. The cell body is labeled 5, and the fiber, oriented upward and to the right, ends in box 1. The results were that the fastest and largest fractional changes (traces 1, 2) occurred near or at the terminal of the cone cell (boxes 1, 2). In locations along the cone fiber approaching the cell body the signals were smaller and slower, while in the cell body itself (box 5) no obvious change in fluorescence was observed: the steady upward slope in the fluorescence trace from the cell body and other regions was caused by the bleaching of fura-2.

During the voltage step to -30 mV, the rise in calcium was approximately linear and probably reflected the steady build-up of calcium through a non-inactivating channel. The slight curvature seen at the top towards the end of the depolarization could reflect the removal of free calcium through buffering or extrusion. At the termination of the voltage step, the free calcium in the terminal began to decline immediately, presumably because the calcium restoration mechanisms had been activated and the calcium entry was turned off. The presence of cobalt (2 mM) in the bathing medium eliminated fluorescence signals during depolarizations (not shown) and suggested that calcium entry was necessary to obtain fluorescence signals.

THRESHOLD VOLTAGE OF FLUORESCENCE CHANGES

Whole-cell patch-clamp recording of solitary monkey cones revealed an activation potential of around -60 mV for a voltage-gated, noninactivating calcium channel (MacLeish, Burrous, and Yagi 1989). A similar experiment was carried out to determine the threshold potential for the detection of fluorescence changes. From a holding potential of -70 mV, the cell received 200-msec voltage steps to -60, -50, and -40 mV, as is shown in figure 2.3, in which only the fiber and terminal of a cone are shown. No changes in fluorescence were seen at -60 or at -50 mV, but at -40 mV a clear signal was observed that was largest and fastest in the terminal region. In fact, no change was detected in the regions in the field away from the terminal at -40 mV. In another cell, detectable fluorescence changes were seen in the terminal at -50 mV.

Therefore, there is fair agreement between the intracellular recording experiments measuring current through the calcium channel and the optical method measuring fura-2 fluorescence for the threshold potential for the activation of calcium entry. As in the previous experiment, the imaging rate was 20 frames per second, which corresponded to a collection time for the CCD camera of 50 msec per frame. This means that the cone is capable of responding well within 100 msec and possibly within 50 msec. More detailed experiments are needed to determine the upper limit on the response time for calcium, but a value of close to 20 msec is expected from flicker fusion frequencies of 50 to 60 Hz if one assumes the involvement of calcium-dependent calcium release in flicker fusion.

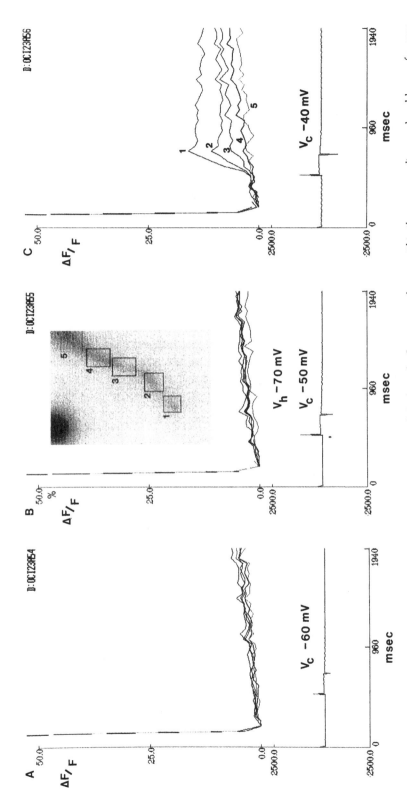

Figure 2.3 Threshold voltage for fluorescence changes. The traces in (A, B, and C) show the fluorescence changes within the corresponding numbered boxes of a cone terminal shown in (B). The voltage was held at −70 mV and stepped to −60 mV, −50 mV, and −40 mV in (A, B, and C), respectively. No changes are seen in A or B but clear-cut responses are observed in (C) at −40 mV. The largest signal was seen near the terminal. Bottom trace is voltage-clamp current. Images were collected at 20 frames per second.

RESPONSES TO 30 mM POTASSIUM IONS

To eliminate any confounding effect of the EGTA in the recording pipette, fluorescence changes were monitored in response to depolarizations by puffs of a solution containing 30 mM potassium ions and in the absence of intracellular pipettes. Thus, the cytoplasm of the cell was not manipulated for these measurements. Figure 2.4 shows that the concentration of free calcium rose rapidly in response to the application of potassium ions and fell at the offset of the pulse. The largest signal was again in the terminal region, while intermediate positions along the fiber showed smaller response. The cell body region showed possibly a small ON response but no clearcut OFF response.

CONCLUSION

Adult retinal cells from the monkey were effectively filled with fura-2 AM without any obvious effects on the light microscopic appearance of the cells. With this preparation, the imaging of fura-2 fluorescence in isolated monkey cones has provided additional information on the dynamics of free intracellular calcium changes in response to voltage changes. Readily detectable fractional changes in fluorescence were observed that differed in amplitude and kinetics depending on the part of the cone from which the signal was being monitored. Invariably, the largest and fastest signals arose in the terminal region but did not always coincide with the most distal part of the cone terminal. For large depolarizations, say to -30 mV, fractional changes in excess of 50 percent were frequently recorded. The signals decreased in amplitude and kinetics in regions approaching the soma, where hardly any change of calcium was observed during the voltage step. A similar finding was reported for the barnacle photoreceptor, in which the most rapid changes in intracellular free calcium were observed in terminal regions (Callaway et al. 1993). Fluorescence changes in the terminal region of monkey cones also showed the lowest threshold to voltage where changes were measurable at a potential of between -50 mV and -40 mV in figure 2.3 and at -50 mV in other cells. In this regard, there is fair agreement between the activation potential for the calcium conductance measured with intracellular pipettes and the threshold potential measured using the present fluorescence approach. The experiments in which potassium was puffed onto cells without intracellular pipette recording indicate that the fluorescence changes arose from intrinsic properties of the intact cone and were not, for example, influenced by the presence and diffusion of the calcium chelator, EGTA, from the patch pipette.

One interpretation of these results is that the calcium channels responsible for calcium entry are preferentially localized to regions near the terminal of the cone cell. If this were the case and if one assumes uniform calcium buffering and extrusion along the process, then the largest and fastest signals would be confined to the terminal region, as was found. It should be pointed out that the ratio of surface area to volume is higher in the terminal than in the cell body, say, and this would favor larger fractional changes in the terminal even

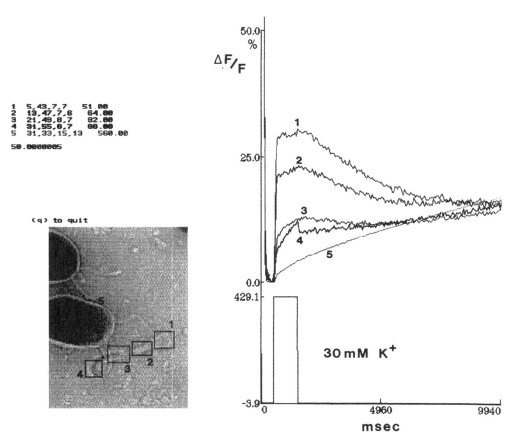

Figure 2.4 Fluorescence changes to 30 mM K$^+$. The potassium was puffed on the cone cell body for the period shown in the bottom timing trace. No intracellular electrical recording was made from this cell. Traces show the fluorescence within corresponding numbered boxes over different parts of the cone. The largest and fastest signals arose near the terminal region.

for a uniform density of calcium channels. We are not suggesting, however, that the density of calcium channels is uniform given the size and kinetics of signals along the process. In fact, there is evidence for local accumulation of calcium channels from freeze fracture experiments, which demonstrated clustering of large particles in the terminal region of cones from turtles (Schaeffer et al. 1982) and monkeys (Raviola and Gilula 1975) resembling putative calcium channels in other systems. Further experiments will be required to definitely determine whether calcium channels are localized to the terminal region and, if they are, to understand the mechanism of localization in normal cones and possible alterations in pathological states.

ACKNOWLEDGMENTS

Thanks to Estela V. O'Brien for collaborating with me in the early experiments, to the members of the Wiesel and Knight laboratories at The Rockefeller University and of the Victor laboratory at Cornell University Medical College for providing monkey eyes at the end of their experiments, to Peter Peirce for photography, and to Vanessa Falgoust for typing the manuscript. Work was supported by NIH Grant EY05201; The St. Giles Foundation, Richard Arkwright, President; and a Jules and Doris Stein Professorship to P.R.M.

REFERENCES

Attwell D, Werblin FS, and Wilson M (1982) The properties of single cones isolated from the tiger salamander retina. J Physiol 328:259–283.

Bader CR, Bertrand D, and Schwartz EA (1982) Voltage-activated and calcium-activated currents studied in solitary rod inner segments from salamander retina. J Physiol 331:253–284.

Barnes S, and Hille B (1989) Ionic channels of the inner segment of tiger salamander cone photoreceptors. J Gen Physiol 94:719–743.

Callaway JC, Lasser-Ross N, Stuart AE, and Ross WN (1993) Dynamics of intracellular free calcium concentration in the presynaptic arbors of individual barnacle photoreceptors. J Neurosci 13:1157–1166.

Grynkiewicz G, Poenie M, and Tsien RY (1985) A new generation of Ca^{2+} indicators with greatly improved fluorescence properties. J Biol Chem 260:3440–3450.

Hamill OP, Marty A, Neher E, Sakmann B, and Sigworth, FJ (1981) Improved patch-clamp techniques for high-resolution current recording from cells and cell-free membrane patches. Pflügers Arch 391:85–100.

Kaneko A and Shimazaki H (1976) Synaptic transmission from photoreceptors to bipolar and horizontal cells in the carp retina. Cold Spring Harbor Symp Quant Biol 40:537–546.

Lam DMK (1972) Biosynthesis of acetylchloine in turtle photoreceptors. Proc Natl Acad Sci USA 69:1987–1991.

Lasser-Ross N, Miyakawa H, Lev-Ram V, Young SR, and Ross WN (1991) High time resolution fluorescence imaging with a CCD camera. J Neurosci Methods 36:253–261.

MacLeish PR, Schwartz EA, and Tachibana M (1984) Control of the generator current in solitary rods of the Ambystoma Tigrinum Retina. J Physiol 348:645–664.

MacLeish PR, Burrous MR, and Yagi T (1989) Voltage-activated calcium current in solitary primate cones. Supplement to Invest Ophthal Vis Sci 30:163.

Maricq AV and Korenbrot JI (1988) Calcium and calcium-dependent chloride currents generate action potentials in solitary cone photoreceptors. Neuron 1:503–515.

Raviola E, and Gilula NB (1975) Intramembrane organization of specialized contacts in the outer plexiform layer of the retina. J Cell Biol 65:192–222.

Schaeffer S, Raviola E, and Heuser JE (1982) Membrane specializations in the outer plexiform layer of the turtle retina. J Comp Neurol 204:253–267.

Schwartz EA (1986) Synaptic transmission in amphibian retinae during conditions unfavorable for calcium entry into presynaptic terminals. J Physiol 376:411–428.

Thoreson WB, and Burkhardt DA (1991) Ionic influences on the prolonged depolarization of turtle cones in situ. J Neurophysiol 65:96–110.

Trifonov YA (1969) Study of synaptic transmission between photoreceptors and horizontal cells by means of electric stimulation of the retina. Biofysika 13:809–817.

Yagi T and MacLeish PR (1989) A large calcium-activated current in solitary primate cones. Invest Ophthal Vis Sci (Suppl) 30:62.

3 Glutamatergic Synaptic Excitation of Retinal Amacrine and Ganglion Cells

David R. Copenhagen, Scott Mittman,
W. Rowland Taylor, and Don B. Dixon

The arrayed retinal photoreceptors convert light from the visual scene into a pixelized neural image. As this neural image, coded initially by electrical potentials in photoreceptors, is transmitted through the retina to ganglion cells, it is selectively amplified, filtered, and modified. The final signal "read" into the ganglion cells is the result of many spatial and temporal interactions of excitation and inhibition. To understand the origin and functional characteristics of the signals that are transmitted to the brain through ganglion cells, it is necessary to dissect the features and parameters of excitation and inhibition. In the study described herein we have begun the process of identifying the temporal, biophysical, and pharmacological bases of the excitation of ganglion cells and amacrine cells in the amphibian retina. Bipolar cells are the predominant source of excitatory input to these cells, and the excitatory neurotransmitter released by the bipolars is most probably glutamate. (Marc et al. 1990; Massey and Redburn 1987; Ehinger et al. 1988; Okada and Tachibana 1990; Slaughter and Miller 1983a).

Pharmacologically, it is possible to distinguish four types of glutamate receptor that mediate glutamatergic synaptic transmission in the nervous system (see Mayer and Westbrook 1987a and Collingridge and Lester 1990). These receptors are differentiated by the selective action of agonists: 2-amino-4-phosphonobutyrate activates the APB type glutamate receptor; N-methyl-D-aspartate activates the NMDA type receptor; kainate, quisqualate, and AMPA activate the non-NMDA type receptor; and quisqualate and ACPD activate the metabotropic type receptor. In the retina, the stimulation of APB, NMDA, and non-NMDA receptors underlies the excitation of bipolar and horizontal cells (Slaughter and Miller 1981; Yang and Wu 1989). Some evidence indicates that amacrine and ganglion cells can be excited by non-NMDA and NMDA glutamate receptors; however, many of these studies concluded that NMDA receptors played little or no role in the generation of light responses in these cells (Slaughter and Miller 1983b; Coleman et al. 1986; Massey and Miller 1988; Coleman and Miller 1988). Here we outline evidence that the light responses of ganglion and amacrine cells are mediated by NMDA and non-NMDA receptors, except for the ON type amacrine cells, which appear to be excited exclusively by non-NMDA glutamate receptors.

Our study was performed in the retinal slice preparation developed by Werblin (1978) and Wu (1987). Patch pipettes used in the whole-cell mode were used to voltage clamp ganglion and amacrine cells while recording their responses to light. The influence of inhibitory neurotransmitters was removed by recording in the presence of bicuculline and strychnine to block GABAergic and glycinergic synaptic inputs, respectively. This study is restricted to ON and ON-OFF cell types since the OFF types were rarely encountered in this preparation.

METHODS

Tiger salamander retinal slices were prepared under dim illumination ($\lambda = 700$ nm) as described by Werblin and Wu. Slices were superfused with saline (104 mM NaCl, 2 mM KCl, 2 mM $CaCl_2$, 1 mM $MgCl_2$, 5 mM glucose, and 5 mM HEPES, adjusted to pH 7.6 with NaOH) at room temperature. The patch pipette, for tight-seal, whole-cell recording, contained 84 mM KF, 3.4 mM NaCl, 400 μM $CaCl_2$, 400 μM $MgCl_2$, 11 mM EGTA and 10 mM NaHEPES, adjusted to pH 7.6 with KOH. The recording bandwidth was 0 to 500 Hz for membrane currents and 0 to 1 kHz for membrane potentials. The membrane potentials have been corrected for the change in the liquid junction at the pipette tip in the whole-cell configuration. Light ($\lambda = 520$ nm) was delivered at a right angle to the long axis of the photoreceptors and illuminated a 680-μm length of the slice, centered on the recorded ganglion cell.

RESULTS

Glutamate Excites ON Ganglion Cells and ON-OFF Amacrine and Ganglion Cells via NMDA and Non-NMDA Receptors

Amacrine and ganglion cells were recorded and identified on the basis of their light responses. Typically, ON cells exhibited a sustained current that lasted for the duration of a light stimulus. ON-OFF cells responded with a transient current at the onset and termination of the light response. Figure 3.1 illustrates the light responses of an ON-OFF and an ON ganglion cell recorded under current clamp (top traces) and under voltage clamp (bottom traces).

Following identification of the cell type, the synaptic transmission to amacrine and ganglion cells was blocked with calcium channel blockers (20 μM cadmium or 5 mM manganese). Under these conditions, light elicited no response in the cells. Figure 3.2A shows the time course over which cadmium blocked the light responses. Typically, glutamate and the glutamate agonists NMDA, quisqualate, or kainate were bath-applied or were ionophoretically puffed onto the cells from tubes or large-lumen pipettes positioned above each slice at the level of the inner plexiform layer. Figure 3.2B shows the responses of an ON-OFF ganglion cell to NMDA. In figure 3.2C the peak

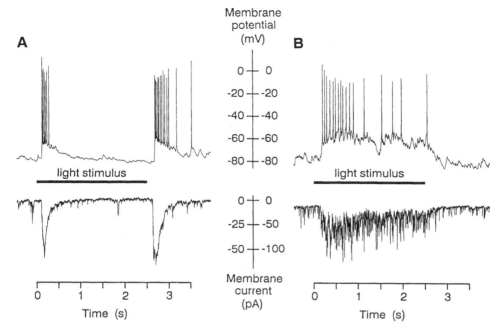

Figure 3.1 Voltage (top traces) and current (bottom traces) responses to light stimulation of an ON-OFF (A) and ON ganglion cell (B). The holding potential was −76 mV. The light stimulus timing is indicated by the bar. The photon densities were 6×10^5 photons $\mu m^{-2}\ s^{-1}$ and 6×10^4 photons $\mu m^{-2}\ s^{-1}$. From Mittman et al. 1990.

current evoked at each holding potential is plotted as a current-voltage (I−V) curve.

The salient features of the I−V curves from ON-OFF amacrine and ganglion cells to NMDA were that the currents reversed near zero mV and were nearly linear for positive holding potentials. Additionally, at holding potentials progressively more negative from zero mV, the inward current increased, reached a peak in the range of −30 to −40 mV, and then declined for further hyperpolarization. This nonlinear behavior, termed a *negative slope region*, in which there is an attenuation of current at progressively larger potentials, is typical of NMDA glutamate receptors. The reduction of current is attributed to a block of the NMDA channels by magnesium (Mayer et al. 1984; Nowak et al. 1984). We found that, if the retina was bathed in magnesium-free saline, the reduction of current at negative potentials was eliminated and the I−V curve became much more linear (Mittman et al. 1990).

The ON-OFF ganglion and amacrine cells also responded to the non-NMDA glutamate agonists kainate and quisqualate. The salient features of these results were that the evoked currents reversed near zero mV and that the I−V curve was nearly linear. These characteristics are typical of responses mediated by non-NMDA glutamate receptors.

The application of glutamate to the ON-OFF amacrine and ganglion cells produced I−V curves that were intermediate between the kainate and NMDA

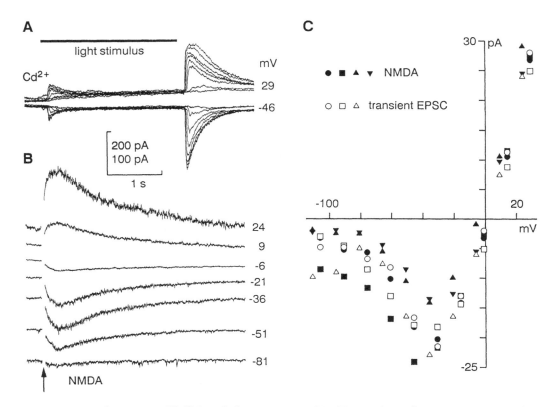

Figure 3.2 NMDA-evoked currents in an ON-OFF ganglion cell. (A) Prior to testing the effects of glutamate-receptor agonists, 20 μM Cd^{++} was added to the superfusing saline to block synaptic activity. The 16 traces show the progressive decline in amplitude of response to 16 light stimuli (6×10^5 photons μm^{-2} s^{-1}) delivered regularly during the first 5 min after addition of 20 μM Cd^{++} to the superfusing saline. In (B) the currents evoked by ionophoresis (5.6 nC) of NMDA are shown. The arrow indicates the timing of the ionophoresis; the stimulus artifacts have been edited out for clarity. Plotted in (C) are the normalized I–V relations of NMDA responses and slow transient EPSCs of four cells. The I–V relations of NMDA responses are plotted with filled symbols (squares and diamonds indicate addition to the superfusing saline, and triangles indicate ionophoretic application). The matched open symbols show the I–V relations of the slow transient EPSC (measured 300 to 432 ms after cessation of light responses) in these same cells. The cell represented by upright triangles had no light responses. All I–V relations were normalized to have a slope of 1 nS between −6 and 29 mV. (From Mittman et al. 1990)

curves. Typically, the current reversed at zero and increased for progressively more negative polarizations of about −30 to −70 mV. The I–V curve was relatively flat from this level to about −70 mV. Our hypothesis is that glutamate simultaneously activates both non-NMDA and NMDA receptors to produce the intermediate I–V curve. Our conclusion from these studies of ON-OFF cells is that glutamate excites these neurons by acting at both NMDA and non-NMDA receptors.

ON ganglion cells were similarly activated by both types of glutamate receptors. The application of glutamate, kainate, or NMDA evoked currents that were similar in form to those described above for the ON-OFF amacrine and ganglion cells (data not shown).

Glutamate Excites ON Amacrine Cells Exclusively via Non-NMDA Glutamate Receptors

Figure 3.3 shows the response of an ON amacrine cell to glutamate, kainate, and NMDA. In a manner similar to that in the above experiments, light responses were blocked with a calcium channel blocker, manganese in this case, and inhibitory inputs were also blocked. Both glutamate and kainate evoked large currents that reversed near zero mV. The I–V curve for these two compounds were nearly identical and showed no evidence of a negative slope region at hyperpolarized holding potentials. NMDA had no effect on these cells. We conclude from these experiments that ON amacrine cells do not express functional NMDA receptors.

The Light Responses of ON-OFF Amacrine and Ganglion Cells and ON Ganglion Cells Are Mediated by NMDA and Non-NMDA Receptors

I–V curves for the light responses of ON-OFF amacrine and ganglion cells were determined. We found that the I–V curve measured before the peak of the light response was monotonic. However, the I–V curve measured after the peak had a distinctive nonlinearity characteristic of NMDA-mediated inputs. We hypothesized on this basis that each light response was composed of a faster non-NMDA and a slower NMDA component. Figure 3.4 shows an example of I–V curves for OFF responses in an ON-OFF ganglion cell computed 180 and 400 msec after the stimulus termination. The open circles, plotting the late I–V, show a distinctive negative slope, which is characteristic of NMDA-mediated inputs. The open squares, plotting the early I–V, are more monotonic. We believe the flat curve at negative holding potentials reflects a mix of non-NMDA and NMDA inputs. The distinct differences in the shapes of the I–V curves measured at early and late times held for both ON-OFF amacrine and ganglion cells (see figure 1, Dixon and Copenhagen 1992). Selective glutamate antagonists were used to better dissect the NMDA and non-NMDA components of light responses in these cells.

Typically, the application of 1 μM 6-cyano-7-nitroquinoxaline-2,3-dione (CNQX), an antagonist to non-NMDA receptors, revealed a slow component of the light responses that had a negative-slope I–V curve at hyperpolarized holding potentials. This slower component is blocked by NMDA antagonists and is therefore thought to be the NMDA part of the light response. The application of 20 μM DL-2-amino-7-phosphonoheptanoate (AP7), a selective NMDA antagonist, revealed a fast component of light responses that had nearly linear I–V curves and reversed near zero mV. We conclude that this faster component of the light response in ON-OFF cells is due to the activation of non-NMDA receptors. Figure 3.5 shows an example of the effects

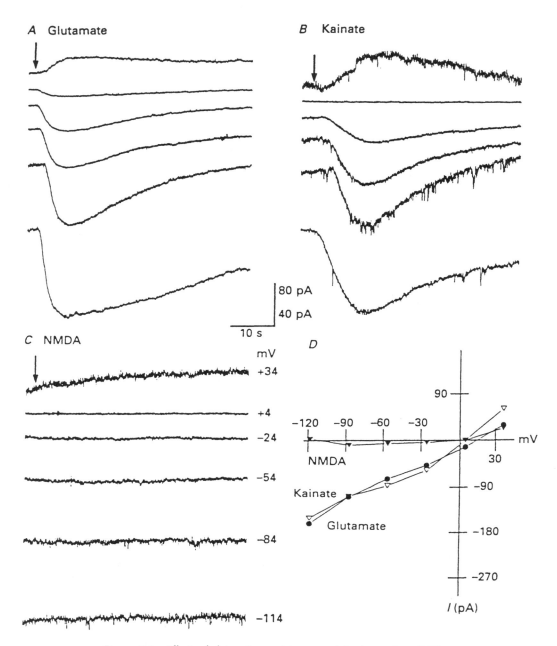

Figure 3.3 Effects of glutamate agonists on a sustained amacrine cell. The agonist concentration in the perfusion pipette was 250 μM; application was for 250 ms at the point indicated by the downward arrow. (A) Responses to glutamate at clamp potentials are indicated in the margin of (C). (B) Responses to kainate. (C) Responses to NMDA. No response could be obtained with NMDA. (D) I–V relations from (A), (B), and (C). Glutamate (closed circles), kainate (triangles), NMDA (filled triangles). For kainate and glutamate microperfusion the light responses were blocked by 20 μM Cd^{2+}. For NMDA microperfusion they were blocked with 5 mM Mn^{2+}. Scale bar: 80 pA (A and B), 40 pA (C). (From Dixon and Copenhagen 1992)

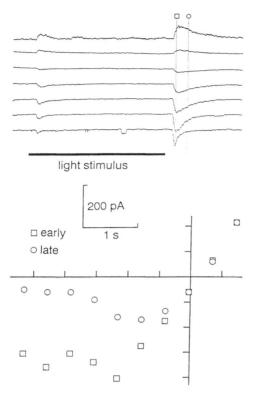

Figure 3.4 I–V curves determined from light responses of an ON-OFF ganglion cell. Light responses were recorded at +29, +14, −1, −16, −31, −46 and −91 mV. The dotted lines labeled by the square and circle mark the times at which transient EPSC I–V relations were determined. The current evoked 184 ms (open squares) or 400 ms (open circles) after cessation of the light stimulus, in 500 nM strychnine and 100 μM bicuculline methobromide, is plotted as a function the membrane potential. The evoked current was calculated as the difference between the membrane current at the indicated time and the membrane current preceding the response. (From Mittman et al. 1990)

of CNQX and AP7 on the OFF response of an ON-OFF amacrine cell. In AP7 (parts A and B) the light response is rapid and has a nearly linear I–V curve. In CNQX (parts C and D) the light response is slower and the I–V has a negative slope below −40 mV. These results indicate that the light response has an NMDA component that is kinetically slower than the non-NMDA component.

The light responses of ON ganglion cells also appear to be mediated by the concurrent activation of NMDA and non-NMDA receptors. Because the light response is continuous for the duration of the stimulus, it was not possible to identify or dissect a slow and fast component of the light responses. However, using CNQX and AP7 it was possible to demonstrate both an NMDA and a non-NMDA component. Figure 3.6 shows the control response of an ON ganglion cell to light stimuli at different holding potentials. Parts B and C show the response in AP7 and CNQX, respectively. In AP7 the response

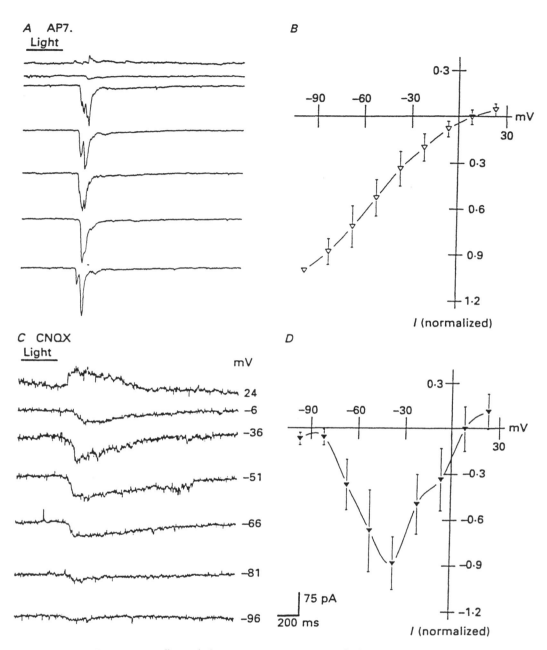

Figure 3.5 Effects of glutamatergic antagonists on the light response of transient amacrine cells. (A) OFF response recorded in AP7 (30 μM). Clamp potentials were identical to those shown in the margin of (C). The prolonged portion of the response that is prominent at membrane potentials positive to -60 mV is absent. (B) Averaged, normalized I–V relation obtained from 5 cells recorded in AP7. The mean peak current at -96 mV was -128.3 p 56.4 pA. The curve is monotonic, with no obvious flattening between -35 and -65 mV. The error bars are standard deviations. (C) OFF response from the same cell recorded in CNQX (2 μM). The fast early portion of the response is eliminated by CNQX. (D) Averaged, normalized I–V relation obtained from 5 cells. The mean peak current at -36 mV was -74.3 p 21.7 pA. A pronounced negatively sloped region was evident between -35 and -80 mV. (From Dixon and Copenhagen 1992)

retains the noisier components but has lower sustained levels than control records at potentials near or above zero mV. The I–V curve (represented by the solid squares in part D) is more linear than in the control. In CNQX, with the non-NMDA receptor blocked, the light response is much smoother and retains the larger sustained component at holding potentials at or above zero mV. The I–V curve (represented by solid circles in part E) has a negative slope region below −30 mV. We conclude that the sustained light response in ON ganglion cells is mediated by continuous activation of both non-NMDA and NMDA receptors. This finding contrasts with the results found for ON amacrine cells.

The Excitatory Response of ON Amacrine Cells Is Mediated Exclusively by Non-NMDA Receptors

Above we showed that glutamate excited ON amacrine cells via non-NMDA receptors only. This same finding held true for the light response. The application of the non-NMDA antagonist CNQX abolished the light responses completely, while the application of the NMDA antagonist AP7 had no effect on these cells. Figure 3.7 shows the light responses of an ON amacrine cell in the control, in AP7, and in CNQX. CNQX eliminated the light response. The I–V curve for the control and AP7 were nearly linear and reversed near zero mV. We conclude from these studies that the light responses of ON amacrine cells do not have an NMDA component. A summary diagram depicting our findings is shown in Figure 3.8. Briefly, the ON and OFF components of the light responses of the ON-OFF amacrine and ganglion cells are mediated via the concurrent activation of non-NMDA and NMDA receptors. ON bipolars release glutamate to activate both types of receptors on the ON ganglion cells but only non-NMDA receptors on the ON amacrine cells.

Bipolar Cells Must Release Glutamate Transiently as Well as Continuously

The transience of the light responses of ON-OFF amacrine and ganglion cells is enigmatic. Bipolar cells, the source of synaptic inputs, maintain a sustained polarization with light stimulation (Werblin and Dowling 1968) and presumably release neurotransmitter continuously. The responses of the ON amacrine and ganglion cells seem consistent with this concept. However, the synaptic inputs to ON-OFF cells are not sustained. This transience cannot be attributed to the desensitization of glutamate receptors, to inhibitory inputs, or to voltage-dependent conductances that truncate the response. The evidence against desensitization is that NMDA receptors typically desensitize with a longer time course than the light responses. The evidence against GABAergic- or glycinergic-mediated inhibition is that the retinas were bathed in bicuculline and strychnine and the transience was preserved. The evidence against voltage-gated conductances is that the cells were recorded under voltage clamp.

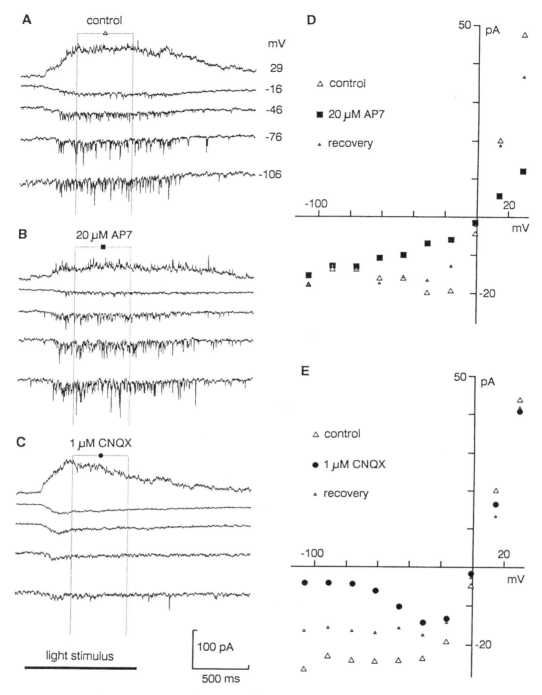

Figure 3.6 AP7 and CNQX each block a component of the sustained EPSC of ON ganglion cells. Light-evoked postsynaptic currents were recorded under three conditions. In (A) the retinal slices were superfused with a control saline. In (B) 20 μM AP7 was added to this control saline, and in (C) 1 μM CNQX was added to the control saline. Traces were recorded at the membrane potentials listed to the right of (A). The dotted lines labeled with the square, circle,

Therefore, we favor the suggestion of Toyoda et al. (1973) that the release of glutamate from bipolar terminals onto ON-OFF cells is transient. Consistent with this idea is the finding of Golcich et al. (1990) that the pharmacological lesioning of amacrine cells in chick retinas does not affect the ON-OFF responses of transient ganglion cells. One implication of this model is that either there are two different classes of ON bipolar cells or that release from one part of the terminal is transient and from another region it is sustained. Further work will be required to verify or rule out these possibilities.

Does the Concomitant Activation of NMDA and Non-NMDA Receptors Linearize Excitatory Synaptic Inputs to ON Ganglion Cells?

Figure 3.6 showed that there was a significant NMDA contribution to the light responses of ON ganglion cells. The I–V curve of the control light response (in figure 3.6, parts D and E) has a near-zero slope from −80 mV to −30 mV. We hypothesize that the near-zero slope conductance results from the combined activity of non-NMDA and NMDA conductances.

We have constructed a simple equivalent circuit model to investigate and assess the functional differences one might expect between a ganglion cell with strictly non-NMDA inputs and one with mixed non-NMDA and NMDA inputs. The efficacy of synaptic input mediated by nonselective cation channels such as the channel gated by the non-NMDA receptor declines with increasing levels of synaptic activity due to the reduction in driving force accompanying depolarization (Martin 1955). With an appropriate mix of NMDA and non-NMDA receptors, however, synaptic efficacy will remain nearly constant until the level of input is sufficient to depolarize the membrane past the range of zero slope-conductance.

To illustrate this point, we calculated the effect of steady-state synaptic inputs on model neurons. Relative synaptic efficacy was calculated by solving the nonlinear simultaneous equations for a resistive network corresponding to a model neuron with an input conductance of 770 pS, a soma diameter of 18 μm, and a trunk 1 μm in diameter and 10 μm in length, giving rise to two dendrites 0.63 μm in diameter and 200 μm in length. The dimensionless electrotonic length (Rall 1977) was 0.34, assuming a cytoplasmic conductivity of 1 S m^{-1}; q was 0.78. The resting membrane potential was −70 mV, and the reversal potential of the synaptic conductances was 0 mV. The non-

and triangle bracket the 500-ms periods over which membrane current was averaged to produce the I–V relations in (D) and (E). (D) The mean I–V relations of two sustained EPSCs were determined before (large square), during (circle), and after (small square) the application of AP7. The evoked current was calculated as the difference between the mean current during a half-second portion of the light response, which is bracketed by the dotted lines in (A–C), and the current in the dark. (E) The mean I–V relations of the same two sustained EPSCs was determined before (large square), during (triangle), and after (small square) application of CNQX. The control I–V relations in the two panels differ because a second control run was recorded between the applications of the two antagonists and because the antagonists were applied in reverse order in the second cell. (From Mittman et al. 1990)

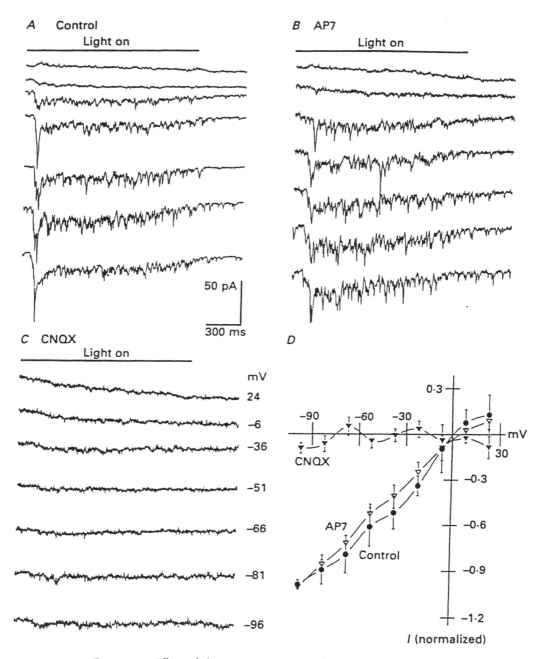

Figure 3.7 Effects of glutamate antagonists on the light responses of sustained amacrine cell. (A) Responses to light in control saline at the holding potentials listed in the margin of (C). (B) Responses in AP7 (30 μM). Compared to the control, the peak and plateau portions of the response were changed minimally, although there was some reduction in the size of the initial peak. The reduction was not typical of all cells recorded in AP7 and could have resulted from a subtle change in the recording conditions. Additionally, the current fluctuations during the response were similar, and the reversal potential was unchanged. (C) Response in CNQX (2 μM). The entire light response was eliminated in CNQX. (D) average, normalized I–V relations for 7 sustained amacrine cells recorded in the control saline (filled circles), AP7 (open triangles), and CNQX (filled triangles). (From Dixon and Copenhagen 1992)

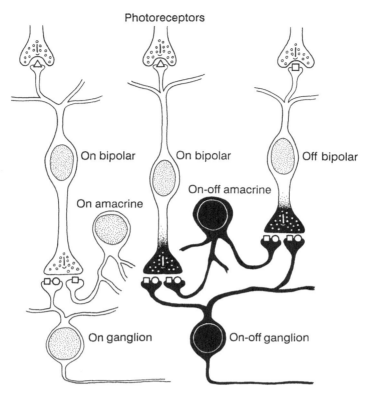

Figure 3.8 Schematic representation of the glutamatergic excitatory pathways in the sala-mander retina. Constant light produces sustained responses in photoreceptors and bipolar cells. In the inner retina some responses become transient, as indicated in this figure by the dark-shaded cell bodies and terminals. The light-evoked response in transient amacrine and in all ganglion cells is mediated by non-NMDA (open squares) and NMDA (open circles) co-activation. Sustained ON ganglion cells also have a mixed non-NMDA and NMDA input, whereas ON sustained amacrine cells have exclusively non-NMDA inputs. Bipolar cell inputs are through the non-NM,DA and AP4 (open triangles) receptor types. (From Dixon and Copenhagen 1992)

synaptic conductances were voltage-independent. The physical and electrical parameters are typical of retinal ganglion cells (present results and R. F. Miller and P. A. Coleman, personal communication), but the conclusions drawn from the model were not changed when simulations were run on neurons with electrotonic lengths of between 0 and 1.

To model the NMDA I–V relation, an interpolating polynomial was fitted to the I–V relation of the CNQX-resistant sustained EPSC in figure 3.6. The I–V relation of the current mediated by the non-NMDA receptor was as-sumed to be a straight line. The mixed I–V relation was obtained by choosing a linear combination of the two I–V relations, giving a shape similar to the control I–V relations of figure 3.6. To generate the curves of part A, synaptic conductance was equally distributed among the 20 dendritic compartments. The current entering the soma as a result of this input is the abscissa of A. The

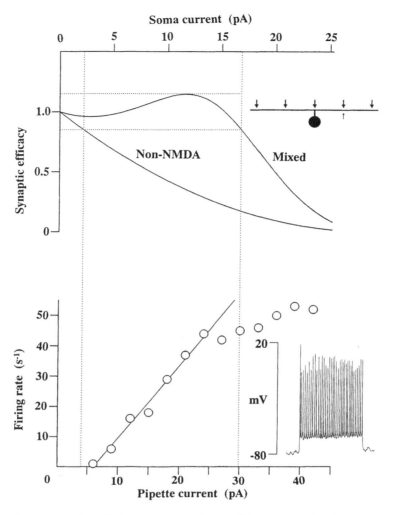

Figure 3.9 Synaptic inputs sum more linearly if inputs are mediated by a mixed population of NMDA and non-NMDA receptors. (A) Efficacy of a small, steady synaptic input applied to the midpoint of a model neuron dendrite (inset, small arrow) as a function of the soma current generated by varying magnitudes of steady synaptic conductance, which are applied uniformly to the dendrites (large arrows). Bottom curve, all input was mediated by non-NMDA receptors. Top curve, all input was mediated by a mixed population of NMDA and non-NMDA receptors. Horizontal, dotted lines mark efficacies of 115 and 85 percent. Vertical, dotted lines mark the currents at which the curves reach 85 percent efficacy. (B) Number of action potentials elicited in an exemplar ganglion cell by a 1-s injection of current through the recording pipette as a function of current magnitude. Although this was an ON-OFF cell, similar results were obtained in two ON cells. The inset shows the response at 21 pA. The line is a least-squares fit to the first 7 points. The abscissae of A and B are related by the equation $i_{soma} = i_{pipette}/(q + 1)$, where q is the ratio of the dendritic and somatic conductances of the model neuron (Rall 1977).

ordinate is the additional current contributed by a small input to the midpoint of one dendrite relative to the current contributed by the same small input in the absence of the distributed input.

Figure 3.9A shows the results for a model neuron (inset) with passive electrical properties similar to those of retinal ganglion cells. The curves plot the normalized change in soma current evoked by a small increment in synaptic conductance (relative synaptic efficacy) as a function of the total soma current in the model neuron. The conductance increment (inset, small arrow) was applied halfway between the soma and the end of a dendrite. The total soma current was varied in the model by varying the magnitude of the synaptic conductance distributed uniformly along the dendrites (inset, large arrows). The lower curve shows the result when synaptic inputs were mediated by non-NMDA receptors. Synaptic efficacy dropped sharply, losing 15 percent of its initial value at a somatic current of only 2.2 pA, equivalent to a depolarization of only 5.2 mV. The upper curve shows the result when synaptic inputs were mediated by a mixed population of NMDA and non-NMDA receptors with an I–V relation similar to that depicted by the triangles in figure 3.6. Synaptic efficacy was much less sensitive to the level of synaptic input; the efficacy of the mixed input remained within 15 percent of its initial value until the somatic current exceeded 17 pA, giving a 39 mV depolarization.

This range of near-constant synaptic efficacy included most of the operating range of a ganglion cell. Figure 3.9B shows that the firing rate of a retinal ganglion cell, like that of some other neurons (Granit et al. 1963; Baylor and Fettiplace 1979) increased linearly with the current injected via the recording pipette, up to about 40 s^{-1}. The abscissae of Figure 3.9A and B are scaled so that the somatic currents of the model can be compared with the currents injected to elicit firing in a real neuron. The dotted vertical lines extending between the two parts of the figure show that, for inputs mediated by non-NMDA receptors alone, synapses began to lose their effectiveness even below the firing threshold. With a mixed population of receptors, however, synapses were almost equally effective over most of the operating range of the neuron.

CONCLUSIONS

Previous work has suggested that NMDA receptor activation may alter the function of postsynaptic neurons by mediating the influx of calcium during maintained postsynaptic depolarization (Mayer and Westbrook 1987; MacDermott et al. 1986) or that neuronal excitability may increase due to the negative slope-conductance of the current gated by NMDA receptors (Mayer et al. 1984; Nowak et al. 1984). Our results suggest an additional role; the synaptic activation of the two receptor types, in the proper ratio, may be a mechanism for achieving more linear summation of synaptic inputs and, hence, maintaining a linear relationship between synaptic input and firing rate.

ACKNOWLEDGMENTS

We thank Tess Noche for the preparation of the manuscript. The work was supported by NIH EY01869 (D.R.C.), GM07618 (S.M.), Fight for Sight (W.R.T. and D.B.D.), the National Society to Prevent Blindness (S.M.), and a Canadian NSERC postdoctoral fellowship (D.B.D.).

REFERENCES

Baylor DA, Fettiplace R (1979) Synaptic drive and impulse generation in ganglion cells of turtle retina. J Physiol 288:107–127.

Coleman PA, Massey SC, Miller RF (1986) Kynurenic acid distinguishes kainate and quisqualate receptors in the vertebrate retina. Brain Res 381:172–175.

Collingridge GL, Lester RA (1989) Excitatory amino acid receptors in the vertebrate central nervous system. Pharmacol Rev 41:143–210.

Dixon DB, Copenhagen DR (1992) Two types of glutamate receptors differentially excite amacrine cells in the tiger salamander retina. J Physiol 449:589–606.

Ehinger B, Otterson O, Storm-Mathisen J, Dowling J (1988) Bipolar cells in the turtle retina are strongly immunoreactive for glutamate. Proc Natl Acad Sci USA 85:8321–8325.

Golcich MA, Morgan IG, Dvorak DR (1990) Selective abolition of OFF responses in kainic acid-lesioned chicken retina. Brain Res 535:288–300.

Granit R, Kernell D, Shortess, GK (1963) Quantitative aspects of repetitive firing of mammalian motoneurones, caused by injected currents. J Physiol 168:911–931.

MacDermott AB, Mayer ML, Westbrook GL, Smith SJ, Barker JL (1986) NMDA-receptor activation increases cytoplasmic calcium concentration in cultured spinal cord neurones. Nature 321:519–522.

Marc R, Liu W-L, Kalloniatis M, Raiguel S, Van Haesendonck E (1990) Patterns of glutamate immunoreactivity in the goldfish retina. J Neurosci 10:4006–4034.

Martin AR (1955) A further study of the statistical composition of the end-plate potential. J Physiol 130:114–122.

Massey SC, Miller RF (1988) Glutamate receptors of ganglion cells in the rabbit retina: evidence for glutamate as a bipolar cell transmitter. J Neurophysiol 405:635–655.

Mayer ML, Westbrook GL (1984) Mixed-agonist action of excitatory amino acids on mouse spinal cord neurones under voltage clamp. J Physiol 354:29– 53.

Mayer ML, Westbrook GL (1987a) The physiology of excitatory amino acids in the vertebrate central nervous system. Prog Neurobiol 28:197–276.

Mayer ML, Westbrook GL (1987b) Permeation and block of N-methyl-D-aspartic acid receptor channels by divalent cations in mouse cultured central neurones. J Physiol 394:501–527.

Mayer ML, Westbrook GL, Guthrie PB (1984) Voltage-dependent block by Mg^{2+} of NMDA responses in spinal cord neurones. Nature 309:261–263.

Mittman S, Taylor WR, Copenhagen DR (1990) Concomitant activation of two types of glutamate receptor mediates excitation of salamander retinal ganglion cells. J Physiol 428:175–197.

Nowak L, Bregestovski P, Ascher P, Herbet A, Prochiantz A (1984) Magnesium gates glutamate-activated channels in mouse central neurones. Nature 307:462–465.

Rall W (1977) Core conductor theory and cable properties of neurons. In Magoun HW (ed), Handbook of Physiology, section 1, Vol 1. Baltimore: William and Wilkins.

Slaughter MM, Miller RF (1981) 2-amino-4-phosphonobutyric acid: a new pharmacological tool for retina research. Science 211:182–185.

Slaughter MM, Miller RF (1983a) Bipolar cells in the mudpuppy retina use an excitatory amino acid neurotransmitter. Nature 303:537–538.

Slaughter MM, Miller RF (1983b) The role of excitatory amino acid transmitters in the mudpuppy retina: an analysis with kainic acid and N-methyl-D-aspartate. J Neurosci 3:1701–1711.

Tachibana M, Okada T (1991) Release of endogenous excitatory amino acids from ON-type bipolar cells isolated from goldfish retina. J Neurosci 11:2199–2208.

Toyoda J, Hashimoto H, Ohtsu K (1973) Bipolar-amacrine transmission in the carp retina. Vision Res 13:295–307.

Werblin FS (1978) Transmission along and between rods in tiger salamander. J Physiol 280:449–470.

Werblin FS, Dowling JE (1969) Organization of the retina of the mudpuppy, Necturus maculosus. II. Intracellular recording. J Neurophys 32:339–355.

Wu SM (1987) Synaptic connections between neurons in living slices of the larval tiger salamander retina. J Neurosci Meth 20:139–149.

Yang XL, Wu SM (1989) Effects of CNQX, APB, PDA and kynurenate on horizontal cells of the tiger salamander retina. Vis Neurosci 3:207–212.

4 You Cannot Inhibit a Good Receptor: GABA Receptor Diversity in the Vertebrate Retina

Malcolm M. Slaughter and Ning Tian

The two primary functions of the vertebrate retina are the transduction of light energy into electrical energy and the translation of visual information into neuronal signals. The first process is accomplished by the outer segments of rods and cones. The second involves the retinal network and culminates in the spike train of ganglion cells. A fundamental element in this process is the decomposition of the visual image into a number of salient components. One of the fascinating achievements of Christina Enroth-Cugell has been the description of an essential building block in this decomposition, the X and Y type ganglion cells.

Decomposition of the visual image begins in the outer retina, where the ON-OFF separation, center-surround inhibition, and color integration begin. This continues in the inner retina and is coupled with such specializations as trigger feature formation. A very successful effort has been made to show the correlations between cell physiology and anatomy in the retina. For example, ON bipolars often make invaginating synapses with photoreceptors, while OFF bipolars make flat contacts, and their axons end in discrete sublamina in the inner plexiform layer (Famiglietti and Kolb 1976). In the inner retina there is a clear separation between linear and nonlinear ganglion cells, and these distinct X and Y physiologies (Enroth-Cugell and Robson 1966) are correlated with discrete anatomies (beta and alpha) as well (Boycott and Wässle, 1974). This indicates that the nervous system must use a combination of anatomical and physiological specializations in concert to perform a particular function in the overall decomposition of the visual image.

In addition to these anatomical and physiological specializations, pharmacological diversity is an essential ingredient in the decomposition of visual images. Although there is a plethora of retinal neurotransmitters, the yeoman's share of synaptic communication is performed by just three: glutamate, the presumed transmitter of photoreceptors and bipolar cells, as well as GABA and glycine, which are used by about two-thirds of the amacrine cells and by some horizontal and interplexiform cells (see the review by Massey and Redburn 1987). This would seem to limit diversity and suggest that pharmacology does not play an important role in creating the variety needed to relay the multiplicity of visual information. But it is becoming apparent that postsynaptic receptor diversity is a key element in this process.

Essentially, several receptors may extract different information from the same neurotransmitter, thereby encoding different aspects of the original signal. This property is well illustrated in the distal retina, where the glutamate released by photoreceptors acts on three discrete receptors in ON bipolars, OFF bipolars, and horizontal cells (Miller and Slaughter 1986). Thus the decomposition of a monotonic photoreceptor light signal into symmetrical signals in ON and OFF bipolars originates in the diversity of glutamate receptors. The unusual properties of the ON bipolar glutamate receptor confer both the sign-inverting polarity and the prolonged synaptic delay that are the hallmarks of the ON bipolar light response (Nawy and Jahr 1990).

A similar receptor diversity exists among inhibitory transmitters in the inner retina, although there is a slight neurotransmitter diversity as well since there are two major transmitters, GABA and glycine. Both inhibitory amino acids are found throughout the inner plexiform layer, although there is an apparent weighting of glycine in the "a" (OFF) sublamina and GABA in the "b" (ON) sublamina. Several studies have been directed at contrasting the effects of GABA and glycine since they both produce a powerful chloride-mediated inhibition through similar mechanisms (Bormann et al. 1987; Cohen et al. 1989). For example, three proposals are (1) that GABA regulates inhibition in the ON system and glycine in the OFF (Frumkes et al. 1981; Ikeda and Sheardown 1983); (2) that glycine mediates phasic inhibition, while GABA generates sustained inhibition (Belgum et al. 1984); or (3) that they mediate different ganglion cell trigger features (Caldwell et al. 1978).

Implicit in these studies was the hypothesis that, since these transmitters acted through similar mechanisms (chloride gating), their unique function must be linked to a sharing of the inhibitory responsibilities. Although there are good experimental data in support of these models, the roles of GABA and glycine are more extensive. The discovery that both inhibitory transmitters act at several different receptors indicates that, like excitatory amino acids, receptor diversity may permit multiple signals to be relayed by one neurotransmitter. In this chapter we discuss the multiplicity of GABA receptors and their possible function in the retina.

METHODS

Studies were performed using two amphibia: the mudpuppy, *Necturus maculosus* and the tiger salamander, *Ambystoma tigrinum*. With respect to the topics addressed in this chapter, no major differences were seen between these two closely related animals. The preparation used was either the superfused retina eyecup (Miller and Dacheux 1976) or the retinal slice (Werblin 1978; Wu 1987). The major differences between these two preparations are that the retinal slice is only a thin segment (approximately 300 μm) of the retina and that it has no attached pigment epithelium. Conventional, high-resistance electrodes were used for current clamp experiments in the eyecup, while low-resistance, whole-cell electrodes were used for current and voltage clamp in the slice.

RESULTS

There are three putative types of GABA receptors: $GABA_A$, $GABA_B$, and $GABA_C$. The $GABA_A$ is the classic, chloride-gating receptor (Krnjevic and Schwartz 1967). The $GABA_B$ receptor acts through second messengers to open potassium channels (Newberry and Nicoll 1984) or close calcium channels (Dolphin and Scott 1986). The $GABA_C$ receptor, although postulated by Johnston et al. in 1975, is the newest putative subtype. There is only limited experimental evidence of this distinct receptor subtype, but the best supporting data come from studies in goldfish retinal bipolar cells (Matthews et al. 1991), where it closes a calcium channel.

Results Using the Retina Eyecup Preparation

GABA activates all three receptors, but there are selective analogs that permit assays of the relative importance of these receptor subtypes. GABA and three such agonists are illustrated in figure 4.1. Figure 4.2 shows the effects of these GABA agonists on a transient ON-OFF third-order neuron. Muscimol (Johnston et al. 1968), the $GABA_A$ agonist, rapidly hyperpolarized the cell and eliminated the light response. In contrast baclofen, a $GABA_B$ agonist (Bowery et al. 1980), produced a smaller hyperpolarization in this particular cell. The light-evoked EPSPs at both onset and offset were enhanced by baclofen. The lower trace shows that a prolonged application of 200 μM CACA (*cis*-4-aminocrotonic acid), the $GABA_C$ agonist (Johnston et al. 1975; Johnston 1986), had little effect on the membrane potential or the light response of this cell. A CACA concentration of 200 μM seems to be near the upper limit of

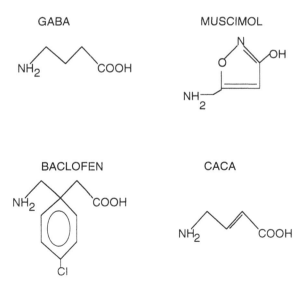

Figure 4.1 The chemical structure of GABA and analogs that are selective for particular receptors: muscimol for $GABA_a$, baclofen for $GABA_b$, and CACA for $GABA_c$.

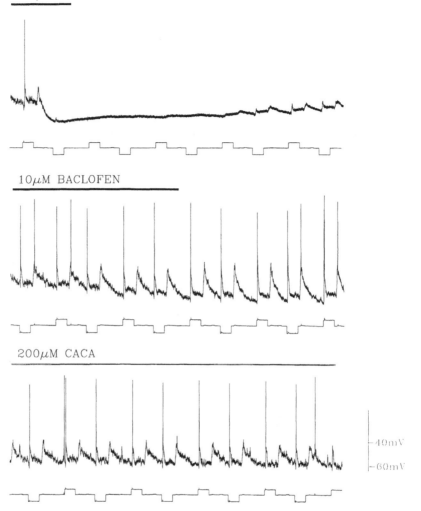

100μM MUSCIMOL

10μM BACLOFEN

200μM CACA

−40mV

−60mV

Figure 4.2 A comparison of the effects of the three GABA analogs illustrated in figure 4.1 on the light responses of a transient ON-OFF cell recorded in the eyecup preparation. The dark bars above the voltage traces indicate the period of drug application, while the square pulses beneath indicate the timing of the light stimuli (upward = diffuse red light; downward = diffuse green light).

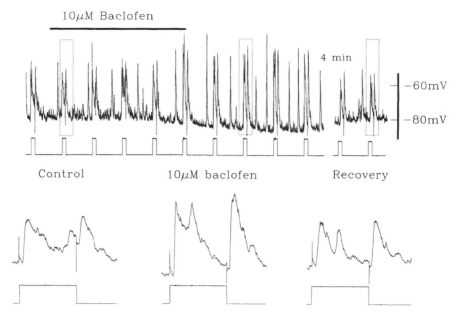

Figure 4.3 The effect of baclofen in the slice preparation. The top trace shows the continuous record during drug treatment, while the three insets below show the responses outlined by the dotted lines in the top trace. A diffuse yellow light stimulus was used.

its selective concentration in the eyecup. When 500 μm CACA is used, a GABA$_A$ effect becomes apparent.

These three different effects are characteristic of our observations in the eyecup preparation. When input resistance changes are monitored, muscimol is found to produce a large decrease in resistance, often 200 to 300 Mohms. In comparison, the change in resistance seen with baclofen is smaller, about 50 Mohms, while no effects are generally observed during CACA application. Muscimol's elimination of the light response is apparently due to this large shunting effect. When GABA is applied to the retina, the effect is similar to that of muscimol, because the effect of GABA$_A$ overwhelms the more subtle actions at other receptor sites.

Results Using the Retinal Slice Preparation

In contrast to results in the retina eyecup preparation, the GABA$_B$ and GABA$_C$ agonists are more potent and more variable in the retinal slice preparation. In the slice, baclofen produces the same effect as it does in the eyecup in about half of our recordings. This is illustrated in the transient ON-OFF cell in figure 4.3. Baclofen caused a hyperpolarization and a decrease in membrane noise, and it also augmented the amplitude of the light response. However, in the other half of the cells recorded, baclofen strongly suppressed all light responses, both transient and sustained. Both effects are seen at baclofen concentrations ranging from 1 to 100 μM, and they do not seem to

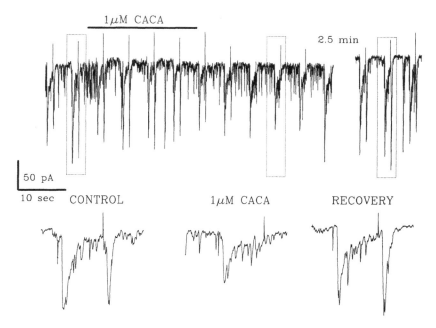

Figure 4.4 The effects of low concentrations of CACA in the slice preparation. The top trace shows the current records from a voltage-clamped ON-OFF transient cell held at −70 mV. The three traces at the bottom are enlarged representations of the boxed areas in the top trace.

depend on dose. Voltage clamp data suggest that this suppression is due to a decrease in presynaptic input, since the currents were also strongly suppressed. Even when baclofen increased the transient voltage responses, the synaptic currents were decreased in third-order neurons.

CACA, which usually has no effect in the eyecup, has a powerful effect in the slice. When CACA is used at concentrations of 100 nM to 1 μM, it tends to suppress the OFF response much more than the ON response. This is illustrated in the voltage clamp recording of the transient ON-OFF cell shown in figure 4.4. Application of 1 μM CACA produced very little change in the holding current (−70 mV holding potential), but produced a diminution of the ON response and an elimination of the OFF response. At concentrations of 10 to 100 μM, CACA suppresses all light responses. The effects of low concentrations of CACA are not blocked by 100 μM bicuculline and are distinctly different from the effects of baclofen, suggesting that they represent actions at a distinct GABA receptor.

The Effects of GABA Receptor Activation

We have previously reported that GABA$_B$ receptor activation tends to enhance the responses of transient cells, such as that shown in figure 4.2, while it suppresses the responses of sustained cells (Slaughter and Bal 1989). In sustained cells, the suppression of the sustained response is accompanied by

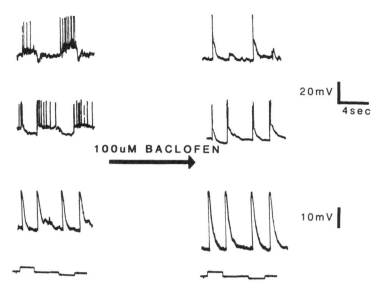

Figure 4.5   The effects of 100 μM baclofen on sustained and transient cells in the mudpuppy eyecup preparation. (From Slaughter and Bai 1988)

the appearance of transient responses. This is illustrated in figure 4.5, which shows the responses of a sustained ON, sustained OFF, and transient ON-OFF cell before and after the application of 100 μM baclofen. These recordings were obtained in the eyecup preparation.

The appearance of transient responses in sustained cells is peculiar and often very dramatic. The light response of the sustained ON cell at the top of the figure is transformed to a response with a large transient ON and small transient OFF response. Similarly, the sustained OFF cell in the middle of figure 4.4 has the light response of a transient ON-OFF cell after the application of baclofen. Current clamp experiments indicate that these transient responses are often present in sustained cells, but masked under normal conditions (Bai and Slaughter 1989). Thus, baclofen is not creating transient responses. Instead, the preexisting transient signals are being enhanced. The simplest explanation is that there is a change in synaptic weighting, resulting in an enhancement of phasic signals at the expense of tonic signals.

Effects of the GABA_B Antagonist CGP35348

Until recently we have been unable to block the GABA_B receptor. Consequently, we could not evaluate the physiological function of endogenous GABA_B receptors. Reputed antagonists, such as phaclofen, saclofen, and 2-hydroxy saclofen (Kerr et al. 1987, 1988, 1989a), were not effective blockers of applied baclofen, nor did they have any consistent effects on light responses. Often they acted like partial agonists at the GABA_B receptor. All of these antagonists were designed using the basic structure of the baclofen molecule and then changing the carboxylic acid moiety (Kerr et al. 1989b).

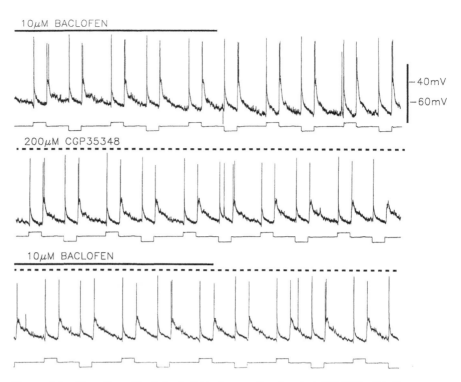

Figure 4.6 The action of baclofen (solid bar) on another transient ON-OFF cell in the eyecup preparation. This figure demonstrates that CGP35348 (dashed line) can block the effects of baclofen.

Recently, using a different approach, an antagonist with a novel structure has been developed that seems to be an effective, although still not very potent, GABA$_B$ antagonist. This agent, developed by Bittinger and colleagues (1990) at Ciba-Geigy, is referred to by the company designation of CGP35348. As shown in figure 4.6, 200 μM CGP35348 blocks the effects of 10 μM baclofen. The three traces are from the same cell, recorded in the eyecup preparation. The top trace shows that baclofen by itself hyperpolarized the cell and augmented the transient ON and OFF responses. After recovery, CGP35348 was applied (middle trace). When baclofen was reapplied in the presence of CGP35348, it had only a very slight effect on the cell (lower trace).

In general, we have found that the effects of CGP35348 are opposite to those of baclofen. When baclofen is applied, it causes a hyperpolarization, a decrease in noise, and an enhancement of the transient components of the response. Figure 4.7, which consists of expanded traces from figure 4.6, shows that CGP35348 increased membrane noise and slowed the light response. CGP35348 also appears to block a delayed inhibition (arrows), similar to that reported for GABA$_B$ receptors in the hippocampus (Dutar and Nicoll 1988). In some retinas the effects of CGP35348 are more dramatic than in others. Generally, an increase in noise is commonly observed. A depolarization and

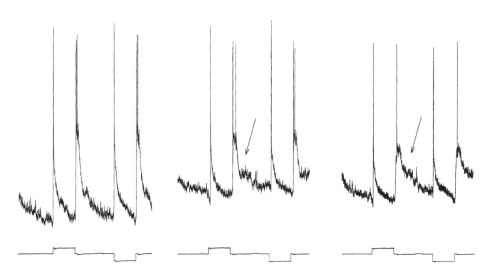

Figure 4.7 An enlargement of select responses from figure 4.6. The control trace is the first pair of light responses in the top trace of figure 4.6, the baclofen records were the first two responses after the termination of baclofen application in the top trace, and the CGP35348 records are from the end of the middle trace. Baclofen produced a large hyperpolarization and made the responses more transient. CGP35348 caused an increase in the membrane noise, slightly reduced the peak amplitude of the responses, and made the light responses more prolonged, especially the OFF responses in this cell (arrows).

transition to a more sustained light response is common, but is not always seen. This variability presumably represents differing steady states of the retinas, but what parameters regulate these states is unknown.

The Detection of Directional Information by GABA_B Receptors

We have proposed that GABA_B receptors play a modulatory role in the retina, setting the synaptic weights of transient and sustained inputs in the inner plexiform layer. One function we have linked to these receptors is the detection of directional information (Barlow and Levick 1965). In the tiger salamander retina, baclofen application enhances directional responses in cells that normally show directionality, and baclofen reveals directionality in many cells that show no directional responses under control conditions (Pan and Slaughter 1991). This effect on nondirectional cells was most apparent when the OFF pathway was isolated by using 2-amino-4-phosphonobutyrate (APB).

An example is shown in figure 4.8. Under control conditions, shown in part A, the cell responded about equally to a moving bar of light regardless of its direction of movement. The responses are shown adjacent to the arrows that indicate the direction of movement. The polygon in the middle maps the peak amplitude of the EPSPs in the various directions. Part B shows the responses

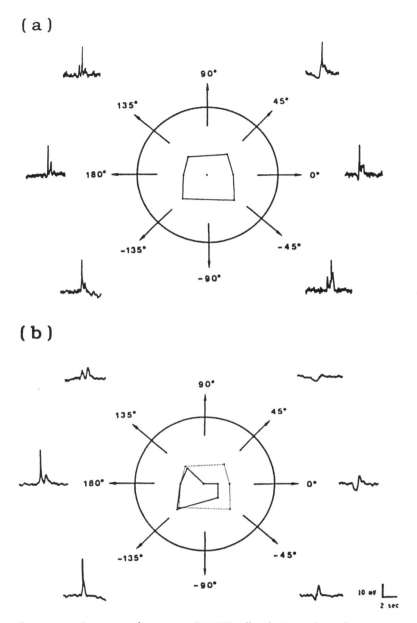

Figure 4.8 Responses of a transient ON-OFF cell in the tiger salamander eyecup to a moving slit of light. The slit was moved at a constant rate in the directions indicated by the arrows. The slit was 100 μM wide, longer than the diameter of the eyecup, and oriented with its long axis orthogonal to the direction of motion. (A) Responses under control conditions. (B) Responses after the application of 100 μM baclofen plus 100 μM APB. (From Pan and Slaughter 1991)

of the cell to the same directions of motion after the application of baclofen and 2-amino-4-phosphonobutyrate. The central polygon with solid lines again maps the peak amplitude of the EPSPs for the different directions. The polygon with dotted lines is a superposition of the control map from part A. The cell shows a distinct directional preference to the same movement paradigm.

DISCUSSION

The functions of the three GABA receptor subtypes in the proximal retina are very different. GABA$_A$ receptors provide a powerful inhibition linked to components of the light response and a weaker, tonic inhibition that may function in a push-pull manner to control the light responses of third-order neurons. Like the inhibitory glycine receptor, the GABA$_A$ receptor acts as a classic inhibitory receptor, producing a large shunt at the postsynaptic membrane. GABA$_A$ receptors are also found presynaptically on bipolar cells. Overall, the GABA$_A$ receptor and associated conductance change far outweigh either of the other two receptors in the proximal retina (Redburn et al. 1989; Slaughter and Bai 1989). The prevalence of GABA$_A$ receptors in the inner plexiform layer has made it difficult to assign a single information processing function to this receptor type.

GABA$_C$ receptors also provide significant inhibition of the light response, but with a bias toward inhibiting OFF responses. This is opposite to the conventional view of the GABAergic system, which is thought to preferentially block ON responses. The action of endogenous GABA on the GABA$_C$ receptor is unknown, since there are no known antagonists. In the fish retina, Matthews et al. (1991) have reported that CACA reduces an L-type voltage-dependent calcium current found in isolated ON bipolar cells (Mbl). A similar mechanism may exist in the amphibian retina, since CACA suppresses the synaptic currents recorded from third-order neurons, suggesting a presynaptic site of action. The voltage clamp records from Dr. Matthews's laboratory indicate that CACA is more effective at suppressing the calcium current evoked in the negative voltage range but, as the potential approaches 0 mV, the blocking action of CACA becomes small. This could explain the relative sensitivity of the OFF system if one assumes that ON bipolar cells are more depolarized than OFF bipolars. CACA was very potent in the slice preparation, but ineffective in the eyecup. We have no explanation for this disparity.

GABA$_B$ receptors in the amphibian retina act to open potassium channels on third-order neurons (Slaughter and Bai 1989) and close calcium channels on a select group of bipolar cells (Maguire et al. 1989b). In the eyecup, GABA$_B$ receptors are responsible for two effects: (1) the production of a small, transient, delayed inhibitory input and (2) a shift toward transient responses. The IPSP is probably due to the opening of potassium channels on third-order neurons, and the delay is probably due to the second messenger system. This is very similar to a synaptic mechanism seen in the hippocampus (Dutar and Nicoll 1988a). The mechanism responsible for the shift to transient responses is still unclear.

Maguire et al. (1989a) suggested that baclofen reduces excitatory bipolar cell input to transient third-order neurons. By suppressing transient responses, the mechanism of Maguire et al. would shift the bias toward sustained responses, which is not what we observed in the eyecup. Our voltage clamp recordings in the slice suggest that baclofen reduces excitatory synaptic inputs to both transient and sustained amacrine and ganglion cells. If baclofen suppressed both inputs, this would favor transient responses only if these signals were less effectively suppressed. This may be the case, since transient signals have a significantly lower saturation threshold than sustained responses. Measurements of acetylcholine release in the rabbit retina indicate that baclofen enhances release (Cunningham and Neal 1983) and suggest that baclofen does not act as a presynaptic inhibitor of GABA release (Neal and Shah 1989). This suggests that baclofen enhances transient responses, since the cholinergic amacrine is a phasically responding cell. In the cat retina, Ikeda et al. (1990) found that baclofen enhanced OFF responses, but not ON responses.

Experiments with $GABA_B$ antagonists indicate that the $GABA_B$ system has a modest modulatory effect on synaptic signaling in the inner retina. CGP35348 increases noise, decreases the light response, and makes the responses more prolonged. These effects are exactly opposite to the actions of exogenously applied baclofen. This comparison indicates that $GABA_B$ receptors are tonically activated in the retina, because blocking the endogenous transmitter has the opposite effect of applied baclofen, which is obviously tonic. This is not surprising, since it is known that there are tonic levels of GABA in the extracellular space and that there is tonic activation of $GABA_A$ receptors.

The effects of 10 μM baclofen suggest that only low levels of $GABA_B$ receptor activation occur under our experimental conditions. Baclofen 10 μM has a dramatic effect in all our experiments, even though it is well below the saturating concentration of baclofen. Since CGP35348 is able to fully block 10 μM baclofen and yet has only a small effect on the light response, this indicates that the endogenous levels of $GABA_B$ activation are low.

In summary, retinal information processing can be well served by the diversity in GABA receptors. They act presynaptically and postsynaptically. They work either directly to gate chloride channels or through second messengers to regulate calcium and potassium channels. They may shape synaptic signals through $GABA_A$ receptors, shift the tonic-phasic balance with $GABA_B$ receptors, pass early signals but block delayed signals using $GABA_B$ receptors, or preferentially suppress OFF signals with $GABA_C$ receptors. The potential variations are far greater than this, since we have not even mentioned the receptor diversity within each class, such as the benzodiazepine enhancement of the $GABA_A$ system that occurs in the amphibian inner retina (Yang et al. 1992), the possibility that there are two types of $GABA_B$ receptors (Dutar and Nicoll 1988b; Scherer et al. 1988) or the carrier-mediated modulation of GABA receptors seen in the distal retina (Yang and Wu 1989). These multiple systems allow for a complex decomposition and modulation of signals that are necessary in a parallel processor such as the retina.

REFERENCES

Bai S-H, Slaughter MM (1989) Effects of baclofen on transient neurons in the mudpuppy retina: Electrogenic and network actions. J Neurophysiol 61:382–390.

Barlow HB, Levick WR (1965) The mechanism of directionally selective units in rabbit's retina. J Physiol (Lond) 178:477–504.

Belgum JH, Dvorak DR, McReynolds JS (1984) Strychnine blocks transient but not sustained inhibition in mudpuppy retinal ganglion cells. J Physiol (Lond) 354:273–286.

Bittinger H, Froestl W, Hall R, Karlsson G, Klebs, K, Olpe, H-R, Pozza MF, Steinmann MW, Van Riezen H (1990) Biochemistry, electrophysiology, and pharmacology of a new GABA$_B$ antagonist: CGP 35348. In: GABA$_B$ receptors in mammalian function (Bowery NG, Bittinger H, Olpe H-R, eds) pp 47–60. New York: Wiley.

Bormann J, Hamill OP, Sakman B (1987) Mechanisms of anion permeation through channels gated by glycine and gamma-aminobutyric acid in mouse cultured spinal neurones. J Physiol (Lond) 385:243–286.

Bowery NG, Hill DR, Hudson AL, Doble A, Middlemiss DN, Shaw J, Turnbull MJ (1980) (−)Baclofen decreases neurotransmitter release in the mammalian CNS by an action at a novel GABA receptor. Nature 283:92–94.

Boycott BB, Wässle H (1974) The morphological types of ganglion cells of the domestic cat's retina. J Physiol (Lond) 240:397–419.

Caldwell JH, Daw NW, Wyatt HJ (1978) Effects of picrotoxin and strychnine on rabbit retinal ganglion cells: Lateral interactions for cells with more complex receptive fields. J Physiol (Lond) 276:277–298.

Cohen BN, Fain GL, Fain MJ (1989) GABA and glycine channels in isolated ganglion cells from goldfish retina. J Physiol (Lond) 418:53–82.

Cunningham JR, Neal MJ (1983) Effect of gamma-aminobutyric acid agonists, glycine, taurine, and neuropeptides on acetylcholine release from the rabbit retina. J Physiol (Lond) 336:563–577.

Dolphin AC, Scott RH (1986) Inhibition of calcium currents in cultured rat dorsal root ganglion neurones by (−)baclofen. Br J Pharmacol 88:213–220.

Dutar P, Nicoll RA (1988a) A physiological role for GABA$_B$ receptors in the central nervous system. Nature 332:156–158.

Dutar P, Nicoll RA (1988b) Pre- and postsynaptic GABA$_B$ receptors in the hippocampus have different pharmacological properties. Neuron 1:585–591.

Enroth-Cugell C, Robson JG (1966) The contrast sensitivity of retinal ganglion cells of the cat. J Physiol (Lond) 187:517–552

Famiglietti EV Jr., Kolb H (1976) Structural basis of 'ON'- and 'OFF'-center responses in retinal ganglion cells. Science 194:193–195.

Frumkes TE, Miller RF, Slaughter M, Dacheux RF (1981) Physiological and pharmacological basis of GABA and glycine action on neurons of mudpuppy retina III. Amacrine-mediated inhibitory influences on ganglion cell receptive-field organization: A model. J Neurophysiol 45:783–804.

Ikeda H, Hankins MW, Kay CD (1990) Actions of baclofen and phaclofen upon ON- and OFF-ganglion cells in the cat retina. Eur J Pharmacol 190:1–9.

Ikeda H, Sheardown MJ (1983) Transmitters mediating inhibition of ganglion cells in the cat retina: Iontophoretic studies in vitro. Neuroscience 8:837–853.

Johnston GAR (1986) Multiplicity of GABA receptors. In: Benzodiazepine/GABA receptors and chloride channels: Structural and functional Properties (Olsen RW, Venter, JC eds) pp. 57–71. New York: Liss.

Johnston GAR, Curtis DR, Beart PM, Game CJA, McCulloch RM, Twitchin B (1975) *Cis* and trans-4-aminocrotonic acid as GABA agonists of restricted conformation. J Neurochem 24: 157–160.

Johnston GAR, Curtis DR, De Groat WC, Duggan AW (1968) Central actions of ibotenic acid and muscimol. Biochem Pharmacol 17:2488–2489.

Kerr DI, Ong J, Johnston GAR, Abbenante J, Prager RH (1988) 2-Hydroxy-saclofen: An improved antagonist at central and peripheral GABA$_B$ receptors. Neurosci Lett 92:92–96.

Kerr DI, Ong J, Johnston GAR, Abbenante J, Prager RH (1989a) Antagonism at GABA$_B$ receptors by saclofen and related sulphonic analogues of baclofen and GABA. Neurosci Lett 107:239–244.

Kerr DI, Ong J, Johnston GAR, Prager RH (1989b) GABA$_B$ receptor mediated actions of baclofen in rat isolated neocortical slice preparations: antagonism by phosphono-analogues of GABA. Brain Res 480:312–316.

Kerr DI, Ong J, Prager RH, Gynther BD, Curtis DR (1987) Phaclofen: A peripheral and central baclofen antagonist. Brain Res 405:150–154.

Krnjevic K Schwartz S (1967) The action of gamma-aminobutyric acid on cortical neurones. Exp Brain Res 3:320–336.

Maguire G, Lukasiewicz P, Werblin F (1989a) Amacrine cell interactions underlying the response to change in the tiger salamander retina. J Neurosci 9:726–735.

Maguire G, Maple B, Lukasiewicz P, Werblin F (1989b) Gamma-aminobutyrate type B receptor modulation of L-type calcium channel current at bipolar cell terminals in the retina of the tiger salamander. Proc Natl Acad Sci USA 86:10144–10147.

Massey SC Redburn DA (1987) Transmitter circuits in the vertebrate retina. Prog Neurobiol 28:55–96.

Matthews G, Ayoub G, Heidelberger R (1991) Inhibition of presynaptic calcium currents via GABA$_C$ receptors. Soc Neuroci Abstr 17:900.

Miller RF, Dacheux RF (1976) Synaptic organization and ionic basis of ON and OFF channels in the mudpuppy retina. I. Intracellular analysis of chloride-sensitive electrogenic properties of receptors, horizontal cells, bipolar cells, and amacrine cells. J Gen Physiol 67:639–659.

Miller RF, Slaughter MM (1986) Excitatory amino acid receptors of the retina: Diversity of subtypes and conductance mechanisms. Trends Neurosci 9:211–218.

Nawy S, Jahr CE (1990) Suppression by glutamate of cGMP-activated conductances in retinal bipolar cells. Nature 346:269–271.

Neal MJ, Shah MA (1989) Baclofen and phaclofen modulate GABA release from slices of rat cerebral cortex and spinal cord but not from retina. Br J Pharmacol 98:105–112.

Newberry NR, Nicoll RA (1984) Baclofen directly hyperpolarizes hippocampal cells. Nature 308:450–452.

Pan Z-H, Slaughter MM (1991) Control of retinal information coding by GABA$_B$ receptors. J Neurosci 11:1810–1821.

Redburn DA, Friedman DL, Massey SC (1989) The function of multiple subclasses of GABA receptors in rabbit retina. In: Neurobiology of the Inner Retina (Weiler R, Osborne NN eds) pp 41–52. Berlin: Springer-Verlag.

Scherer RW, Ferkany JW, Enna SJ (1988) Evidence for pharmacologically distinct subsets of $GABA_B$ receptors. Brain Res Bull 21:439—443.

Slaughter MM, Bai S-H (1989) Differential effects of baclofen on sustained and transient cells in the mudpuppy retina. J Neurophysiol 61:374—381.

Slaughter MM, Miller RF (1981) 2-Amino-4-phosphonobutyric acid: A new pharmacological tool for retina research. Science 211:182—185.

Werblin FS (1978) Transmission along and between rods in the tiger salamander retina. J Physiol (Lond) 280:449—470.

Wu S-M (1987) Synaptic connections between neurons in living slices of the larval salamander retina. J Neurosci Meth 20:139—149.

Yang C-Y, Lin Z-S, Yazulla, 5 (1992) Localization of $GABA_A$ receptor subtypes in the tiger salamander retina. Vis Neurosci 8:57—64.

Yang X-L, Wu SM (1989) Effects of prolonged light exposure, GABA, and glycine on horizontal cell responses in tiger salamander retina. J Neurophysiol 61:1025—1035.

5 Can We Ever Understand How the Retina Communicates with the Brain?

Ken-ichi Naka and Hiroko M. Sakai

Few men think;
Yet all will have opinions.
—Bishop Berkeley (1685–1753)

One of the goals of neurophysiology is to decipher the messages carried by nerve fibers and to relate their message to network functions, which may include the storage and retrieval of information. Our particular goal is to decipher the messages carried by optic nerve fibers to the brain—in other words, to determine what the retina is telling the brain. Adrian (1931) discovered that sensory messages, including those carried by optic nerve fibers, are coded by a train of spike discharges. Adrian demonstrated that the message is encoded into a point process in which only the timing of each discharge carries relevant information. In studies of the transmission as well as the transformation of information, it is the relative timing of each spike discharge that is relevant and not the complex physicochemical processes that underlie spike generation. The problem is therefore to discover how the visual world is encoded into a series of spike discharges. As the information-carrying capacity of a spike train is limited (because of noise), and as the ever-changing visual world contains a vast amount of information, the encoding of signals processed in the retinal neuron network into a spike train must involve sophisticated transformation. Since Adrian's discovery, there have been numerous reports dealing with spike discharges from optic nerve fibers. However, the all-important question of how the visual world is encoded into spike trains has rarely been addressed. It seems to us that all visual physiologists have opinions on this issue, but only a few have really thought about it. Had we really thought about this problem twenty years ago, we would have pursued a very different line of research.

We would like to review here our past efforts that were designed to untangle the neuron network in the retina of the catfish, *Ictalurus punctatus*, using a methodology based on Wiener's theory of nonlinear analysis. Studies of network functions, including the deciphering of messages carried by optic nerve fibers, represent long-term projects because of the multivariate nature of the nervous system. Moreover, in any long-term endeavor it is appropriate to reflect, from time to time, upon the way in which the results that we have obtained and the conclusions that we have reached relate to our ultimate goal. In our case, the goal is to discover how catfish really see. Unless we take time to ponder the past, our efforts will eventually lose their bearings and, after years of work, we may discover to our dismay that we are not far from where we originally started in spite of the vast amount of knowledge that we have accumulated during those years; we are forced to concede that this is indeed the case. In addition, in these times of massive production and high-speed processing of data, a leisurely detour from daily routines seems to be appropriate.

BACKGROUND

Any study of a visual system, whether that of a man or a fish, must begin with the presentation of a visual stimulus. Then we can observe and examine the way in which elements in the system respond to the stimulus. In our case, we examine the relationship between the stimulus and spike discharges from the optic nerve fibers and try to guess what kinds of message are carried by the fibers to the brain. There are three categories of methodology that are used to study the messages. Unfortunately, these methodologies are not merely experimental means, but are intimately interwoven with the researchers' preconceived ideas about how the visual system functions.

A Black-Box Approach: Spike Discharges Are a Signaling Device

The black-box approach is the traditional approach used to find the type of visual stimulus that produces some response in the visual system. Simple stimuli used in earlier experiments, such as a spot or an annulus of light, have become progressively more complex, culminating in such complex and esoteric stimuli as the face of a grandmother or a fellow monkey. With this approach, only a qualitative relationship is sought between a stimulus and the resulting response. The spike discharges are a signaling device, and the visual system detects particular features of the stimulus. The neuron networks that process the input and produce a particular response are represented as a black box. It is inevitable that ideas such as that of a key stimulus or an ethologically meaningful stimulus will emerge from this approach.

A Quantitative Approach: Spikes Are a Point Process

In this case, spike discharges are recognized as a point process, and quantitative measurements are made of the process. An important parameter is the timing of spike discharges. Spike-interval histograms and instantaneous spike-firing frequencies are two typical measures. Autocorrelations and cross-correlations of trains of spike discharges are also made. Poststimulus time histograms provide one method for converting a point process into an analog form so that an intuitive appreciation of the process is possible. These measures are useful, but they cannot be directly related either to the stimulus or to network function. The classic classification of ganglion cells into X and Y cells by Enroth-Cugell and Robson (1966) falls in this category.

A Cross-Correlation Approach: Excitation by Random Signal

This approach can be viewed as a modification of the second approach. Here a visual stimulus is modulated by a stochastic (chaotic) signal, and a correlation can be made between the input and the resulting spike discharges. This approach was first proposed by de Boer and Kuyper (1968), who referred to this method as "reverse correlation" because each spike discharge was used to seek out the waveform of the particular part of the (past) stimulus that triggered a given discharge. The accumulation of such waveforms describes the optimal stimulus waveform that triggers a discharge.

In 1958 Norbert Wiener formulated a theory, known as *Wiener's nonlinear analysis* or *white noise analysis*, that allows for the identification of a system by exciting it with a white noise signal (Wiener 1958). In his theory, a system is characterized by a series of kernels or *Wiener kernels*. In the 1970s Marmarelis and Naka (1972) computed kernels from spike trains, which were transformed into an analog form, but interpretation of their kernels was problematic. Victor and Shapley (1979) replaced the white noise with a sum of sinusoids, a very efficient signal. They discovered important differences in the spatial non-linearity between the X and Y cells in the cat. However, the interpretation of their kernels was also problematic.

THE RELATION OF SPIKE KERNELS TO THE INTRACELLULAR RESPONSE

Significant progress was made when Sakuranaga et al. (1987) noted the similarity between two sets of kernels, one set computed from a ganglion cell's intracellular potential (postsynaptic potential or PSP), and the other set computed from the cell's spike discharges. Korenberg et al. (1989) further showed that the slight discrepancy between the two sets of kernels could be accounted for by a filter in the spike generation process. In these analyses spike kernels were computed from a light stimulus and spike discharges, a point process, which were transformed into short pulses. The kernels relate only to the stimulus, and they are therefore the optimal stimulus waveform for the production of a spike discharge. However, our analysis has shown that the spike kernels are similar to those computed from the PSP. Therefore, the PSP represents that part of the light stimulus whose waveform is optimal for triggering a spike discharge. Our studies have also shown that the major parts of the first- and second-order components of a ganglion cell's response originate in the outer and inner retinal layer, respectively. Thus spike kernels are related not only to the stimulus, but also to the network functions in the retina. Therefore, the slow-potential kernels and the spike kernels from a same ganglion cell are related to one another through a proportionality factor.

Marmarelis and Naka (1974) extended Wiener's original theory to multiple-input systems, the simplest form of which is two-input white noise analysis. The inputs were in the form of a spot of light located centrally and a concentric annulus of light. Both the spot and the annulus were modulated by two independent white noise signals. Cross-correlations were made between the two light inputs and one output, and the spike discharges from a ganglion cell were transformed into PST histograms (Marmarelis and Naka 1972). In a sense, their analysis represents a variation of the classical Wiener analysis.

More recently Sakai and Naka (in preparation) performed similar two-input experiments in which they directly cross-correlated two inputs with the spike discharges themselves, and the spike discharges were transformed into unitary pulses. They obtained two sets of first-order kernels. In an ON-center cell, the spot produced a depolarizing (spike frequency increasing) kernel, and the annulus produced a hyperpolarizing (spike frequency decreasing) kernel. In the OFF-center cells the polarity of the kernels was reversed. In both the ON- and OFF-center ganglion cells, the spot and annular inputs produced first-order kernels of opposing polarity, whereas both stimuli produced similar second-order kernels. Thus the concentric receptive field organization is encoded by the first-order kernels, and changes occurring anywhere in a receptive field are encoded by the second-order kernels. Therefore, a spike train simultaneously carries four kinds of information; in other words, the spike train is a carrier of multiplexed signals. Cross-correlation decomposes multiplexed messages into separate components that are produced by the action of each input on the different parts of the retinal network. Second-order components are recovered through a second-order correlation—namely, the time relationship between a discharge and two points within the stimulus.

IMPLICATIONS

Our results from recent studies in the catfish have produced the first concrete evidence that a train of spike discharges contains and communicates complex information to the brain. The spike discharges are therefore not a simple signaling device that lets the brain know that the retina has seen a spot or grandmother's face. Measures such as instantaneous firing frequency or spike intervals also fail to encompass the complex nature of the message carried by the spike train. The current view of the functional organization of the retinal network that is derived from these two measurements is bound to be over-simplified, although it may not actually be misleading.

In contrast to the other two approaches, white noise analysis is based on sound mathematical theory. For example, the idea of functional identification of a time series, of which neural responses are a typical example, was advanced at the turn of the century by a group of mathematicians that included Volterra (1930). Theoretically, a system can be characterized by a series of Volterra kernels, although no practical method has been devised to compute these kernels. Arguably, the study of stochastic processes is one of the finest achievements of the human mind during the first half of this century. No other mathematical notion has been defined more rigorously than that of stochastic processes, which include Brownian motion and its derivative, white noise (Wiener 1938). It was Wiener (1958), an extraordinary mathematician, who combined the idea of functional identification with excitation of a system by a white noise signal. White noise analysis is therefore based on sound mathematical theory that can be taken to represent truth in an absolute sense (compared with biological observations). Admittedly, many problems arise when these mathematical theories are translated into formulas that can be executed in a computing machine, and there are many problems associated with the performance of white noise experiments in the laboratory. For example, Jonathan D. Victor (personal communication) argues that a rigorous computation of a Wiener kernel is not possible and that the white noise used in experiments is not really as "white" as prescribed by theory. Experimental time is also limited to tens of seconds, far from the infinite that is expected in theory. Results from (experimentally executed) white noise analyses are therefore not exact in a mathematical sense, but represent approximations. However, we believe that these errors and approximations are not serious enough to totally negate our conclusions.

Problems arise because of the actual nature of the way in which we study nervous systems. If we really think about them, the conclusions that we have reached from our white noise analysis of spike trains are not quite right, and we find this insight disturbing. There is something unsettling about the conclusions. For example, in the analysis we know exactly what the inputs and outputs are, and we derive the correlation between the inputs and the resulting spike discharges using a computing machine that may take several minutes to complete the process of correlation. It is only then that our results are displayed as first- and second-order kernels. It is obvious that the catfish brain is not analyzing a spike train the same way that we analyze the spike train in our experimental system. Catfish have no access to the input, and the goal of neural processing in the catfish neural network is to process signals in such a way that the fish is able to suvive in a hostile and ever-changing environment. For the fish, response to visual stimuli has to be almost instantaneous. Many kinds of messages carried by a spike train have to be decoded on line, without reference to the inputs, and the visual world of the catfish is much more complex than a simple random modulation of a spot or an annulus of light. Therefore, it seems to us that the results of our analysis have, in fact, little to do with what is really going on in the visual system of the catfish. Our results are therefore an artifact, not in the sense that they are erroneous, but in the sense that results are based on our thought process, which ultimately originates from our innate faculty to appreciate the abstract concepts of time, space, and causality. And it is our own nervous system that processes such abstract ideas. The catfish has no notion of "multiplexed signals" or of "cross-correlation"; these notions are ours. Indeed, it was Lee and Schetzen (1965) who showed that Wiener's kernels could be computed by cross-correlation between the input and output, while the fish had already survived millions of years.

Animals live in a world of intuition; we humans are endowed with a mental capacity to abstract. It is exactly our ability to appreciate abstract ideas that enables us to produce a system of knowledge about the intuitive world. This is science—namely, the interpretation of the external world on the basis of our ability to abstract. In our immediate world, research into channels or transmitters is direct and intuitive. Such research may require the dexterity of experimenters or the sophistication of techniques, but the research is not derived from an abstract idea, nor does it have a mathematical foundation (although mathematical methods may be used), because the goal of such research is to define something intuitive. In contrast, attempts to identify network functions or to decipher the messages carried by a spike train are not intuitive, as our past effort has shown, but are aimed at discovering the way in which information is processed in the retinal network and the nature of the information that is carried by a spike train. And information so discovered is delineated by our capacity to abstract; the conclusions are ours, and not those of the catfish.

In years to come, we will be able to advance our knowledge of the material aspects of retinal neuron networks. Perhaps we will be able to define all the neurotransmitters, putative or real, and also all the ionic channels. With Herculean effort, we may even be able to define all the synapses and produce a three-dimensional model of the neuron network that can be rotated on a multicolored computer display. But all that we discover is as lifeless and stark as the pictures sent from Mars. Matter is essential in the transformation of information, but matter is not information itself, just as chips are essential to a computer but are really sets of instructions that turn a computer into a computing machine. Such instructions will never be found by dismembering the computer.

The analysis of spike trains from optic nerve fibers has to be the first and easiest step in attempts to understand the complex functions of visual systems and ultimately of the brain. However, our past experience with the analysis of spike trains casts serious doubts on our intellectual ability to understand the function of a nervous system. It is doubtful, for example, that we will ever determine how the brain decodes complex messages carried by the spike trains that originate from the retina. Simply put, our mental faculties are inadequate for these task. The neuron network in the catfish tectum must decode (even this term may not be applicable) the messages that are carried by the optic nerve fibers in a fashion that is unfathomable to us, just as a four-dimensional world is foreign to us. We may erect a system of knowledge about a nervous system that is based upon sound logic and mathematically defined methodologies, but such a system of knowledge is bound to be artificial and all too human. The system based on white noise analysis of the catfish retinal neuron network that we are striving to construct is one humble example of a human-based, and therefore limited, perspective. After all, things are as they are because we are.

CONCLUSION

Lord Adrian (1959) wrote, "Though we can record the impulses, there are still a good many problems to be settled before we can reach a clear understanding of how the full description of the stimulus is handed on to the brain." Lord Adrian's statement still holds true after numerous papers have been published on the impulses from optic nerve fibers during the last 30 years. It is significant that he emphasized understanding. The current tendency is to explain an observation without understanding it.

ACKNOWLEDGMENTS

We thank Susan Stone and Daniel Tranchina for reading this essay. Preparation of this essay has been supported by NEI Grants 07738 and 08848 and NSF Grants DIR 8718461 and BNS 891993. K.-I. Naka thanks Research to Prevent Blindness, Inc., for his Jules and Doris Stein Professorship.

REFERENCES

Adrian, E. D. (1931). Croonian Lecture. The messages in sensory nerve fibres and their interpretation. Proc. R. Soc. Lond. Ser. B. 109: 1–18.

Adrian, E. D. (1959). Sensory mechanisms—introduction. Section I. Neurophysiology. In Handbook of Physiology. Ed. H. W. Magoun, Washington, D.C.: Amer. Physiol. Soc.

De Boer, E. and Kuyper, P. (1968). Trigger correlation. IEEE Trans. Biomed. Eng., BME-15: 169–179.

Enroth-Cugell, C. and Robson, J. G. (1966). The contrast sensitivity of retinal ganglion cells of the cat. J. Physiol. (London), 187: 517–552.

Korenberg, M. J., Sakai, H. M., and Naka, K.-I. (1989). Dissection of the neuron network in the catfish inner retina. III. Interpretation of spike kernels. J. Neurophysiol., 61: 1110–1120.

Lee, Y. W. and Schetzen, M. (1965). Measurements of the Wiener kernels of a non-linear system by cross-correlation. Int. J. Control., 2: 237–254.

Marmarelis, P. Z. and Naka, K.-I. (1972). White-noise analysis of a neuron chain: an application of the Wiener theory. Science 175: 1276–1278.

Marmarelis, P. Z. and Naka, K.-I. (1974). Identification of multi-input biological systems. IEEE Trans. Bio. Med. Eng., BME-21: 88–101.

Sakuranaga, M., Ando, Y.-I., and Naka, K.-I. (1987). Dynamics of the ganglion cell response in the catfish and frog retinas. J. Gen. Physiol., 90: 229–259.

Victor, J. D. and Shapley, R. M. (1979). The nonlinear pathway of Y ganglion cells in the cat retina. J. Gen. Physiol., 74: 671–687.

Volterra, V. (1930). Theory of Functional and Integral and Integrodifferential Equations. London: Blackwell Scientific.

Wiener, N. (1938). The homogeneous chaos. Am. J. Math. 60: 897–936.

Wiener, N. (1958). Non-linear Problems in Random Theory. New York: John Wiley.

II Retinal Ganglion Cells

The output of the retina to the brain is composed of the axons of retinal ganglion cells. These neurons link the retina with all visual processing areas in the brain. As such, they have attracted many investigators who wish to understand the function of the retina.

This section begins with a review of the theory of retinal receptive fields in mammalian retina, composed by John Troy. A chapter by Robert Shapley, Ehud Kaplan, and Keith Purpura follows. It is concerned with retinal light adaptation, a critical process in the regulation of contrast sensitivity. The problem raised in that chapter is the site and nature of retinal light adaptation. It is followed by a provocative chapter by R. W. Rodieck, R. K. Brening, and M. Watanabe about the retinal origin of parallel pathways or parallel channels from the retina to the brain. These authors use quantitative neuroanatomical techniques to analyze the nature of retinal function. This section ends with the Helmerich Award Lecture by Christina Enroth-Cugell. Here Dr. Enroth-Cugell gives a historical review of the receptive field concept and the history of recording single- and multi-cell activity from retinal ganglion cells.

6 Modeling the Receptive Fields of Mammalian Retinal Ganglion Cells

J. B. Troy

Since the publication of the classic paper entitled "The contrast sensitivity of retinal ganglion cells of the cat" by Enroth-Cugell and Robson (1966), quantitative models of the receptive fields of retinal ganglion cells and the study of contrast sensitivity have been intimately entwined. Many studies have followed. However, I do not propose to attempt to review the body of subsequent modeling of the receptive fields of mammalian retinal ganglion cells in this paper. Neither do I intend to subject the reader to a myopic summary of my own work in this area. Rather what I hope to accomplish is a general overview of why I believe that models of ganglion cell receptive fields are essential for us to understand the retina's representation of visual images. In so doing, I will attempt to place the published work of a number of groups within a general theoretical framework. Although much of what I write has been presented elsewhere, I believe that I have included here some novel components that should be of interest. However, before I start, I must acknowledge that among the authors of this volume are two people who have produced the quantitative receptive field models that laid the foundation for most subsequent receptive field modeling. These are R. W. Rodieck and Robert Shapley. Rodieck's (1965) *difference of Gaussians* model for center-surround receptive fields and Hochstein and Shapley's (1976) *subunit model* for the Y cell receptive field have proven durable and are widely used.

USES OF RECEPTIVE FIELD MODELS

There have been two major reasons for modeling receptive fields quantitatively. First, there has been interest in the neural circuitry that accounts for the receptive field and the belief that modeling can help us to better understand and describe these circuits. Second, there has been interest in the receptive field from the perspective of sensory information processing. Modeling has been useful in this area as a way of characterizing the information processing function of the receptive field succinctly and of enabling us to consider how these models conform with the predictions of different theories of retinal information processing. My principal interest lies in the second area, and it is in this context that I will discuss receptive field modeling. Since the subject of this book is contrast sensitivity, I will discuss the retinal processing of achromatic visual images and the part played by ganglion cells in performing this task. I will consider how models of ganglion cell receptive fields help us to describe this process. As noted earlier, I will not talk about results from our laboratory, but rather offer a perspective on observations published by others. Only spatial models will be considered.

RETINAL REPRESENTATION OF VISUAL IMAGES

The representation of achromatic images by the mammalian retina may be summarized by the chain of events diagramed in figure 6.1. The eye fixates a point in a scene whose luminance distribution is defined as $L(r, \theta)$, where r is the radial distance from the point of fixation and θ is the angular displacement from a meridian of the imaginary surface that is optically conjugate to the viewer's retina. An image, $I(\rho, \phi)$, of the scene is formed on the retina, where ρ is the radial distance from the center of the fovea (in primates) or the area centralis (in cats) and ϕ is the angular displacement from a meridian of the eye running from the fovea or the area centralis.

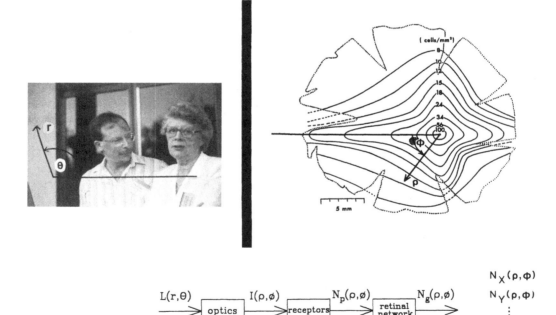

Figure 6.1 Chain of processing in the generation of the retinal visual image. The luminance distribution in a scene, $L(r, \theta)$, is blurred by the optics of the eye, sampled by the photoreceptors, and processed by the retinal circuitry to give the ganglion cell or set of ganglion cell representations. Points in the image are defined relative to the point of fixation in polar coordinates. The isodensity lines on the retinal whole-mount are from the work of Wässle et al. (1975) and represent densities of α (Y) cells.

As indicated in the figure, $I(\rho, \phi)$ is generally considered to be an optically blurred (filtered) transformation of $L(r, \theta)$. However. additional nonoptical blurring also results from image slip due to eye, head, or body movements of the viewer or from motion in the scene that occurs within the capture period of an image. Fluctuations in accommodation (Campbell, Robson, and Westheimer 1959) or pupil size will also influence image quality, but their combined effects during a capture period are probably negligible.

The second transformation in the processing chain is from $I(\rho, \phi)$ to $N_p(\rho, \phi)$. This is the stage of photoreceptor sampling. The light-collecting properties of the photoreceptor (e.g., the inner-segment aperture. the Stiles-Crawford effect) modify $I(\rho, \phi)$ and this modified image is point-sampled by the array of photoreceptors. N is used to signify that the image is now a *neural image*, and the subscript p distinguishes this *photoreceptor image* from the *ganglion cell image*, $N_g(\rho, \phi)$, to be introduced next.

The next stage in the chain is the transformation from $N_p(\rho, \phi)$ to $N_g(\rho, \phi)$, which symbolizes the processing of the photoreceptor image by the retinal network. The output is expressed by the activity of the array of retinal ganglion cells. At the level of the retinal ganglion cells the neural image is represented by the activities of a number of cell classes. For the cat, the mammal whose retina has been best described, there are known to be at least nine physiologically distinct classes of ganglion cells (Cleland and Levick 1974a,b; Stone and Fukuda 1974), four of which have center-surround organized receptive fields that have both ON-center and OFF-center subtypes (Kuffler 1953). Hence, it proves useful to consider the final stage in the chain as a set of parallel operations. The two classes of cat retinal ganglion cells that have been studied most extensively are the X and Y cells, and the remainder of this paper is principally concerned with these cells. It may help to consider that part of $N_g(\rho, \phi)$ represented by the X and Y cells as two separate neural images, $N_X(\rho, \phi)$ and $N_Y(\rho, \phi)$.

Hypothetical Forms of $N_x(\rho, \phi)$ and $N_y(\rho, \phi)$

The neural images $N_X(\rho, \phi)$ and $N_Y(\rho, \phi)$ are assumed to be *point process* representations. This means that the images are defined at only those discrete points in space given by the retinal locations of the receptive field midpoints of X or Y cells, respectively. In the language of communications engineering, the sets of positions of the X and Y cell receptive field midpoints are *carriers* (Black 1953), and the instantaneous discharge rates of these cells are *amplitude modulations* in the images $N_X(\rho, \phi)$ and $N_Y(\rho, \phi)$.

Continuous X and Y Images

It helps to consider two continuous spatial signals just prior to the point-sampling stage that creates $N_X(\rho, \phi)$ and $N_Y(\rho, \phi)$, one a continuous X image and the other a continuous Y image. These imaginary signals conveniently represent the output of the retinal network after all of the optical and neural processing of the visual scene that precedes X and Y cell sampling. For the next part of this discussion, it is important to understand that the hypothetical X and Y images are bandwidth-limited in spatial frequency, determined by (1) the blurring of the luminance distribution of the scene, $L(r, \theta)$, that results from optical and other factors; (2) photoreceptor sampling; and (3) processing of $N_p(\rho, \phi)$ by the retinal network. As we will see, the bandwidth limits are critical to the positioning of the receptive field midpoints of X and Y cells on the retina. In order to explain this I must digress slightly and give the reader some background.

Spatial Frequencies

Figure 6.2A is the reproduction of a sinusoidal luminance grating. Luminance is a sinusoidal function of distance in the horizontal direction and is constant in the vertical direction. In the context of this chapter, the grating has three important characteristics. One is the grating's spatial frequency, which is the number of pairs of light and dark bars per unit of horizontal distance. Distance is usually given units of angle of subtense at the eye or, equivalently, of retinal curvature. The second is the grating's orientation. In this case the orientation

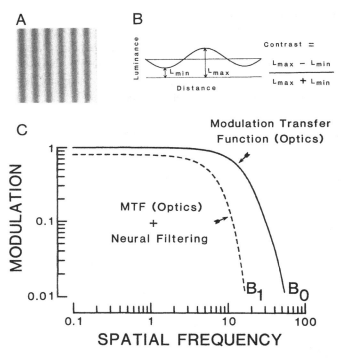

Figure 6.2 Bandwidth limiting the ganglion cell neural image. The image is first limited to spatial frequency B_0 by the eye's optics and, second, to a lower spatial frequency, B_1, by the spatial summation of signals within retinal circuits (C). The reproduction of a sinusoidal luminance grating is shown in (A), and a diagramatic definition of contrast is given in (B).

is vertical. The third is the grating's contrast, which is the luminance modulation divided by the mean luminance of the grating (figure 6.2B).

It is useful to consider the orientation of the grating in a slightly different way. The grating can be considered a planar wave formed from the product of two sinusoidal modulations, one in the vertical and one in the horizontal direction. In this grating the modulation in the vertical direction is at a spatial frequency of 0 cycles degree^{-1}. However, if the spatial frequency in the vertical direction is increased, another planar sinusoidal grating is generated. This grating no longer has a vertical orientation; it is angled obliquely. The orientation will swing more and more to the horizontal the higher the spatial frequency of the vertical component. Hence, the orientation and spatial frequency of the grating will depend on the spatial frequencies of the horizontal and vertical components. Thus, one can consider an oriented grating of some (resultant) spatial frequency as decomposable into two (component) spatial frequency dimensions (Jones and Palmer 1987). This will be important later.

SAMPLING

Now consider again the final stage in the processing chain of figure 6.1, where the hypothetical continuous X and Y images are transformed into sampled representations. Provided that the receptive field midpoints (i.e., the sample locations) of neighboring cells of the same class (X or Y) are spaced closely enough together, it is possible for the information content of the imaginary continuous signals and of $N_X(\rho, \phi)$ and $N_Y(\rho, \phi)$ to be the same. In fact, the imaginary signals could be realized from $N_X(\rho, \phi)$ and $N_Y(\rho, \phi)$. Sampling theory dictates the relationship required between the spatial frequency bandwidths of the imaginary signals and the spacing between cells to achieve this goal. Therefore the bandwidths of the X and Y images determine how closely the receptive field midpoints of X and Y cells, respectively, must be spaced. Unfortunately. the application of sampling theory to the retina is far from trivial.

Sampling One-Dimensional Signals

To understand sampling theory it is helpful to first consider the case of sampling a one-dimensional signal. An example of a one-dimensional signal with which most vision scientists will be familiar is the b wave of the human rod electroretinogram, which is shown schematically as (a) in figure 6.3. The b wave is an electrical potential that is evoked by a brief flash of light. It has an amplitude that changes with time. If one multiplies the b wave by the sine and cosine waves of different temporal frequencies and integrates the products over all time, some of the integrations will result in nonzero values. One can plot the sum of the squares of the integrated cosine and sine products versus temporal frequency. With the b wave's biphasic form, the magnitude of this function will decrease with increasing temporal frequency. The square root of this function as it might appear on double logarithmic axes is plotted as (b). It

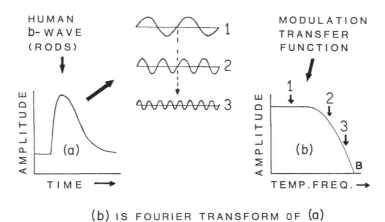

Figure 6.3 Sampling one-dimensional signals. A schematic representation of the b wave of the human rod electroretinogram is shown as (a). The amplitude part of the Fourier transform of the b wave is shown and called the modulation transfer function (MTF); it is plotted on double logarithmic axes as (b). The MTF represents the amplitude of modulation of different temporal frequency components of (a). The lowest rate of sampling of (a) that will not introduce aliasing distortion is 2B, where B is the highest temporal frequency of the measurable amplitude in (b).

is referred to as the *modulation transfer function* (MTF) and represents the amplitude part of the Fourier transform of the b wave. It provides the measure of how much of the amplitude of the b wave (a) can be ascribed to each temporal frequency of (b). Sampling theory says that, in order to capture all of the information in the b wave, we must sample it in time at least twice as frequently as the highest temporal frequency with a measurable amplitude in the modulation transfer function. This is the bandwidth limit. (For MTFs that are band-pass—not low-pass, as this one is—bandwidth limiting occurs at both high and low frequencies).

Bandwidth Limit   The reason that the hypothetical continuous X and Y images are bandwidth-limited in spatial frequency is simple. These images result from weighting the luminance distribution of the visual scene by the spatial sensitivity profiles of X and Y cell receptive fields. The receptive fields filter spatial frequencies from the scene. This occurs because of the spatial summation of signals within the receptive field that results from the optical spreading of light from points in the scene and from the spatial integration of neural signals in the retina (see figure 6.2C). For any field of finite extent within which signals are summed, there will always be a grating of spatial frequency high enough that the weighted integration of its modulation (and that of all higher spatial frequencies) throughout the field is effectively zero (in the sense that the cell's output is indistinguishable from its noise level). This argument holds no matter how small various subunits of a receptive field may be as long as they have a finite size. Obviously, physical reality necessitates that all fields and their subunits, however small, have some finite size. Hence,

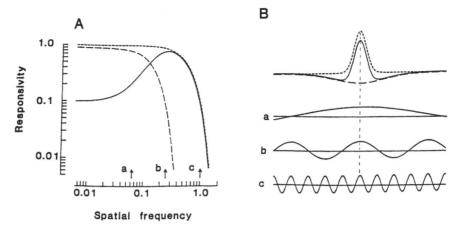

Figure 6.4 The line-weighting function (LWF) and modulation transfer function (MTF) of Rodieck's (1965) difference of Gaussians model for center-surround receptive fields. At the top of (B; solid curve) is shown the LWF of the difference of Gaussians receptive field. The LWF is the difference of two Gaussian LWFs, one representing the receptive field's center mechanism (short dashes), the other the field's surround mechanism (long dashes). (A) Plots, on double logarithmic axes, the amplitude part of the Fourier transform of the LWF of the receptive field. This is the amplitude part (i.e., MTF) of the receptive field spatial frequency response. In this case, the phase part of the transform is actually constant at zero degrees for all spatial frequencies (i.e., the Fourier transform is all cosine). Amplitudes are given in terms of normalized responsivity. The spatial frequency axis is also normalized. Three spatial frequencies (a, b, and c) are indicated on the plot in (A). They correspond to the three cosine waves in (B). Cosine wave a is an effective stimulus for both center and surround receptive field components. Cosine wave b is a poor stimulus for the surround, but a good stimulus for the center mechanism. Cosine wave c is a less effective stimulus for the center and an ineffective stimulus for the surround. This can be seen in (A) where the responsivities of the center (short dashes) and surround components (long dashes) are plotted versus spatial frequency. (Adapted from EnrothCugell and Robson 1984)

there will always be a set of spatial frequencies that are "invisible" to an X or Y cell receptive field. The lowest of these is considered the bandwidth limit of the X or Y image, respectively (if we ignore bandwidth limiting at low spatial frequencies due to surround anatagorism [figure 6.4]). The bandwidth limit is important because, as I have noted, it determines the spacing needed between the midpoints of X and Y cell receptive fields for the X and Y images to be represented without aliasing distortion.

Rodieck's Difference of Two Gaussians Model The spatial frequency content of the X and Y images results from the product of the spatial frequency content of the scene and the spatial frequency responses of the X and Y cell receptive fields. Let us consider these spatial frequency responses and how they are related to receptive field models. We take as an example Rodieck's (1965) difference of Gaussians model for center-surround receptive fields. It is a reasonable choice for both X and Y cells. The solid curve at the top of figure 6.4B is the line-weighting function (LWF) of Rodieck's model.

The line-weighting function measures the receptive field's sensitivity to luminance, integrated along a line perpendicular to a diameter of the receptive field, as a function of distance along that diameter. The receptive field's LWF results from the difference between a broad Gaussian function (long-dashed curve, which represents the LWF of the surround mechanism) and a narrow Gaussian function (short-dashed curve, which represents the LWF of the center mechanism); hence, a difference of Gaussians.

Part A plots, on double-logarithmic axes, the amplitude part of the Fourier transform of the difference of Gaussians LWF. This is the amplitude part (i.e., the MTF) of the receptive field spatial frequency response. For this case, the phase part of the spatial frequency response is actually constant at zero degrees for all spatial frequencies (i.e., the Fourier transform is all cosine). The amplitudes are given in terms of normalized responsivity (i.e., the gain of the cell's response to contrast over a range in which the response amplitude scales linearly with contrast and the response phase does not change). The spatial frequency axis is also normalized. Three spatial frequencies (a, b, and c) are indicated on the plot in A. They correspond to the three cosine waves of B. Cosine wave a is an effective stimulus for both center and surround receptive field components. Cosine wave b is a poor stimulus for the surround, but a good stimulus for the center mechanism. Cosine wave c is a less effective stimulus for the center and an ineffective stimulus for the surround. This can be seen in panel A, where the responsivities of the center (short dashes) and surround components (long dashes) are plotted versus spatial frequency.

It is clear from the preceding discussion that the receptive fields of ganglion cells themselves bandwidth limit the neural image and, from the close coincidence of the short-dashed and solid curves in A, that the limit is principally set by the MTF of the receptive field center mechanism (the low temporal frequency attenuation in responsivity is less significant). However, as noted above, the bandwidth limit in the image will be the product of the receptive field's spatial frequency response and the Fourier transform of the scene, $L(r, \theta)$. We may conclude that it is never greater than the bandwidth limit of the receptive field's spatial frequency response. We may also be certain that the bandwidth limit of the X image is greater than that of the Y image since the center mechanism of Y cell receptive fields is broader.

Having considered how frequently time functions must be sampled to avoid aliasing and how visual images are bandwidth limited. we will now examine how images should be sampled to avoid aliasing.

Sampling Two-Dimensional Space-Invariant Signals

Images are two-dimensional signals and, while samples can be evenly spaced in only one way over the one time dimension, there are many ways to achieve even spacing in two dimensions. Nonetheless, sampling of space-invariant two-dimensional signals is relatively well understood. Consequently, the application of sampling theory to visual images has been quite rigorous to the extent that they can be treated as space-invariant. In the context of X and

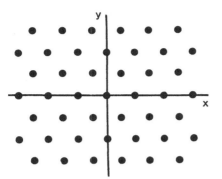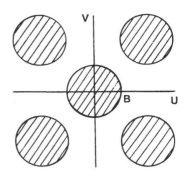

Figure 6.5 Relationship between sampling with a triangular (or hexagonal) sampling lattice and the representation of an image in the two-dimensional spatial frequency plane (U, V). The image is circularly bandwidth-limited on the spatial frequency plane to a spatial frequency of (B; right-hand panel). When sampled by the triangular lattice (left-hand panel) there are multiple representations of the image spaced about the spatial frequency plane. The five hatched circles represent examples. Aliasing occurs if the different representations of the image overlap. The separation between the hatched areas is inversely proportional to the spacing between the elements in the sampling array. The most efficient distortion-free sampling is when the hatched areas abut one another but do not overlap.

Y cells, *space-invariant* means that the spatial filtering properties of the receptive fields of each cell type do not change across the retina. This is obviously not true, and we will consider the implications of this shortly. Nevertheless, on a sufficiently local scale, retinal signals may be considered approximately space-invariant.

Let us now reconsider an oriented grating as a point on the two-dimensional spatial frequency plane. Figure 6.5 (right-hand side) shows the two-dimensional (U, V) spatial frequency plane. The Fourier transform of a receptive field's LWF gives the spatial frequency response only for gratings perpendicular to a receptive field diameter. In other words, it gives the spatial frequency response along a straight line passing through the origin of the spatial frequency axes. If the receptive field is circularly symmetric, as has been frequently assumed, the spatial frequency response over the whole plane can be determined by simply rotating the spatial frequency response along this line about the origin. The bandwidth limit then becomes a circularly symmetric limit on the two-dimensional spatial frequency plane. Recall from the earlier discussion that the bandwidth limit of an image filtered by such receptive fields can never be greater than the bandwidth limit of the cell's spatial frequency response.

For space-invariant two-dimensional signals that are bandwidth-limited in a circularly symmetric fashion in the two-dimensional spatial frequency plane, say to a spatial frequency of B, the spacing between neighboring cells arranged in a triangular (or hexagonal) lattice must be no greater than $(B\sqrt{3})^{-1}$ (Snyder and Miller 1977; Dudgeon and Mersereau 1984; Williams, 1985). The left-hand side of figure 6.5 shows a triangular sampling lattice. The neural image is represented only at these points of the *x-y* plane. In the spatial frequency domain, the image has multiple representations. Five examples are shown hatched on the right-hand side of the figure under the assumption that the image is bandwidth-limited in a circularly symmetric fashion to a spatial frequency of B. Aliasing occurs if the different representations of the image overlap. The separation between the hatched areas is inversely proportional to the spacing between the elements in the sampling array. The most efficient distortion-free sampling is when the hatched areas abut one another but do not overlap. Triangular spacing of samples provides the most efficient means of sampling circularly bandwidth-limited signals and, if one presumes the retina to be exquisitely optimized, it is reassuring that retinal ganglion cell sampling lattices appear to be pseudotriangular (e.g., Wässle, Boycott, and Illing 1981).

Figure 6.6A shows a sample of a cat retina from the work of Wässle et al. (1981) with an array of β (X) cells. Cell bodies and proximal dendrites are drawn. An estimate of the size of a full dendritic tree is provided by the speckled area around the cell in the lower right-hand corner. Only β cells whose dendritic trees arborize within the outer portion of the retina's inner plexiform layer are shown. They are presumed to be the off-center cells (Nelson, Famiglietti, and Kolb, 1978). In part B of the figure are marked only the positions of the cell bodies. This indicates the sampling positions of the presumed off-center X cells under the assumption that the midpoints of their

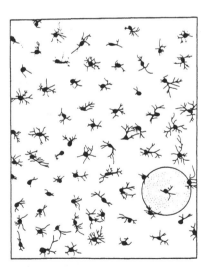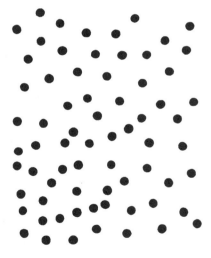

Figure 6.6   The β (X) cell sampling array from Wässle et al. (1981). (Left) Positions of β cell bodies and the proximal parts of their dendritic trees. The full dendritic tree of a β cell would occupy the area indicated by the speckled region. Only β cells whose dendritic trees arborize within the outer portion of the inner plexiform layer are shown. They were presumed to be off-center cells. (Right) Only the positions of the cell bodies are marked. This indicates the sampling positions of OFF-center X cells under the assumption that the midpoints of their receptive fields coincide with the locations of the cell bodies.

receptive fields coincide with the locations of the cell bodies, which is an over-simplification (Peichl and Wässle 1983; Schall and Leventhal 1987). It is apparent from inspection that parts of the lattice in part B show close to triangular symmetry. There is obviously some disorder, too.

Restating a point made earlier, the penalty of failing to meet the spacing criterion is that the sampling process will produce aliasing. The penalty of surpassing the criterion too generously is redundancy in the representation and an inefficient overload of neural tissue throughout the visual system. Although the sampling lattices for X and Y cells are approximately triangular in one location, we cannot assume that aliasing does not occur. Based on a comparison of the retinal densities of α cells (the morphological counterparts of Y cells) and β cells (the morphological counterparts of X cells) and the spatial frequency bandwidth limits of Y and X cells from the same locations, Hughes (1981b) has suggested that there is undersampling. However, she compared data from different animals, and the spatial frequency bandwidth limits used for X and Y cells were unusually high. Moreover, she took no account of the spatial frequency content of the scenes that a cat might be expected to view or of blurring due to eye, head, and body movements.

Space-Variant Sampling

A complication with the images $N_X(\rho, \phi)$ and $N_Y(\rho, \phi)$ is the fact that the density of sampling varies with position on the retina for both X and Y cells. There is a gradient of declining density with eccentricity, and the rate of decline is not the same for all values of ϕ. This point is exemplified by the isodensity lines for α (Y) cells drawn on a retinal whole-mount by Wässle, Levick, and Cleland (1975) and shown in figure 6.1.

It is well known that the uneven distribution of ganglion cells used to represent the retinal visual image leads to a distortion of that image, with greater emphasis placed on detail close to the point of fixation and less on peripheral details. This treatment of information is something akin to the confused geography that often afflicts undereducated children, and is presented humorously from a Chicagoan's perspective in figure 6.7. Chicago and Illinois are grossly over-represented.

The space-variant form of retinal sampling can be interpreted as a mapping from retinal space to a new space where distance is compressed reciprocally in proportion to the spacing between retinal ganglion cells. Since the primary visual cortex allots its neural processing volume in proportion to numbers of retinal ganglion cells (Tusa, Palmer, and Rosenquist 1978; Wässle, Grünert, Röhrenbeck, and Boycott 1989; Curcio and Allen 1990) and cortical thickness is constant, the cortical surface is actually organized geometrically according to this new space. Therefore, the characterization of this mapping is of great functional significance. On theoretical grounds and from an analysis of cortical visual field maps (Daniel and Whitteridge 1961; Cowey 1964; Allman and Kaas 1971; Tusa et al. 1978), it has been suggested that the transformation in the radial direction, ρ, is logarithmic (Schwartz 1980; Braccini, Gambardella,

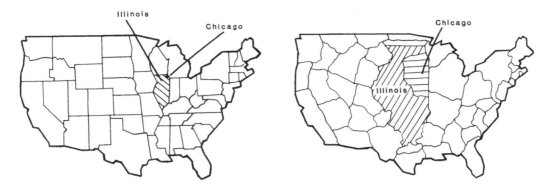

Figure 6.7 Two maps of the United States. The one on the right is distorted, with Chicago and Illinois much larger than they really are. Distortion of this general nature occurs in the visual system. More information per square millimeter is gathered in the center of the retina than peripherally.

Sadini, and Tagliasco 1982). This would mean that the spacing between sampling points would grow exponentially with eccentricity. To date, distortion in the angular coordinate has been ignored in all theoretical analyses, simply assuming that sampling is radially symmetric.

Using data from a number of published works, I have roughly characterized the general form of the dependence of spatial scale on retinal eccentricity for the cat. The results are shown in figure 6.8, where normalized measures of the spatial frequency resolution of lattices (Wässle, Levick, and Cleland 1975; Wässle 1981), cells (Cleland, Harding, and Tulunay-Keesey 1979), or cats (Pasternak and Horn 1991) are plotted versus eccentricity. The anatomical data were corrected for the varying retinal magnification factor that is a consequence of the departure of the eyeball from a true sphere (Hughes 1976; Holden Hayes and Fitzke 1987).

An exponential dependence of spatial frequency resolution on eccentricity would be a straight line in this plot, and the line's slope would give the exponential rate of change. As the data include measurements taken along many meridians (many values of ϕ), the data should fan out with eccentricity as indicated (in exaggerated fashion) by the dashed lines. The results are somewhat equivocal, and Cleland et al. (1979) found that their data were actually better fitted by a hyperbolic function. Nonetheless, since the exponential relationship is approximately correct, I explored the implications of this relationship for the correct application of sampling theory to the retina.

First suppose that sampling of the retinal image is space-invariant. If the sample points are spaced δ apart in a perfect triangular lattice, the spatial frequency bandwidth limit will be $(\delta\sqrt{3})^{-1}$, as noted earlier. If the sampling lattice is now stretched radially so that the distance between sample points increases exponentially, one can ask how the spatial frequency bandwidth limit should be adjusted to accommodate the new sampling lattice. Intuitively, one would guess that the bandwidth limit should decrease in proportion to the increased spacing between sample points. Some theoretical work suggests

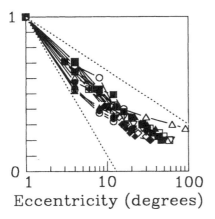

Eccentricity (degrees)

Figure 6.8 The general form of the dependence of spatial scale on retinal eccentricity for the cat. Normalized measures of the spatial frequency resolution of lattices (Wässle et al. 1975; Wässle 1981), cells (Cleland et al. 1979), and cats (Pasternak and Horn 1991) are plotted vs. retinal eccentricity. The anatomical data were corrected for the varying retinal magnification factor that is a consequence of the departure of the eyeball from a true sphere (Hughes 1976; Holden et al. 1987). An exponential dependence of spatial frequency resolution on eccentricity would be a straight line in this plot, and the line's slope would give the exponential rate of change. The data include measurements taken along many meridians (many values of ϕ in figure 6.1) and should fan out with eccentricity as indicated (in exaggerated fashion) by the dashed lines.

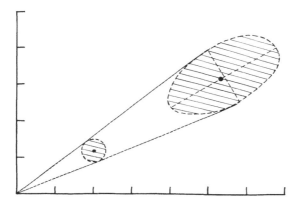

Figure 6.9 Projection of a circular field that would satisfactorily bandwidth-limit a triangular array of samples onto a new surface in such a way that it would cover the same set of samples. The circular field is mapped into a pseudo-elliptical field. A few interesting features of this "receptive field" are evident. First, it is close to elliptical in shape and has its major axis oriented towards the center of the sampling lattice. Second, the midpoint of the elliptical field (intersection of the major and minor axes) does not coincide with the projected midpoint of the circular field (black spots). Another consequence of this unequal stretching is that the LWF of this field will be asymmetric about the center, except for the case in which the midline of the weighting function passes through the lattice origin. Hence, the projection of a center-surround field might be expected to generate an offset between the center and surround midpoints. Note also that the mapping will not have the form illustrated when the circular field includes the central point of the lattice ($\rho = 0$). These features are characteristics of the receptive fields of cat retinal ganglion cells (see figure 6.10).

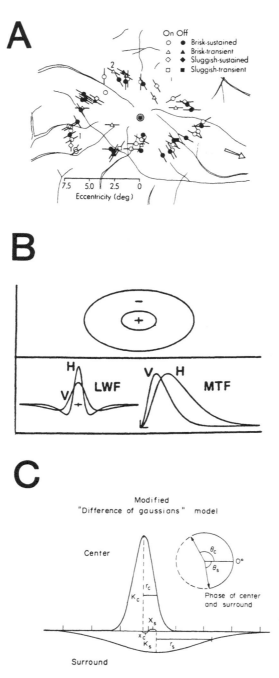

Figure 6.10 Anisotropies of X and Y cell receptive fields reported by various investigators. Levick and Thibos (1980) showed that the preferred orientation of the receptive field was oriented along a line joining the midpoint of the receptive field with the center of the area centralis. In (A) the receptive field locations are indicated by the symbols in the key, and the lines through the symbols are the preferred orientations of the receptive fields. The spoked wheel symbol gives the location of the area centralis. The X cells are probably brisk-sustained cells, and the Y cells are probably brisk-transient cells. (B) Levick and Thibos (1982) analyzed

that this intuition is correct for a smoothly varying function such as the relationship between spacing and eccentricity (Sawchuk 1973, 1974; Marks, Walkup, and Hagler 1976). However, I believe that more theoretical work is needed. In any event, the relationship just given is closely related to the assumption often used in the vision science literature that lattices can be treated as space-invariant on a local scale (Coletta and Williams 1987; Hirsch and Miller 1987).

What, then, is the consequence of a decrease in the bandwidth limit in proportion to the increasing spacing between sample points? Figure 6.9 shows the projection of a circularly symmetric field that would have the appropriate bandwidth limit for a regular triangular lattice transformed into a pseudo-elliptical field that would have the appropriate bandwidth limit to match the triangular lattice after it had been stretched exponentially. A few interesting features of this "receptive field" are evident. First, it is close to elliptical in shape and has its major axis oriented towards the center of the sampling lattice. These features agree with published data on X and Y cell receptive field centers (Hammond 1974; Levick and Thibos 1980, 1982; Leventhal and Schall 1983; Soodak, Shapley, and Kaplan 1987). Second, the midpoint of the elliptical field (intersection of the major and minor axes) does not coincide with the projected midpoint of the circular field (black spots). This occurs because points that are farther from the center of the lattice are stretched more.

Another consequence of this unequal stretching is that the line weighting function of this field will be asymmetric about the center, except for the case in which the midline of the weighting function passes through the lattice origin. Hence, the projection of a center-surround field might be expected to generate an offset between the center and surround midpoints similar to that sometimes observed by Dawis, Shapley, Kaplan, and Tranchina (1984). Note also that the mapping will not have the form illustrated in figure 6.9 when the circular field includes the central point of the lattice ($\rho = 0$). This may explain Levick and Thibos's (1982) observation that orientation bias is less evident for cells with receptive fields near to the area centralis. In summary, this model qualitatively satisfies many of the features reported for X and Y cell receptive fields. A number of these features are shown in figure 6.10.

Whether this currently qualitative model can be made to agree quantitatively with measurements on X and Y cells remains to be seen. Some more theoretical work is needed that is specifically tailored to the question of space-variant sampling by the retina, particularly consideration of the effects on

the orientation bias of X and Y cell receptive fields. This panel indicates how the horizontal (H) and vertical (V) line-weighting functions (LWF) and the corresponding modulation transfer functions (MTF) for horizontally oriented (H) and vertically oriented (V) gratings would appear for the receptive field shown. Note that the bandwidth limit is greater for horizontally oriented gratings. (C) Dawis et al.'s (1984) "mod DOG model," which permits midpoints of the center and surround Gaussian weighting functions to be displaced from one another, here by $x_c + x_s$. This model was needed to account for some spatial frequency responses that they measured from X retinal ganglion cells.

receptive field shape of asymmetric stretching for different values of ϕ. However, the general modeling approach outlined in this chapter seems to hold some promise. Moreover, even if (or should I say when?) the theory proves to be wrong, we will learn something important about retinal representations of visual images. We would not even address such questions if we did not try to model.

ACKNOWLEDGMENTS

The preparation of this manuscript was supported by NIH R01 EY06669 and a grant from the Whitaker Foundation. J. B. Troy is a Sloan Research Fellow.

REFERENCES

Allman JH, Kaas J (1971) Representation of the visual field in striate and adjoining cortex of the owl monkey brain. Brain Res 35:89–106.

Black HS (1953) Modulation Theory. New York: Van Nostrand.

Braccini C, Gambardella G. Sandini G, Tagliasco V (1982) A model of the early stages of the human visual system: functional and topological transformations performed in the peripheral visual field. Biol Cybern 44:47–58.

Campbell FW, Robson JG, Westheimer G (1959) Fluctuations of accommodation under steady viewing conditions. J Physiol (Lond) 145:579–594.

Cleland BG, Levick WR (1974a) Brisk and sluggish concentrically organized ganglion cells in the cat's retina. J Physiol (Lond) 240:421–456.

Cleland BG, Levick WR (1974b) Properties of rarely encountered types of ganglion cells in the cat's retina and an overall classification. J Physiol (Lond) 240:457–492.

Cleland BG, Harding TH, Tulunay-Keesey U (1979) Visual resolution and receptive field size: examination of two kinds of cat retinal ganglion cell. Science 205:1015–1017.

Coletta NJ, Williams DR (1987) Psychophysical estimate of extrafoveal cone spacing. J Opt Soc Am A 4:1503–1513.

Cowey A (1964) Projection of the retina onto striate and prestriate cortex in the squirrel monkey, *saimiri sciureus*. J Neurophysiol 27:366–393.

Curcio CA, Allen KA (1990) Topography of ganglion cells in human retina. J Comp Neurol 300:5–25.

Daniel M, Whitteridge D (1961) The representation of the visual field on the cerebral cortex in monkeys. J Physiol (Lond) 159:203–221.

Dawis S, Shapley R, Kaplan E, Tranchina D (1984) The receptive field organization of X-cells in the cat: spatiotemporal coupling and asymmetry. Vision Res 24:549–564.

Dudgeon DE, Mersereau RM (1984) Multidimensional digital image processing. Englewood Cliffs, NJ: Prentice-Hall.

Enroth-Cugell Ch. Robson JG (1966) The contrast sensitivity of retinal ganglion cells of the cat. J Physiol (Lond) 187:517–552.

Enroth-Cugell Ch, Robson JG (1984) Functional characteristics and diversity of cat retinal ganglion cells. Invest Ophthal 25:250–267.

Hammond P (1974) Cat retinal ganglion cells: size and shape of receptive field centres. J Physiol (Lond) 242:99–118.

Hirsch J, Miller WH (1987) Does cone positional disorder limit resolution? J Opt Soc Am A 4:1481–1492.

Hochstein S. Shapley RM (1976) Linear and nonlinear spatial subunits in Y cat retinal ganglion cells. J Physiol (Lond) 262:265–284.

Holden AL, Hayes BP, Fitzke FW (1987) Retinal magnification factor at the ora terminalis: a structural study of human and animal eyes. Vision Res 27:1229–1235.

Hughes A (1976) A supplement to the cat schematic eye. Vision Res 16:149–154.

Hughes A (1981a) Population magnitudes and distribution of the major modal classes of cat retinal ganglion cell as estimated from HRP filling and a systematic survey of soma diameter spectra for classical neurones. J Comp Neurol 197:303–339.

Hughes A (1981b) Cat retina and sampling theorem: the relation of transient and sustained brisk-unit cut-off frequency to α and β-mode cell density. Exp Brain Res 42:196–202.

Jones JJ, Palmer LA (1987) An evaluation of the two-dimensional Gabor filter model of simple receptive fields in cat striate cortex. J Neurophysiol 58:1233–1258.

Kuffler SW (1953) Discharge patterns and functional organization of mammalian retina. J Neurophysiol 16:37–68.

Leventhal AG, Schall JD (1983) Structural basis of orientation sensitivity of cat retinal ganglion cells. J Comp Neurol 220:465–475.

Levick WR, Thibos LN (1980) Orientation bias of cat retinal ganglion cells. Nature 286:389–390.

Levick WR, Thibos LN (1982) Analysis of orientation bias in cat retina. J Physiol (Lond) 329:243–261.

Marks RJ II, Walkup JF, Hagler MO (1976) A sampling theorem for space-variant systems. J Opt Soc Am 66:918–921.

Nelson R, Famiglietti EV Jr, Kolb H (1978) Intracellular staining reveals different levels of stratification for on- and off-center ganglion cells in cat retina. J Neurophysiol 41:472–483.

Pasternak T, Horn K (1991) Spatial vision of the cat: variation with eccentricity. Vis Neurosci 6:151–158.

Peichl L, Wässle H (1983) The structural correlate of the receptive field centre of α ganglion cells in the cat retina. J Physiol (Lond) 341:309–324.

Rodieck RW (1965) Quantitative analysis of cat retinal ganglion cell response to visual stimuli. Vision Res 5:583–610.

Sawchuk AA (1973) Space-variant system analysis of image motion. J Opt Soc Am 63:1052–1063.

Sawchuk AA (1974) Space-variant image restoration by coordinate transformation. J Opt Soc Am 64:138–144.

Schall JD, Leventhal AG (1987) Relationships between ganglion cell dendritic structure and retinal topography in the cat. J Comp Neurol 257:149–159.

Schwartz EL (1980) Computational anatomy and functional architecture of striate cortex: a spatial mapping approach to perceptual coding. Vision Res 20:645–669.

Snyder AW, Miller WH (1977) Photoreceptor diameter and spacing for highest resolving power. J Opt Soc Am 67:696–698.

Soodak RE, Shapley RM, Kaplan E (1987) Linear mechanism of orientation tuning in the cat retina and lateral geniculate nucleus of the cat. J Neurophysiol 58:267–275.

Stone J, Fukuda Y (1974) Properties of cat retinal ganglion cells: a comparison of W-cells with X- and Y-cells. J Neurophysiol 37:722–748.

Tusa RJ, Palmer LA, Rosenquist AC (1978) The retinotopic organization of area 17 (striate cortex) in the cat. J Comp Neurol 177:213–236.

Wässle H (1981) Morphological types and topographical distribution of ganglion cells in the cat retina. In Szentágothai J, Hámori J, Palkovits M (eds.) Advances in Physiological Sciences. Vol. 2. Regulatory Functions of the CNS. Subsystems, pp. 245–254.

Wässle H, Boycott BB, Illing R-B (1981) Morphology and mosaic of on- and off-beta cells in the cat retina and some functional considerations. Proc R Soc Lond B 212:177–195.

Wässle H, Grünert U, Röhrenbeck J, Boycott BB (1989) Cortical magnification factor and the ganglion cell density of the primate retina. Nature 341:643–646.

Wässle H, Levick WR, Cleland BG (1975) The distribution of the alpha type of ganglion cells in the cat's retina. J Comp Neurol 159:419–438.

Williams DR (1985) Aliasing in human foveal vision. Vision Res 25:195–205.

7 Contrast Sensitivity and Light Adaptation in Photoreceptors or in the Retinal Network

Robert Shapley, Ehud Kaplan, and
Keith Purpura

Sensitivity to contrast is one of the most important attributes of the visual system of humans and other animals. This chapter is about some of the reasons for the dependence of visual responses on contrast and about the neural machinery in the retina that makes it possible.

One of the questions that has recurred in this field is this: to what extent does light adaptation depend on processes that take place within single photoreceptors, and to what extent does spatial interaction within the retinal network contribute to visual adaptation? In this chapter, in honor of Christina Enroth-Cugell's Helmerich Award, we consider old and new evidence about receptoral adaptation, in particular the evidence about light adaptation in primate cone photoreceptors. This has recently become an area of intense interest because of apparently conflicting evidence about this fundamental issue. Our goal in this paper is not to resolve the conflicts definitively—that will require sharper experiments—but to present the points of disagreement and to suggest possible means of reaching a definitive answer.

Before delving into the receptor adaptation issue, we review classic evidence about the function of adaptation, recapitulating some of the ideas in the massive review that Christina Enroth-Cugell and one of us composed (Shapley and Enroth-Cugell, 1984). Visual adaptation has been one of Christina Enroth-Cugell's lasting research interests, and she and her colleagues have made many contributions to our understanding of retinal adaptation in the retina of the cat. The question regarding the role of photoreceptors in adaptation remains to vex us all.

Visual adaptation is inextricably linked to the perception of brightness. Although it seems that perception of the brightness of objects is effortless, visual scientists know that complex neuronal computations are required to perform the task. The perception of brightness is not simply a matter of counting photons. The primary determinant of brightness perception is local contrast, the local difference between luminances on either side of a boundary normalized by the (local) average luminance (Heinemann 1955, 1972; Shapley and Enroth-Cugell 1984).

CONTRAST, CONTRAST SENSITIVITY, AND CONTRAST GAIN

Contrast is a physical property of the visual stimulus. When studying the visibility of aperiodic objects such as uniform disks or bars or rectangles on a background, an investigator would naturally define contrast as

$$C = (L_0 - L_B)/(L_B) \tag{7.1a}$$

where L_0 is the luminance of the object and L_B the luminance of the background. $L_0 - L_B$ is usually called ΔL, and so equation 7.1a is usually written as

$$C = \Delta L/L_B \tag{7.1b}$$

At high mean luminance, and for test stimuli of large area and long duration, psychophysical sensitivity follows Weber's Law, as shown empirically below. Then we can write

$$\Delta L_T/L_B = k \tag{7.2a}$$

$$C_T = k \tag{7.2b}$$

where k is a constant, the threshold contrast. The threshold contrast C_T is also referred to in the psychophysical literature as the *Weber fraction*. Equation 7.2 says, in words, that, when Weber's law is obeyed, the visual system's criterion for detection is that the stimulus contrast must equal a fixed value, k, the threshold contrast.

There is a second definition of contrast that is used for periodic spatial patterns like sine gratings.

$$C_R = (L_{max} - L_{min})/(L_{max} + L_{min}) \tag{7.3}$$

The two different definitions, equations (7.2) and (7.3) are related because they refer to a single physical quantity: the relative variation of a modulated component referred to (or normalized by) a steady-state component.

Contrast sensitivity is the reciprocal of the psychophysical threshold contrast. Contrast gain (Shapley and Enroth-Cugell 1984) is neural response divided by stimulus contrast in the limit as contrast approaches zero, and will be expressed in units of mV/unit contrast or (impulses/sec)/unit contrast. Contrast gain and contrast sensitivity depend directly on the process of light adaptation, as shown below.

BRIGHTNESS, CONTRAST SENSITIVITY, AND ADAPTATION

Animals evolved in a world of reflecting surfaces. What characterizes a reflecting surface visually is its reflectance. The reflectance is determined by the physical properties of the surface of the object. Reflectance is therefore invariant with respect to illumination. The luminance of an object is proportional to the product of the object's reflectance and illumination. Over a wide range of illumination, the brightness of a reflecting object is constant even though its luminance may vary widely. Land and McCann (1971) explained the purpose of brightness constancy by asserting that the visual system was designed to calculate reflectance. We know now that this is not correct, but it is on the right track.

The early stages of vision compute contrast, not reflectance. One can view contrast as *relative reflectance*, the comparison of the reflectance of an object with its background. The response of retinal, geniculate, and some primary cortical neurons is dependent on contrast. Constancy of neuronal response with contrast may be achieved for stimuli that activate only the center mechanism of the receptive field (Enroth-Cugell and Robson 1966; Shapley and Enroth-Cugell 1984). This means that the responsiveness of the visual system to contrast is not simply a result of center-surround interaction or of lateral inhibition (as in the standard textbook accounts, e.g., Cornsweet 1970). Rather, contrast dependence is primarily a result of the automatic gain control that produces light adaptation (Whittle and Challands 1969; Shapley and Enroth-Cugell 1984). The automatic gain control that regulates the contrast sensitivity of a receptive field center is localized to the center, and thus contrast is computed only locally (Shapley and Enroth-Cugell, 1984).

CONTRAST VS. REFLECTANCE: SIMULTANEOUS CONTRAST

An example of the power of contrast to determine perception is the elaboration of the classic picture of equally luminant circles on a nonuniform background, as in figure 7.1. The figure shows sixteen equally luminant circles placed on six rectangular strips that vary in luminance. This could be interpreted as a scene with sixteen equally reflective disks placed on a cloth with six different rectangular regions of reflectance. If the visual system is computing local contrast, then the disks should all appear different in brightness because their contrasts are not all the same. If the visual system were computing reflectance as Land and McCann (1971) suggested, then all sixteen disks should look the same shade of grey. It is obvious to every observer that they look different and so, at least qualitatively, the quantity computed by the visual system must be closer to contrast than to reflectance.

Land and McCann (1971) anticipated this refutation of their theory (the 1971 Retinex) in a footnote to their 1971 paper in which they asserted that pictures such as those in figure 7.1 were unnatural because the objects were completely surrounded by their backgrounds. This is a weak argument, since in nature isolated objects on backgrounds are the rule rather than the exception. But, accepting the Land and McCann argument as valid for the moment, we can put it to the test by constructing a "Mondrian"-like pattern (which Land and McCann considered more natural) and then looking again at equally reflective objects on nonuniform backgrounds. This is shown in figure 7.2, which I have reproduced from an earlier paper (Shapley 1986). It can be seen that the circle and square, though equally luminant, are not equally bright. An explanation is that neurons are computing local contrast and the visual system is basing its estimate of brightness on contrast-dependent neural responses. Reid and Shapley (1988) measured the magnitude of such brightness induction

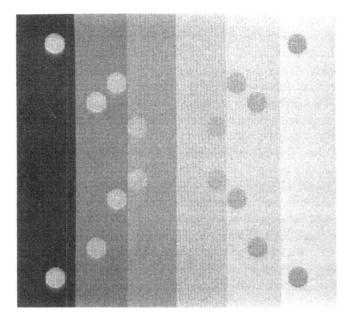

Figure 7.1 Sixteen equiluminant circles on a luminance staircase. This pattern was created on a CRT display with a computer-controlled instrument. Each rectangular area in the staircase is of a fixed uniform luminance. The luminance of the circles—all of which have the same luminance—is the same as the mean luminance of the staircase.

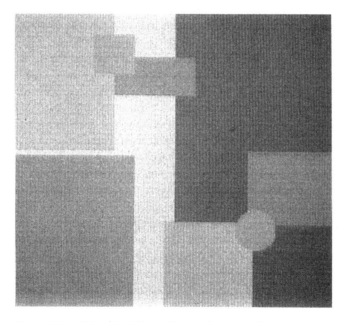

Figure 7.2 "Mondrian"-like pattern with an equally luminant square and circle. The local areas of contrast around the square and circle are different and opposite in sign, so the square appears dark while the circle appears light.

in Mondrian-like patterns like that in figure 7.2, and it was virtually identical to that seen in more conventional displays, such as that in figure 7.1.

Psychophysical Evidence

Constant contrast sensitivity is the ideal toward which retinal light adaptation must strive if it is to achieve its main goal: perceptual invariance of reflecting surfaces with changes in background illumination. To the extent that psychophysics approaches Weber's law, this major goal has been met. A graph of threshold contrast versus background retinal illumination shows a clear break between rod and cone function (for example, see Blackwell 1946). The minimal contrast threshold for the rods, at the high end of the scotopic range of backgrounds, is about 0.08, which approximately corresponds to a contrast sensitivity of 12. There is a clear jump in performance when the cones come in, with contrast thresholds declining asymptotically to 0.005 in the high photopic range.

In the regime of Weber's law, contrast sensitivity is constant as in equation (7.2); a graph of contrast sensitivity vs. mean illumination would be a flat line. In fact, human contrast sensitivity increases as the square root of mean luminance over most of the scotopic range, though it is beginning to level off toward behavior described by Weber's law for the largest targets at the high end of the scotopic range (Blackwell 1946).

THE REGULATION OF PHOTOPIC CONTRAST SENSITIVITY

The cone system (photopic system) is like the rod system in yielding results in line with Weber's law under some circumstances and in line with the square root law under others. In human vision the cones take over at threshold from the rods above 0.1 to 1 troland (td) in background retinal illumination (Wyzecki and Stiles 1982). The increment threshold curves in the literature tend to show a cone plateau from 0.1 up to about 10 td. Above 10 td one usually observes results in line with Weber's law for a bipartite field or a moderate-sized test spot (diameter $> 0.5°$). For most targets, and in particular for moderate-sized spots with sharp edges, on a large background, Weber's law holds from 10 td to 10^5 td, i.e., throughout the photopic range of backgrounds (Whittle and Challands 1969). The mechanisms that cause Weber's law to apply in human photopic vision are therefore also achieving the goal of brightness constancy, i.e., illumination-invariant appearance by making responses proportional to contrast.

The concept of light adaptation in photoreceptors comes from psychophysical investigations of color vision. For example, the success of the two-color method of Stiles for isolating chromatic mechanisms provides some support for the independent adaptation of different photoreceptors (Wyszecki and Stiles 1982). More recently, the extensive investigations of chromatic detection by Stromeyer and colleagues have been framed in terms of the Weber contrast in each cone type (for example, see Stromeyer et al. 1985).

The coherence of the account of chromatic detection in terms of cone contrast supports the concept of cone adaptation in the human visual retina. For instance, Stromeyer and colleagues found that chromatic detection thresholds fell on a straight line in Weberian cone contrast coordinates, indicating that signals proportional to L cone contrast are simply subtracted from signals proportional to M cone contrast in the detection of chromatic targets.

However, recent experiments by Krauskopf and Gegenfurtner (1992) on color discrimination seem to suggest that cone adaptation is not required to account for their results at retinal illuminations of 500 td or below. They found that the chromatic modulation threshold, on different chromatic backgrounds that were fixed in luminance, did not depend upon the color of the background, but only on background luminance. The predictions of independent cone adaptation were not confirmed. These experimental findings thus raise again the question of whether there is light adaptation in human cones. In our view the crucial findings in this area concern the link between dynamics and gain control in light adaptation, which we will present now.

THE DYNAMICS OF PSYCHOPHYSICAL LIGHT ADAPTATION

A clue to the mechanisms of adaptation, and a crucial adumbration of later physiological work on photoreceptor light adaptation, was provided by the psychophysical study of the dynamics of light adaptation. The temporal frequency of a stimulus influences the dependence of sensitivity on mean level. This has been shown in psychophysical experiments, mainly by Kelly (1972). At low spatial frequency and low to intermediate temporal frequency, he obtained results described by Weber's law. At high spatial frequency and low to intermediate temporal frequencies he observed results described by the square root law. At very high temporal frequencies he discovered that sensitivity was more or less independent of mean level. This is what Kelly called the "linear" region of temporal frequencies, because the visual system appears to be behaving in a linear manner in that the sensitivity for a modulated stimulus is not affected by the presence of different steady levels.

An explanation for Kelly's results has emerged from recent work on the dynamics of light adaptation in photoreceptors and retinal ganglion cells, though there are some contradictory results that require consideration. We will refer back to Kelly's findings when considering the dynamics of retinal adaptation. In the context of our previous discussion of contrast and brightness constancy, it is interesting to note that brightness induction and the stable estimation of brightness fail at moderate temporal frequencies (DeValois et al. 1986). Thus, stable brightness perception seems to work only in the low temporal frequency region within which Weber's law holds.

CONTRAST GAIN IN PRIMATE RETINAL GANGLION CELLS

There are several types of retinal ganglion cells in the retinas of macaque monkeys, close evolutionary relatives of man. Two different types of ganglion cells project to the lateral geniculate nucleus (LGN) of the thalamus. These types, called P cells and M cells (Shapley and Perry 1986), resemble human ganglion cells in morphology (Rodieck 1988), and therefore it is reasonable to suppose that they might also resemble human ganglion cells physiologically. Quite a lot is now known about the contrast gain of these neurons. The P cells have low contrast gain (Kaplan and Shapley 1986) like their parvocellular targets (Shapley et al. 1981; Kaplan and Shapley 1982; Hicks et al. 1983; Derrington and Lennie 1984) within the macaque's LGN. P cells are color-opponent neurons and probably constitute the front end for chromatic perception. M cells project to the magnocellular layers of the LGN. Like magnocellular neurons, M cells have high contrast gain (Shapley et al. 1981; Kaplan and Shapley 1982; Hicks et al. 1983; Derrington and Lennie 1984; Kaplan and Shapley 1986). M cells have a broad-band spectral sensitivity and may be the neural basis for "luminance" perception.

The dependence of contrast gain on mean level is always informative, so we have studied this function in macaque ganglion cells (Purpura et al. 1988). Some of our results are shown in figure 7.3 as contrast gain vs. mean illumination. There it can be seen that M cell contrast gain is higher than P cell contrast gain at all light levels. Furthermore, many P cells have an unmeasurably small contrast gain when the mean illumination is lowered into the scotopic range where rods determine neural responses. This suggests that scotopic pattern vision depends on the responses of M cells that are relayed

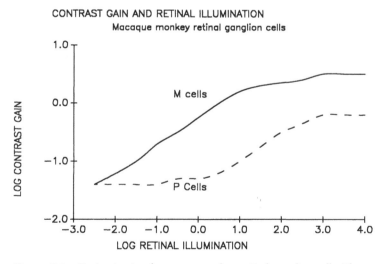

Figure 7.3 Contrast gain of macaque monkey retinal ganglion cells. These are averages of the contrast gains of the data presented by Purpura et al. (1990). The stimuli were drifting sine gratings at around 3 c/deg spatial frequency and 4 Hz temporal frequency. The stimuli were achromatic patterns on a "white" screen. Contrast gain is the slope of the response vs. contrast function and has units of (impulses/sec)/percent contrast. Mean retinal illumination is in macaque trolands (td). One macaque troland is equivalent to a retinal illumination of 200 quanta/cone sec incident on the retina, and about 50 quanta/cone sec absorbed by the cone and effective in transduction (estimated).

through the LGN to the visual cortex. Finally one can see that the contrast gain of macaque ganglion cells does not reach the flat line of Weber's law until the cells are exposed to medium to high photopic levels of illumination, as in human observers. It is interesting that in the cat, a nocturnal animal, many retinal ganglion cells reach the flat, Weber-law asymptote under scotopic conditions (Shapley and Enroth-Cugell 1984; Shapley 1991).

There is a close correspondence between the contrast gain functions of retinal ganglion cells and the contrast sensitivity of human observers. This suggests that the basic mechanisms of contrast sensitivity are located in the retinal network. These basic mechanisms include the local gain controls of light adaptation, spatial and temporal filtering by the photoreceptors and interneurons that provide input to the ganglion cells, and amplification of receptor signals.

The Dynamics of Retinal Adaptation

The site of light adaptation in the retina and the mechanisms of retinal adaptation have been studied extensively. It is beyond the scope of this paper to discuss the subject fully. In an earlier article (Shapley and Enroth-Cugell 1984), Christina Enroth-Cugell and one of us reviewed the already large body of literature on the subject and concluded that there were multiple, hierarchically organized mechanisms for light adaptation. The multiplicity of retinal mechanisms is a consequence, we think, of the multiple neural channels that are set up by the functional connections of the retinal network. For instance, in the macaque monkey retina there are P and M ganglion cells and they have different numbers of functional connections to photoreceptors (Rodieck 1988). More cones make functional connections with M cells than with P cells, and the cone connections to P cells may be quite specific. Therefore, gain controls for preventing response saturation and for making responses invariant with levels of illumination may have to exist in single cone photoreceptors and also in retinal interneurons within which cone signals are pooled.

The characteristic "signature" of cone photoreceptor adaptation is the differential effect of mean illumination on cone dynamics, as illustrated in figure 7.4. This is redrawn from figure 2 in Sneyd and Tranchina (1989) and illustrates the temporal frequency response of a cone photoreceptor from the retina of a turtle. These data on cones resemble quantitatively the earlier results obtained by Tranchina et al. (1984) on turtle horizontal cells and by Naka et al. (1987) in their study of turtle cones, and they are qualitatively very much like the psychophysical results reported for human observers by Kelly (1972), cited above. Weber's law is observed for low temporal frequencies only. At intermediate temporal frequencies, the dependence of gain on mean illumination has a shallower slope on log-log coordinates, and so the contrast gain vs. mean illumination will also have a slope between 0 and 1. At high temporal frequency there is no dependence of gain on mean illumination, so contrast gain at high frequencies grows proportionally with mean light level in these photoreceptors.

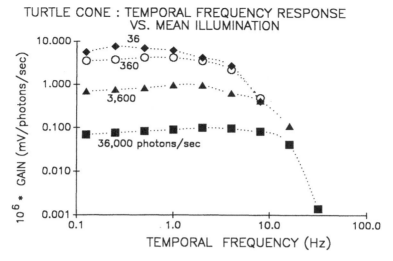

Figure 7.4 Temporal frequency responses of a turtle cone at different background illuminations, redrawn from Sneyd and Tranchina (1989). Retinal illumination of the background for each data set is written next to the curves. These are not theoretical curves but merely splines through the data.

It is surprising and significant that monkey ganglion cells of the P variety reveal the same sort of dynamic dependence on mean illumination as do turtle cones. This seems to us to indicate that photoreceptor adaptation is the predominant influence on these neurons. Figure 7.5 shows some of the data on this point, redrawn from Purpura et al. (1990). It is also significant that, at higher mean illumination levels, a similar link between gain and dynamics is seen in M ganglion cells, as demonstrated in figure 7.6. The background illuminations for the monkey ganglion cell data are given in terms of quanta/cone sec. This is done to facilitate comparison with the turtle cone adaptation data in figure 7.4. It is remarkable that the dynamic changes in the temporal frequency responses and the corresponding vertical shifts, indicative of corresponding gain changes, are very similar between these two different data sets.

The peculiar and highly structured dynamic dependence of temporal frequency response on mean illumination constrains theoretical models of photoreceptor function. The earliest mathematical models of photoreceptor adaptation were designed to explain the link between gain and dynamics in a transducer with an automatic gain control (e.g., Fuortes and Hodgkin 1964). However, there were no satisfactory phenomenological models of photoreceptor function prior to the theory advanced by Tranchina et al. (1984), in part because the dynamic dependence of frequency responses on mean illumination had not previously been measured. In the admittedly black-box theory advanced in Tranchina et al. (1984), the cone's temporal frequency response is written as

$$R(f) = \frac{A(f)}{1 + I_0 B(f)} \tag{7.4}$$

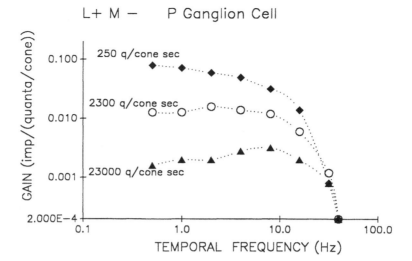

Figure 7.5 Temporal frequency responses at different mean illuminations for a P retinal ganglion cell from macaque monkey, redrawn from Purpura et al. (1990). Achromatic sine gratings were used as stimuli. Spatial frequency was 3 c/deg. Gain is given in impulses/(quanta/cone). Mean retinal illumination in quanta/cone sec is given alongside the data sets.

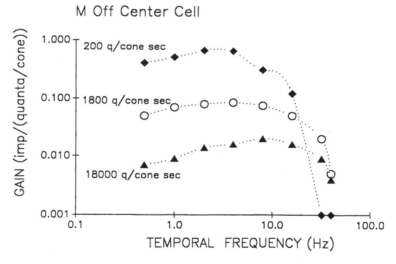

Figure 7.6 Temporal frequency responses at different mean illuminations for an M retinal ganglion cell from macaque monkey, redrawn from Purpura et al. (1990). Achromatic sine gratings were used as stimuli. Spatial frequency was 3 c/deg. Gain was derived from the response vs. contrast function. Gain is given in impulses/(quanta/cone). Mean retinal illumination in quanta/cone sec is given alongside the data set.

where R is the frequency response of the cone, A and B are the frequency responses of (low-pass) stages of neural transduction and temporal integration, and I_0 is the mean illumination level. One could criticize this formula as being no more than a formal description of the data, because there is no valid mechanistic theory to explain the functional form. Tranchina and Peskin (1989) elaborated this model and made it plausible in terms of possible mechanisms. However, a conceptual advance has recently been made by Sneyd and Tranchina (1989) in their article on a kinetic theory of cone photoreceptor transduction, which is based on the known biochemistry of photoreceptors. These authors show that the characteristic frequency response data of figure 7.4 can be accounted for very well using a model that includes calcium-dependent feedback in the biochemical cascade from activated rhodopsin to channel closing in the photoreceptor. Therefore, the ganglion cell data in figures 7.5 and 7.6 also presumably can be explained with similar biochemical kinetic mechanisms at work in the cones of the monkey retina. There is ample physiological evidence of the role of calcium in photoreceptor light adaptation (Lamb and Pugh 1990). Tranchina et al. (1991) present the most elaborate version of the model. The heart of the adaptation mechanism is the (highly nonlinear) regulation by calcium of the production of cyclic GMP, the internal transmitter in photoreceptors, by an enzyme called guanylate cyclase.

It would seem that the physiological evidence is all on the side of cone light adaptation, and the psychophysical results of Krauskopf and Gegenfurtner (1992) must be accounted for in terms of some postreceptoral mechanism. However, the recently reported results of Schnapf et al. (1990) on light adaptation in primate cones suggest that the picture is darker. Their results on the photocurrent of isolated monkey cones recorded with suction electrodes indicated that gain was not reduced until the retinal illumination was about 3×10^5 quanta/cone sec. This is about 300 times more illumination than one expects based on the monkey ganglion cell recordings, and much higher than is expected from human psychophysics. Previous work on photoreceptor mass responses in the monkey retina is equivocal. Valeton and Van Norren (1983) found light adaptation in primate foveal ERG to begin at a mean illumination between the high level reported by Schnapf et al. and the lower level implied by the data of Purpura et al.

One striking difference between the responses of monkey ganglion cells and cone responses concerns the dynamics of dark-adapted cones. Human psychophysics, monkey ganglion cells, and turtle cones were all low-pass in temporal frequency tuning when dark-adapted. However, Schnapf et al. (1990) reported the remarkable result that the temporal impulse response of dark-adapted cones was biphasic, implying by linearity that the temporal frequency response of these cones would be band-pass in temporal frequency tuning. It is possible that a low-pass filter between cones and ganglion cells could reshape the cones' temporal frequency response to resemble that of the ganglion cells. However, the existence of such a filter would imply that the retina would be attenuating most of the signal strength of the cones under dark-adapted conditions. This seems implausible on functional grounds. Furthermore, according to this hypothesis the dynamic changes with light adaptation in ganglion cell responses observed by Purpura et al. would have to be produced by postreceptoral circuits.

The state of the field at this point is confusing and contradictory on a fundamental functional point—whether cone photoreceptors of the primate retina adapt to light at the beginning or only at the high end of the photopic range of vision. Future experiments on the basis of visual perception must address this fundamental issue. One could imagine further experiments on light adaptation in retinal ganglion cells and in retinal interneurons as techniques improve for recording from primate retinas in vitro. Better studies of the role of second-site adaptation within the retina will also clarify the nature of the processes that control gain downstream from the photoreceptors. It seems that cone adaptation will have to be investigated again using extracellular and intracellular recording techniques in order to resolve the contradictions in the present data. This further research is needed because the perception of brightness and color depends upon the regulation of contrast sensitivity within the retina. It is surprising and humbling that such a basic issue remains unsettled. But it is also encouraging that there is important work yet to be done!

ACKNOWLEDGMENTS

Thanks to Christina Enroth-Cugell for starting us on this path. Special thanks to Dan Tranchina for his contributions to the research. R. M. S. thanks Jim Gordon and John Krauskopf for many helpful discussions. Our research and the preparation of this article have been supported by grants from the National Eye Institute (EY 1472, EY 4888, and EY 188) and the National Science Foundation (BNS 8708606) and by a MacArthur Fellowship.

REFERENCES

Blackwell, H. R. (1946) Contrast thresholds of the human eye. J. Opt. Soc. Am. 36: 624–643.

Cornsweet, T. (1970) Visual Perception. p. 273, also Chapter 2. Academic Press, New York.

Derrington, A. M. and Lennie, P. (1984) Spatial and temporal contrast sensitivities of neurones in the lateral geniculate nucleus of macaques. J. I Physiol . 357: 219–240.

De Valois, R. E., Webster, M. A., De Valois, K. K., and Lingelbach., B. (1986) Temporal properties of brightness and color induction. Vis. Res. 26: 887–898.

Enroth-Cugell, C. and Robson, J. G. (1966) The contrast sensitivity of retinal ganglion cells of the cat. J. Physiol. 187: 517–552.

Fuortes, M. G. F. and Hodgkin, A. L. (1964) Changes in time scale and sensitivity in the ommatidia of *Limulus*. J. Physiol. 156: 179–192.

Heinemann, E. G. (1955) Simultaneous brightness induction as a function of inducing- and test-field luminances. J. Exp. Psychol. 50: 89–96.

Heinemann, E. G. (1972) Simultaneous brightness induction. In: Handbook of Sensory Physiology (D. Jameson and L. M. Hurvich, eds) Vol . VII/4, pp. 146–169. Springer, Berlin.

Hicks, T. P., Lee, B. B., and Vidyasagar, T. R. (1983) The responses of cells in the macaque lateral geniculate nucleus to sinusoidal gratings. J. Physiol. 337: 183–200.

Kaplan, E. and Shapley, R. (1982) X and Y cells in the lateral geniculate nucleus of macaque monkeys. J. Physiol. 330: 125–143.

Kaplan, E. and Shapley, R. (1986) The primate retina contains two types of ganglion cells, with high and low contrast sensitivity. Proc. Nat. Acad. Sci. USA 83: 2755–2757.

Kelly, D. H. (1972) Adaptation effects on spatio-temporal sine-wave thresholds. Vis. Res. 12: 89–102.

Lamb, T. D. and Pugh, Jr., E. N. (1990) Physiology of transduction and adaptation in rod and cone photoreceptors. Semin. Neurosci 2, 3–13.

Land, E. H. and McCann, J. J. (1971) Lightness and retinex theory. J. Opt. Soc. Am. 6: 1–11.

Naka, K., Itoh, M., and Chappell, R. (1987) Dynamics of turtle cones. J. Gen. Physiol. 89: 321–337.

Purpura, K., Kaplan, E., and Shapley, R. M. (1988) Background light and the contrast gain of primate P and M retinal ganglion cells. Proc. Natl. Acad. Sci. USA 85: 4534–4537.

Purpura, K., Tranchina, D., Kaplan, E. and Shapley, R. M. (1990) Light adaptation in the primate retina: analysis of changes in gain and dynamics of monkey retinal ganglion cells. Vis Neurosci. 4: 75–93.

Reid, R. C. and Shapley, R. (1988) Brightness induction by local contrast and the spatial dependence of assimilation. Vis. Res. 28: 115–132.

Rodieck, R. W. (1988) The Primate Retina. Comp. Primate Biol. 4: 203–278.

Schnapf, J., Nunn, B., Meister, M. and Baylor, D. A. Visual transduction in cones of the moneky *Macaca fascicularis*. J. Physiol. 427: 681–713.

Shapley, R. (1986) The importance of contrast for the activity of single neurons, the VEP and perception. Vis. Res. 26: 45–61.

Shapley, R. (1991) "Neural mechanisms of contrast sensitivity." In Spatial Vision, ed. D. M. Regan, MacMillan, Vol. 10 of Vision and Visual Dysfunction series.

Shapley, R. and Enroth-Cugell, C. (1984) Visual adaptation and retinal gain controls. In Progress in Retinal Research Vol. 3, ed. N. Osborne and G. Chader, pp. 263–346, Pergamon, Oxford.

Shapley, R., Kaplan, E. and Soodak, R. (1981) Spatial summation and contrast sensitivity of X and Y cells in the lateral geniculate nucleus of the macaque. Nature 292: 543–545.

Shapley, R. and Perry, V. H. (1986) Cat and monkey retinal ganglion cells and their visual functional roles. Trends neurosci. 9: 229–235.

Shapley, R. and Victor, J. D. (1979) The contrast gain control of the cat retina. Vision Res. 19: 431–434.

Sneyd, J. and Tranchina, D. (1989) Phototransduction in cones: an inverse problem in enzyme kinetics. Bull. Math. Biol. 51: 749–784.

Stromeyer, C., Cole, G., and Kronauer, R. (1985) Second site adaptation in the red-green chromatic pathways. Vis. Res. 25: 219–237.

Tranchina, D., Gordon, J. and Shapley, R. (1984) Retinal light adaptation—evidence for a feedback mechanism. Nature 310: 314–316.

Tranchina, D. and Peskin, C. S. (1988) Light adaptation in the turtle retina: embedding a parametric family of linear models in a single nonlinear model. Vis. Neurosci. 1: 339–348.

Tranchina, D., Sneyd, J., and Cadenas, I. (1991) Light adaptation in turtle cones. Biophys. J. 60: 217–237.

Valeton, M. and Van Norren, D. (1983) Light adaptation of primate cones; ana anlysis based on extracellular data. Vis. Res. 23: 1539–1547.

Whittle, P. and Challands, P. D. C. (1969) The effect of background luminance on the brightness of flashes. Vis. Res. 9: 1095–1110.

Wyszecki, G. and Stiles, W. S. (1982) Color Science: Concepts and Methods, Quantitative Data and Formulas, 2nd Edition. Wiley, New York.

8 The Origin of Parallel Visual Pathways

R. W. Rodieck, R. K. Brening, and M. Watanabe

The retina sends a variety of different messages to the brain, each conveyed by a spatial array of ganglion cells of a given type. In mammals there appear to be between thirteen and twenty different ganglion cell types, and their messages are distributed among about twenty different zones on each side of the brain. Different types exhibit different functions, forms, spatial densities and distributions, retinal connections, and central projections. Many if not most of the messages conveyed by these types do not contribute directly to visual consciousness. Some are used to stabilize gaze toward a fixed target as the head moves, track a moving target, synchronize the circadian rhythm of the body to the diurnal rhythm of light and dark, control pupil size, etc.

The origin of these pathways depends upon one's frame of reference. This chapter assumes that the ganglion cells are the origin and summarizes what is known of this aspect of visual circuitry in cats and primates. In order to better appreciate and to place in context what is known in this restricted domain, it is useful to set the stage by briefly considering two other frames of reference: evolutionary origins and functional origins.

EVOLUTIONARY ORIGINS

The eye has figured in our quest for origins for some time. The theologian William Paley in his widely read book *Natural Theology* (1802) argued the case for the existence of God on instances of the manifestations of design found in nature. He used as his prime example the eye, which he described in detail, pointing out that its optical properties compared favorably with those of the best telescopes then produced. One could conceive how nature alone might produce a rock but, when it comes to a watch or an eye, one is forced to concede that some presence other than nature is required.

In *The Origin of Species* (1859) Charles Darwin dealt extensively with the eye in the section on Organs of Extreme Perfection and Complication in the chapter "Difficulties with the Theory." Although he did not refer to Paley directly, Darwin attempted to deal with Paley's argument point by point. Asa Gray, a botanist at Harvard and a frequent and supportive correspondent with Darwin, received an early copy of this book and wrote to Darwin that the weakest part dealt with the eye. Darwin replied, "About the weak points I agree. The eye to this day gives me a cold shudder, but when I think of the fine known gradations, my reason tells me I ought to conquer the cold shudder" (from F. Darwin 1896).

Darwin's concerns were almost wholly with the optical properties of the eye. At the time almost nothing was known of the retina. Cajal (1937), contemplating the retinas of vertebrates and the optic lobes of insects, finally sided with Paley. Thus the ignorance of retinal structure at the time of Darwin's book may have been a godsend; he could have come down with pneumonia.

About the only thing we know of the precursors of the vertebrate eye is that the ancestors of vertebrates, not surprisingly, had eyes. The unifying observation is that the protein portion of the visual pigment is homologous throughout the animal kingdom (Nathans 1987; Goldsmith 1990). Vertebrates first appeared about 530 million years ago, some 70 million years after the explosion of life forms that marks the start of the Cambrian period.

Among our most distant relatives with well-developed eyes is the ratfish (*Chimaera monstrosa*); the last common ancestor of humans and ratfish lived some 410 to 480 million years ago. Despite the fact that we have been separated from ratfish for some 80 to 90 percent of the age of vertebrates, our retinas are remarkably similar to those of the fish. Indeed, at the cellular level the dopaminergic amacrine cell of the ratfish is essentially identical in size, morphology, and level of stratification of its processes to our own dopaminergic amacrines (figure 8.1; compare with Nguyen-Legros et al. 1984). Thus some retinal cell types, including starburst amacrine cells (Brandon 1991),

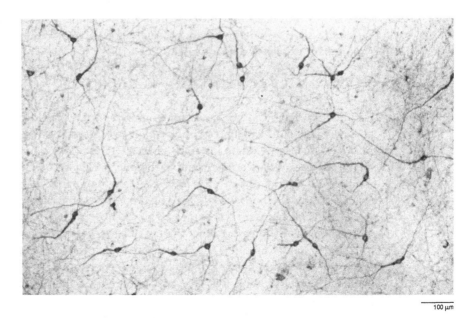

100 µm

Figure 8.1 Whole-mount of ratfish retina, reacted with an antibody to tyrosinehydroxylase conjugated to HRP. (From an unpublished collaborative work with K. Keyser and H. Karten)

date back to the earliest vertebrates, if not before. Furthermore, vertebrates possess similar targets for ganglion cell axons, including an accessory optic system, pretectum, optic tectum, and terminal fields in the dorsal and ventral thalamus (Ebbesson 1970, 1972).

The evolutionary pressures that shaped the visual system of a species must at some stage have included the introduction of new cell types. Most commonly, this involved the conversion of an old cell type whose function no longer enhanced survival (Darwin's "conversion of function in anatomical continuity"), although gene duplication may have played a role in increasing the total number of neural types. Other types, whose function either had been supplanted, or no longer enhanced survival, may have been discarded along certain evolutionary pathways. Furthermore, each type of retinal ganglion cell in each species has been shaped by the visual environment of that species and its interactions with that environment in terms of population size, retinal distribution, retinal connections, central projections, the functions of other types, and so on.

Evolutionary pressure, however, hinges only on the survival and reproduction of the organism. Thus the way in which evolution shapes the properties of a cell type is fundamentally different from the way in which it shapes a species (Rodieck and Brening 1983). Put simply, *cooperation* between cell types within an organism acts to enhance the successful *competition* of that organism with others in the struggle for survival; furthermore, the competition is not only for *efficiency* in the established niche, but for *exploration* to find a new niche or adapt to the consequences of a climatic change. Thus a random variation that results in a minor improvement in some cortical function can, from generation to generation, also modify one or more ganglion cell types to further improve this function, just as useful variations in a property of some ganglion cell type can act to modify central visual circuitry. In all of this, there is never the opportunity to redesign and rebuild the system from scratch (Partridge 1982), and the result seems closer to a breadboard circuit than a printed one; as Francois Jacob (1982) said, "This process resembles not engineering but tinkering, *bricolage* as we would say in French."

Thus, in comparing parallel visual pathways of cats and primates, consideration of evolutionary origins suggests a foundation of highly conserved features, some shared by all vertebrates, which has been tinkered with over the last 100 million years or so since primates and carnivores diverged.

FUNCTIONAL ORIGINS

Ganglion cell types sensitive to contrast typically pay little heed to the direction of movement of an object, and those sensitive to the direction of movement tend to ignore contrast and color. Perhaps because it is common to refer to a ganglion cell as *coding* one of these properties, there has been some interest in how synapses of various sorts might be arranged along the ganglion cell dendrites to somehow encode some property from the underlying matrix of more primitive and less specialized signals (e.g., Koch, Poggio, and Torre 1982). It is possible that mammalian ganglion cells operate in this way, but there appears to be no direct evidence for it. Considering the fact that their dendrites do not appear to be presynaptic to any other processes, such circuits would have to make do without presynaptic feedback mechanisms.

An alternative hypothesis is that ganglion cells do not in themselves code for anything in particular. Instead, they may do no more than sum the signals that characterize their observed response properties (e.g., they might sum directionally selective signals to the movement of a dark edge in some preferred direction with signals to the movement of a light edge in the same direction). To the degree that this is so, the dendritic morphology reflects little more than the spatial grain and extent of the sampling area in the regions of the inner plexiform layer in which the processes lie, process thickness being one of the parameters that determines the extent of electronic spread. Otherwise ganglion cell morphology may be of little functional significance.

There is a sufficient number of amacrine cell types to encode all the special features (e.g., directional selectivity and local edge detection) that cannot easily be accounted for by simple summation of bipolar signals (Kolb, Nelson, and Mariani 1981; Rodieck 1988; Dacey 1989, 1990; Mariani 1990). Thus as-yet-unknown amacrine cell types may prove to be the true functional origins of some parallel pathways. If the hypothesis is correct that midget ganglion cells contact midget bipolar cells, whereas parasol cells contact diffuse bipolars (figure 3 of Rodieck 1988; Boycott and Wässle 1991), then the origin of the midget and parasol pathways may best be viewed as the cone-bipolar synapse.

Thus, in comparing parallel visual pathways of cats and primates, a consideration of functional origins suggests that the morphologic features of ganglion cells per se need not reflect qualitative functional attributes, and thus provide no firm basis for trans-species comparisons. Nevertheless, as discussed below, the morphologies of certain ganglion cell types in the cat are remarkably similar to those in primates.

CENTRAL PROJECTIONS OF CAT GANGLION CELLS

Figure 8.2 is a semischematic diagram of the regions on the left side of the cat brain that receive a direct retinal input. There are about forty such zones in the brain, twenty on each side. As in other mammals, the lateral geniculate nucleus (LGN) is a nuclear complex that contains a number of distinct retinorecipient zones, as does the pretectum. As will be discussed, different zones receive from different ganglion cell types.

In all vertebrates, the ganglion cells that lie in the nasal retina project contralaterally. In nonmammalian vertebrates this is true for the ganglion cells in the temporal retina as well. In mammals, however, the central projection from the temporal retina is species-dependent. In the cat temporal retina, beta cells and almost all alpha cells project ipsilaterally. Collectively, they compose

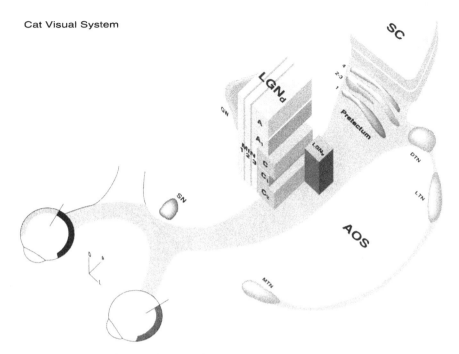

Figure 8.2 Semischematic diagram of the retinal recipient zones in the left half of the cat brain. The relative sizes of the zones are not to scale, and some have been moved slightly so that all the zones can be seen from this perspective. Abbreviations and principal sources are as follows: SN, suprachiasmatic nucleus (Berman 1968); LGN$_d$, dorsal lateral geniculate nucleus (Sanderson 1971; Guillery et al. 1980); MIN, medial interlaminar nucleus (Sanderson 1971); GW, geniculate wing (Guillery et al. 1980); LGN$_v$, ventral lateral geniculate nucleus; pretectum (Koontz, Rodieck, and Farmer 1985); SC, superior colliculus (Behan 1981);AOS, accessory optic system (DTN, dorsal terminal nucleus; LTN, lateral terminal nucleus; MTN, medial terminal nucleus) (Hayhow 1959; Berman 1968; Gregory and Giolli 1985).

about half the ganglion cells in the temporal retina. Of the remaining half, half of them also project ipsilaterally, and the remainder (i.e., a quarter of the total) project contralaterally.

It is possible to determine the morphology of the ganglion cell types that project to different regions of the brain by injecting a small amount of a fluorescent dye into one of the recipient zones of the brain. When the dye has been retrogradely transported to label the ganglion cells that project to that region, the animal is sacrificed and the retina is removed and placed in an in vitro chamber where the labeled cells may be intracellularly injected with a substance such as horseradish peroxidase (HRP), which is able to reveal the full morphology of the cell. By this means we have been able to elucidate the morphology of the ganglion cell types that project to a number of different regions in the brains of cats and monkeys. The following is a brief summary of our findings.

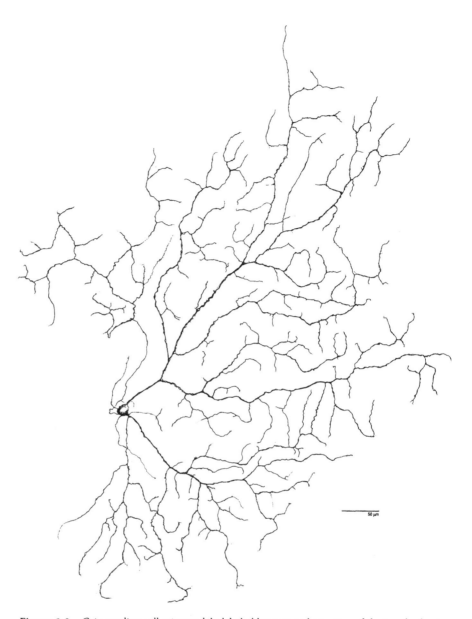

Figure 8.3 Cat ganglion cell retrogradely labeled by a central injection of dextranrhodamine to the contralateral medial terminal nucleus and then intracellularly injected with HRP in an in vitro preparation. Eccentricity 3.8 mm, temporal retina (Rodieck and Watanabe unpublished).

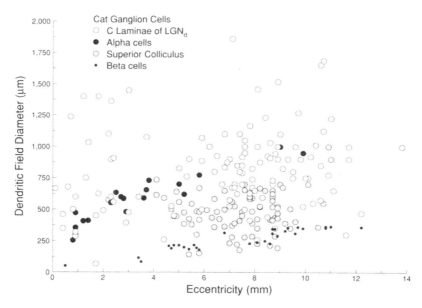

Figure 8.4 Dendritic field sizes of cat ganglion cells labeled by means of a central injection of a retrograde marker and injected with HRP in an in vitro preparation. The alpha and beta cells were labeled via injections to lamina C. (Data from Brening and Rodieck 1986 and Rodieck and Watanabe 1986)

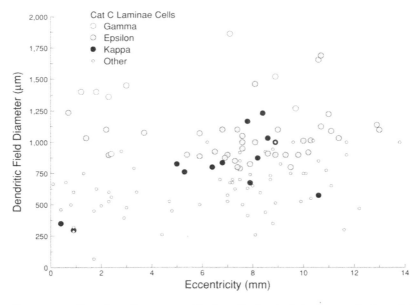

Figure 8.5 Data from figure 8.4, with the cells that had the largest dendritic fields distinguished by type.

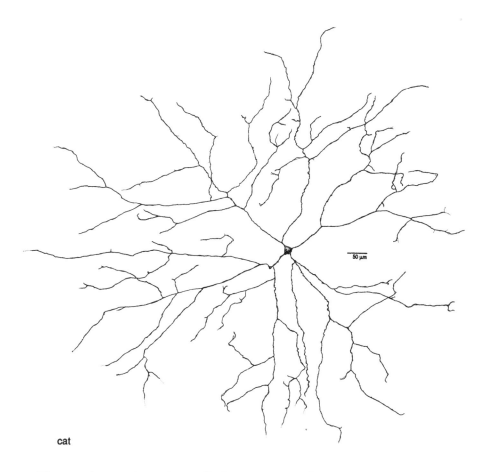

cat

The population of ganglion cells that projects to the accessory optic system (AOS) is unique in that every cell projects contralaterally. This is a special group of directionally selective cells whose signals are used to adjust the gain of the vestibulo-ocular reflex to stabilize the direction of gaze during head movements (Simpson 1984). Figure 8.3 is a drawing of a cat ganglion cell that projects to the medial terminal nucleus (MTN) of the AOS. These cells have the same morphology as those that project to the rabbit MTN (Buhl and Peichl 1986; Amthor, Takahashi, and Oyster 1989). As far as is known, they do not project to recipient zones outside the AOS.

The ganglion cell type or types that project to the suprachiasmatic nucleus (SN) are known only from central injections of HRP (Murakami, Miller, and Fuller 1989); the filling of the somata and primary dendrities was sufficient to demonstrate that the labeled cells were neither alpha nor beta cells, but it was insufficient to further characterize them morphologically. This projection is used to synchronize the circadian rhythm of the body to the diurnal rhythm of light and dark (Moore 1983). This is one of the few functions of the visual system that involves ambient light intensity per se (the only other that we are aware of is the steady component of pupil size).

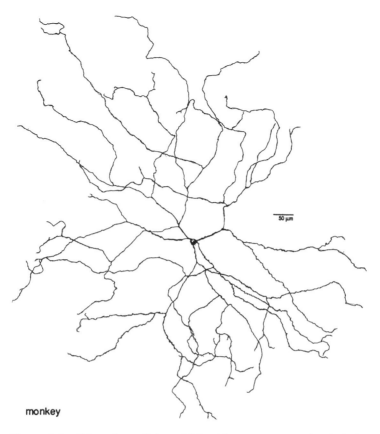

monkey

Figure 8.6 Cat epsilon cell (eccentricity 10 mm, upper nasal retina), from Rodieck and Watanabe (1986), and macaque epsilon-like cell (eccentricity 13 mm, lower nasal retina), from Rodieck and Watanabe (1988). Cat epsilon cells project to the C laminae of the LGNd and to the geniculate wing. The central destination of macaque epsilon-like cells is unknown.

The A laminae of the cat LGNd appear to receive only from alpha and beta cells (Kelly and Gilbert 1975; Illing and Wässle 1981). Figure 8.18A is a scatter plot that shows the dendritic field size of these cell types plotted against retinal eccentricity. Alpha cells also project to the superior colliculus (SC), and some project to the medial interlaminar nucleus (MIN) of the LGNd, the upper portion of lamina C of the LGNd, and the pretectum (reviewed by Rodieck 1979). The primary projection of beta cells is to the A laminae, but a few also project to the MIN, the upper portion of lamina C, the pretectum, and the superior colliculus (Rodieck 1979; Koontz, Rodieck, and Farmer 1985; Wässle and Illing 1980).

Figure 8.4 is a scatter diagram that plots dendritic field size against retinal eccentricity for ganglion cells that project to either the C laminae of the LGNd or to the superior colliculus. A few of the labeled alpha and beta cells that projected to the C laminae were also injected and are shown for reference. It is apparent from the dendritic field sizes alone that the two regions receive from different populations of ganglion cells. In double-label experiments, we

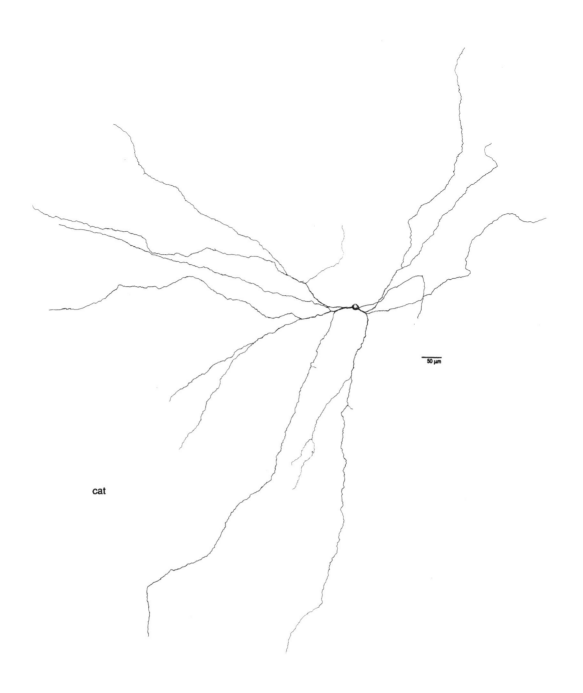

cat

50 μm

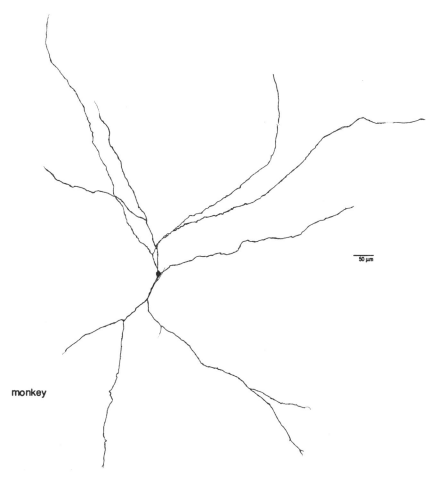

monkey

Figure 8.7 Cat gamma cell (eccentricity 9 mm), from Rodieck and Watanabe (1986), and macaque gamma-like cell, from Rodieck and Watanabe (1988). Cat gamma cells project to the C laminae of the LGNd and to the medial interlaminar nucleus. The central destination of macaque gamma-like cells is unknown.

have thus far failed to observe cells other than alpha and beta cells that project to both the LGNd and the SC.

Each population in figure 8.4 consists of a number of different ganglion cell types; however, their detailed description lies beyond the scope of this review. We will briefly describe the ganglion cells with the largest dendritic fields that project to the C laminae. Figure 8.5 shows the dendritic field sizes of these cells, partially distinguished by type. A characteristic feature of these cells is that, unlike others, they show little variation in dendritic field size with retinal eccentricity. A drawing of an epsilon cell is shown in figure 8.6. The dendrites of these cells lie in the innermost portion of the inner plexiform layer, and the horizontal orientation of their primary dendrites gives the soma a somewhat scalloped form. These cells also project to the geniculate wing (GW) of the LGNd, where they were first described (Leventhal, Keens, and

Törk 1980). Another group is the cat gamma cells, an example of which is shown in figure 8.7; these cells also project to the complex of the medial interlaminar nucleus.

Are the C Laminae Specialized for Nocturnal Vision?

The large dendritic fields of many of the ganglion cells that project to the C laminae are puzzling. Whatever the job they do, could not the far more abundant alpha and beta cells do it better? In this spirit, one possibility is that they are merely the residua of earlier pathways, serving no particular purpose in their modern forms, but not yet fully dispensed with. However, if one considers the ability of the visual system to operate at very low light levels, then another possibility arises.

We can see at retinal illuminances as low as about 10^{-4} trolands. Assuming a photon catch rate of 3 photons per rod per second for each troland (Westheimer 1966), each rod captures a photon only about once every hour. Over at least the first log unit or so above absolute threshold, visual acuity throughout the retina is set by the sparseness of photons rather than ganglion cell density. An area centralis or visual streak is of no particular use under these conditions. Those ganglion cells that operate effectively at these low light levels must sum over a sufficiently large pool of rods in order to obtain a reliable signal. The ganglion cells that project to the C laminae have the largest dendritic fields found in the cat retina. Their dendritic fields are sparse, but they may well collect from cells or paths with a finer spatial grain. Their invariance in dendritic field size with eccentricity is consistent with a system operating in a sparse photon environment.

In contrast to the cells in the A laminae of the LGNd, those in the C laminae are insensitive to monocular deprivation (Spear, McCall, and Tumosa 1989). This observation is consistent with cells of the C laminae subserving a role in very dim conditions since, under these conditions, detection is more important than acuity, and competition between the signals from the two eyes would not improve matters. In primates, which have similar ganglion cells (see figures 8.6 and 8.7), severe monocular deprivation causes to the deprived eye to show the rod action spectrum at all light levels (Harwerth et al. 1981). This surprising observation could be simply interpreted in terms of this hypothesis by proposing that the monocular deprivation successfully blocked the major pathways from the parasol and midget cells for the deprived eye, leaving only the signals from the ganglion cells that are specialized for dim nocturnal vision.

CENTRAL PROJECTIONS OF PRIMATE GANGLION CELLS

Figure 8.8 is a semischematic diagram of the regions of the primate brain to which the retinal ganglion cells project. The retinorecipient zones are basically the same as those in the cat, although the patterns of lamination in the LGN differ.

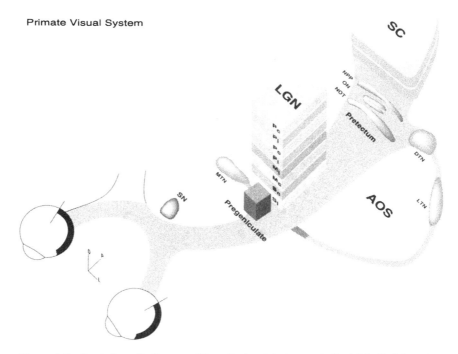

Figure 8.8 Semischematic diagram of the retinal recipient zones in the left half of the primate brain. The relative sizes of the zones are not to scale, and some have been moved slightly so that all the zones can be seen from this perspective. Abbreviations and principal sources are as follows: SN, suprachiasmatic nucleus (Winters, Kado, and Adey 1969); LGN, lateral geniculate nucleus (M, magnocellular laminae; P, parvicellular laminae; S, S laminae; i, ipsilateral projection; c, contralateral projection) (Kaas et al. 1978); pretectum (NOT, nucleus of the optic tract; ON, olivary nucleus; NPP, posterior pretectal nucleus) (Benevento and Standage 1983; Hutchins and Weber 1985); SC, superior colliculus (Szabo and Cowan 1984; Winters, Kado, and Adey 1969); AOS, accessory optic system; DTN, dorsal terminal nucleus; LTN, lateral terminal nucleus; MTN, medial terminal nucleus, (Weber and Giolli 1986; Cooper and Magnin 1987; Fredericks et al. 1988).

Figure 8.9 shows the dendritic field diameters of macaque ganglion cells that project to the pretectum and the superior colliculus (SC) compared with those of midget ganglion cells (which project to the parvicellular laminae of the macaque LGN) and those of parasol ganglion cells (which project to the magnocellular laminae of the macaque LGN). The four clusters are by and large separate; in fact, the few cells labeled by the pretectal injection that overlap the SC cluster show the morphology of cells that project to the SC, and they may have been labeled because their axons passed through the injection site on their way to the SC. In any case, this diagram shows that there is a strong central segregation of ganglion cell types. Thus far, with one minor exception, we have not observed any primate ganglion cell type that projects to more than one of the six major recipient zones of the brain. The

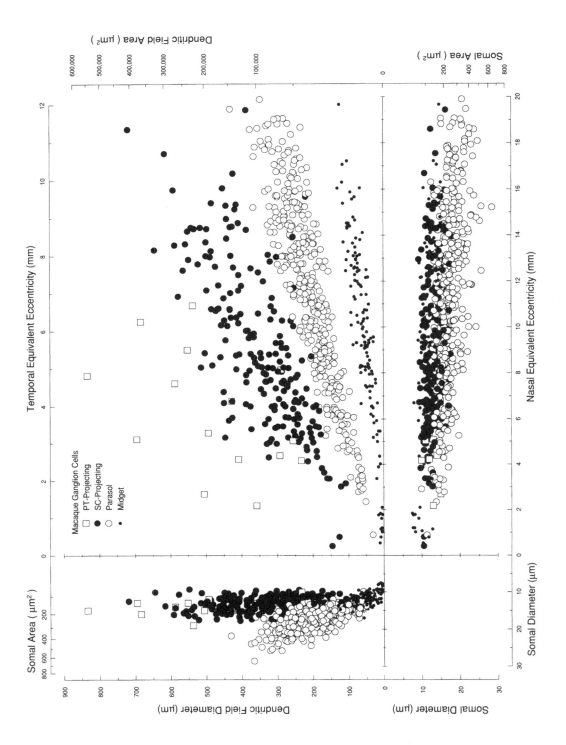

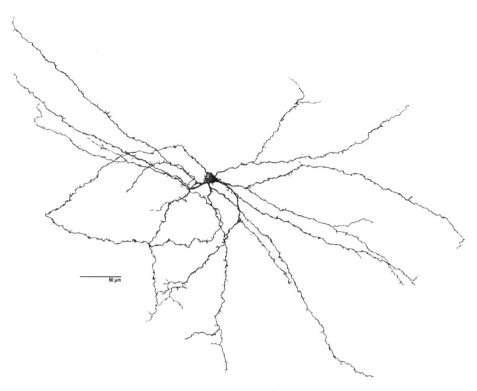

Figure 8.10 Macaque ganglion cell labeled using an injection of a retrograde marker to the pretectal complex and injected in vitro with HRP. Eccentricity 4 mm, lower nasal retina. (From Rodieck and Watanabe 1988)

exception has to do with a very sparse projection of parasol cells to the SC, which we estimate is not more than one in a thousand SC-projecting ganglion cells and interpret as developmental error.

Figure 8.10 is a drawing of a cell that projects to the pretectum. All the pretectal-projecting cells shown in figure 8.9 were labeled from a single injection and, except for the few found in the SC cluster, all had a morphology similar to that shown in figure 8.10. The primate pretectum, however, contains a number of different recipient zones (figure 8.8), so the pretectum may well receive from other ganglion cell types. Perry and Cowey (1984) injected

Figure 8.9 Dendritic field and somal sizes of retinal ganglion cells, plotted as a function of equivalent eccentricity. The data for parasol cells (364) and midget ganglion cells (147) are taken from Watanabe and Rodieck (1989) and are included here in order to provide comparisons with the properties of injected cells labeled following injections to the superior colliculus and the pretectal complex. Three scatter diagrams are shown. The one at the upper right shows dendritic field size plotted against equivalent eccentricity. The diagram at the lower right plots somal size (increasing in the downward direction) as a function of equivalent eccentricity, whereas the diagram at the upper left plots somal size against dendritic field size. Every plotted cell (747) appears in all three plots. The three two-dimensional scatter plots may be viewed as different shadow casts of a single three-dimensional scatter plot, and they are thus similar to a draftsman's orthogonal rendering of a three-dimensional object (Rodieck and Watanabe 1988).

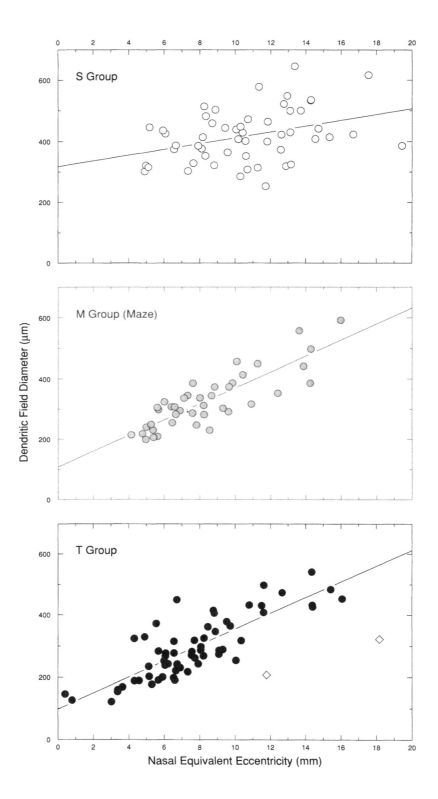

HRP into the primate pretectum, and the labeled cells they observed differed sufficiently from those we observed (e.g., many had their somata displaced to the inner plexiform layer) to support the notion that the pretectal zones collectively receive from more than one ganglion cell type.

The macaque superior colliculus appears to receive from at least twelve ganglion cell types. The distinctions between these cell types represent a complex issue that is outside the scope of this review. Briefly, it is convenient to divide these cells into three groups, termed S, M, and T. Figure 8.11 replots the data for SC projecting ganglion cells shown in Figure 8.9, with these groups distinguished. The S group consists of cells with sparse dendritic fields, and the sizes of the dendritic fields of the population show only a small change with eccentricity (it is possible that some of the cell types subsumed within this group show no change at all). The M group consists of a single type, which we term *maze* cells; these cells have strongly monostratified dendritic fields and a morphology suggestive of a maze (figure 8.12). The T group contains a number of types that are partially or fully bistratified, one of which is shown in figure 8.13.

Midget ganglion cells project to the parvicellular laminae and parasol cells to the magnocellular laminae of the primate LGN, as summarized in figure 8.14. The parvicellular laminae of the primate LGN receive from at least two additional cell groups (figure 8.15). In addition to midget ganglion cells, which are monostratified and form the major projection, there are bistratified ganglion cells with dendritic fields about the same size, or slightly larger than those of parasol cells, which we have termed *PB* (*parvicellular bistratified*) cells (figure 8.16). The PB group may signal color (Rodieck 1991). In addition, the parvicellular region receives from ganglion cells with very large and monostratified dendritic fields, which we have termed *PG* (*parvicellular giant*) cells (figure 8.17).

In primate retinas in which the ganglion cells were not labeled, we have injected all of the primate cell types that we have observed by injecting ganglion cells labeled via central injections. In addition we have observed ganglion cell types that have not yet been observed from central injections. In particular, there are ganglion cells that strongly resemble in morphology and size both cat epsilon cells, as shown in figure 8.6, and cat gamma cells, as shown in figure 8.7.

Figure 8.11 Scatter diagrams of the ganglion cell parameters of the different cell groups that project to the macaque superior colliculus. The slopes of the regression lines for all three groups (the T group does not include diamond symbols, as discussed below) are positive at a high level of significance ($p < 0.01$). However, the slopes for the T group (25.7 μm/mm) and the M group (26.2 μm/mm) were considerably larger than for the S group (9.4 μm/mm). The two diamond symbols in the lowest diagram represent the only parasol cells labeled following the injection of a retrograde tracer to the superior colliculus in a search for such cells (Rodieck and Watanabe 1988).

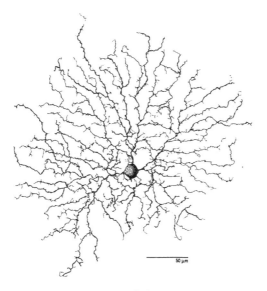

Figure 8.12 Monostratified macaque ganglion cell, termed a *maze* cell, labeled following the injection of a retrograde tracer to the superior colliculus and injected in vitro with HRP. Eccentricity 3.7 mm, lower temporal retina (Rodieck and Watanabe 1988).

A COMPARISON OF GANGLION CELL POPULATIONS IN THE CAT AND MONKEY

The cat retina contains about 150,000 to 200,000 ganglion cells (Hughes and Wässle 1976; Illing and Wässle 1981; Chalupa, Williams, and Henderson 1984; Williams et al. 1986), of which about 45 percent are beta cells and 5 percent alpha cells. The remaining 50 percent (ca 90,000 cells) comprise a number of additional types (Rodieck 1973; Hughes and Wässle 1976). These additional types show as great a variation in their dendritic morphology and size (Brening and Rodieck 1986) as do the macaque cells described and illustrated in this paper. They have sometimes been collectively referred to as "gamma" cells when speaking of their morphology (as distinct from the usage that refers to a specific cell type) or as "W" cells when speaking of their function (Rodieck 1973). However, these terms appear to be little more than mental constructs without empirical support (Farmer and Rodieck 1980; Rodieck and Brening 1983), and their usage has been discouraged (Rodieck 1979).

The macaque retina contains about 1.5 to 1.8 million ganglion cells (Potts et al. 1972). Perry, Oehler, and Cowey (1984) estimate that 10 percent are parasol cells, 10 percent (ca 165,000 cells) project to the SC and comprise a number of types not including midget and parasol cells, and the remaining 80 percent are midget ganglion cells.

Note that the number of ganglion cells reported as "additional types" is roughly comparable in cats and monkeys. Furthermore, the "epsilon" and

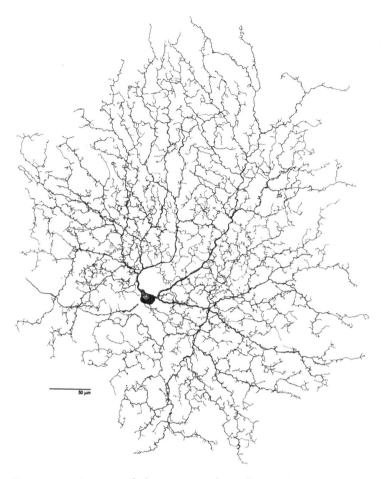

Figure 8.13 Monostratified macaque ganglion cell, termed a *thorn* cell (one of the cell types that compose the T group), labeled following the injection of a retrograde tracer to the superior colliculus and injected in vitro with HRP. Eccentricity 7.1 mm, upper nasal retina (Rodieck and Watanabe 1988).

"gamma" types of cells in both cats and primates are not only strikingly similar in morphology, but they also have dendritic fields of about the same sizes. There are also strong similarities between the morphology and sizes of ganglion cells in the cat that project to the SC (Brening and Rodieck 1986) and those in the primate, which are described here. Put another way, thus far we have been unable to find any notable differences between the "additional types" of cells in cats and primates.

Parts A and B of figure 8.18 show the logarithm of dendritic field diameter plotted against eccentricity for cat alpha and beta cells (from Boycott and Wässle 1973) and macaque parasol and midget ganglion cells (from Watanabe and Rodieck 1989). The clusters of cat alpha and beta cells are similar in form, but they are separated vertically by a factor of about 3 in the periphery. The

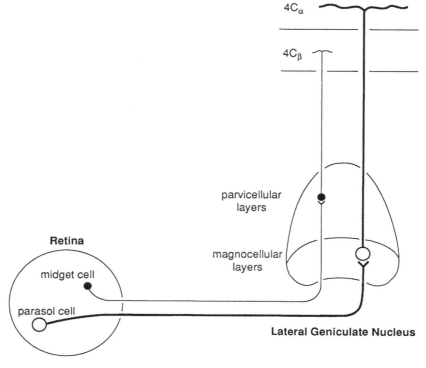

Striate Cortex

$4C_\alpha$

$4C_\beta$

parvicellular
layers

magnocellular
layers

Retina

midget cell

parasol cell

Lateral Geniculate Nucleus

Figure 8.14 Schematic diagram of the pathways of parasol and midget ganglion cells from the retina to the striate cortex (Rodieck et al. 1985).

clusters of macaque parasol and midget cells are likewise similar in form, and also separated by a factor of about 3 in the periphery.

To a first approximation, the macaque cell clusters appear similar to those of the cat, but shifted downward. An attempt to bring the monkey pair into alignment with the cat pair by means of a vertical shift (i.e., scaling of dendritic field diameter) is shown in part C of the figure. The vertical shift between species for best fit at large eccentricities is a scaling factor of 3.0 (the fact that this value also happens to be the vertical scaling factor for the two clusters within each species is presumably fortuitous).

Although the alignment is satisfactory for large eccentricities, it clearly fails near the central area. However, this first approximation suggests that an additional horizontal shift to the right could bring the cell clusters of the cat into alignment with those of the macaque. The result is shown in part D. The horizontal shift for best fit is 2.5 mm, and this yields a good alignment at all but the smallest eccentricities (where the cat clusters lie within the shifted macaque clusters but appear to increase more steeply with eccentricity). Put another way, as a rule of thumb, given a cat alpha cell of a given dendritic field diameter and eccentricity, a parasol cell at a temporal eccentricity 2.5 mm

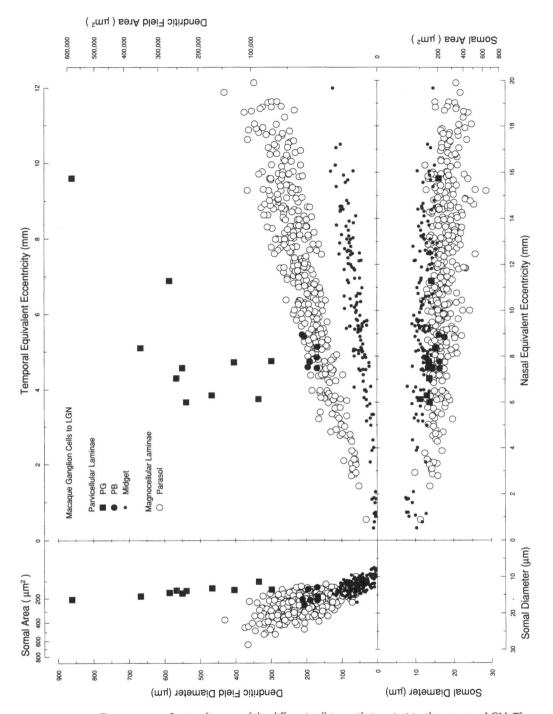

Figure 8.15 Scatter diagram of the different cell types that project to the macaque LGN. The midget and parasol cells are the same as those shown in figure 8.9. The PG and PB cells were labeled and injected in the nasal portion of the contralateral retina following a single injection to the parvicellular laminae of *M. fascicularis* (Rodieck and Watanabe 1988).

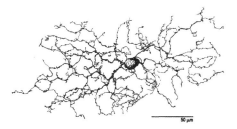

Figure 8.16 Macaque PB (parvicellular bistratified) cell in the nasal retina, labeled following an injection to the parvicellular laminae of the contralateral LGN and injected in vitro with HRP. Eccentricity 7.2 mm, upper nasal retina (Rodieck and Watanabe 1988).

greater will have a dendritic field diameter approximately one-third that of the alpha cell. The same rule converts the parameters for cat beta cells to the parameters for macaque midget ganglion cells.

Rodieck, Binmoeller, and Dineen (1985) and Rodieck (1988) have argued that, at the level of cell type, midget ganglion cells are homologous with cat beta cells, and likewise for parasol and alpha cells. Because of certain similar functional properties, Shapley et al. (1981) and Kaplan and Shapley (1982) have argued that cat beta cells are homologous with primate parasol cells and that, between cats and primates, midget ganglion cells are unique to primates and alpha cells are unique to cats. This issue, however, need not be resolved in order to make the following point. If the overlap factor (the product of dendritic field area and spatial density) for each type is to be roughly the same for all cell types, then the spatial density of each type should vary inversely as the square of the dendritic field diameter. For example, the ratio of the number of beta cells to alpha cells in the cat is about 9, and the square of the ratio of their diameters is also about 9, as for the midget and parasol cells of primates. But since the primate pair have diameters smaller than the cat pair by a factor of about 3, there would have to be about 9 times more of them in order to preserve the overlap factor.

Based upon the values cited above, the current best estimate of the total number of alpha and beta cells in the cat retina is about 90,000. As discussed above, in order to bring the cat cell clusters into alignment with those of macaques they must be shifted 2.5 mm to the right. In other words, the macaque cells with eccentricities less than 2.5 mm should not be included when comparing cat and monkey cells. Based upon measurements and calculations made from figure 2C in Wässle et al. (1990), the number of ganglion cells in this region is about 600,000. Thus the remaining retina contains about 1,000,000 ganglion cells, of which about 90 percent or 900,000 are estimated by Perry Oehler and Cowey (1984) to be midget and parasol cells. Thus, using these estimates, there are about 10 times more cells in the midget + parasol group as in the beta + alpha group, which can be compared to a predicted value of 9 if the same overlap factor is assumed.

Interestingly, Perry, Oehler, and Cowey's (1984) estimate for the fraction of midget ganglion cells neglects the PB cells which, based upon dendritic

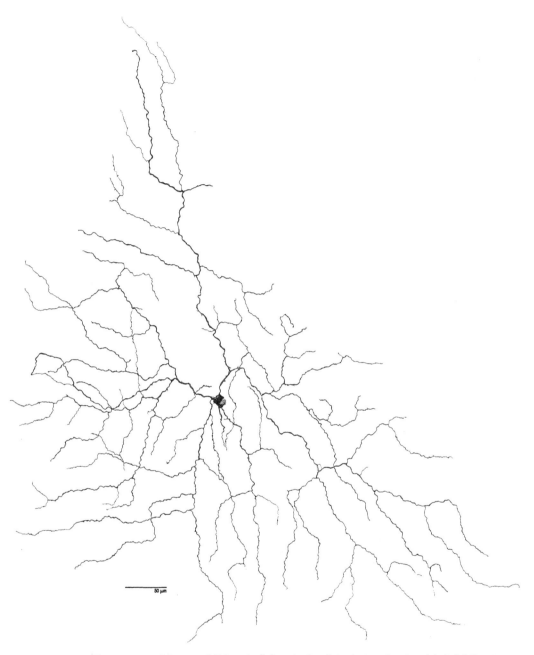

Figure 8.17 Macaque PG (parvicellular giant) cell in the nasal retina, labeled following an injection to the parvicellular laminae of the contralateral LGN and injected in vitro with HRP. Eccentricity 10.8 mm, lower nasal retina (Rodieck and Watanabe 1988).

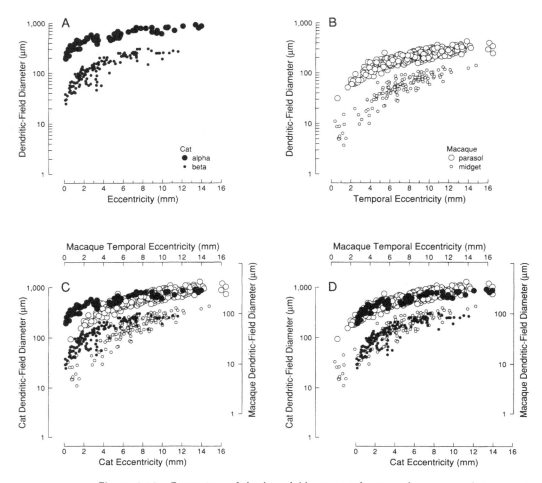

Figure 8.18 Comparison of dendritic field size as a function of eccentricity between cat alpha and beta cells (A) and macaque parasol and midget ganglion cells (B). The cat data are taken from figure 7 of Boycott and Wässle (1974), and the macaque data from figure 9 of Watanabe and Rodieck (1989). (C) Cat and macaque data superimposed, with the macaque data shifted vertically upward by a factor of 3 with respect to the cat data. (D) Similar to (C) but shows the cat data shifted to the right by 2.5 mm with respect to the macaque data. This combination of horizontal and vertical offsets brings the data clusters from the two species into alignment.

field size, coverage factor, and other issues discussed by Rodieck (1991), may have a spatial density near that of parasol cells. Their inclusion would reduce the number outside the central region by about 80,000 or so, yielding a value even closer to the predicted one of 9. It is also worth noting that color-coding cells in the cat retina have dendritic field sizes similar to those of alpha cells (see the legend of table 1 in Rodieck 1979 for references), just as PB cells have dendritic field sizes similar to those of parasol cells (figure 8.15). If cat color-coding cells have about the same overlap factor and thus density as alpha cells, then the ratio of color acuity to achromatic acuity in the cat (subserved by color and X [beta] cells) could be similar to the same ratio in the macaque (subserved by PB and tonic [midget] cells).

The range of the various estimates used is larger than the difference between predicted and observed values, so the closeness of these measures is somewhat fortuitous. Furthermore, we have implicitly assumed that the coverage factor of midget ganglion cells is based upon their coding of achromatic stimuli, and thus that they are composed of essentially only two types (ON- and OFF-center cells), just as for cat beta cells. This is a hypothesis one of us supports (Rodieck 1991), but one that has not yet become widely accepted.

To summarize this section on trans-species comparisons, the difference between the ganglion cell populations in cats and macaques appears as a first approximation to be quantitative rather than qualitative, with the major difference being the dendritic sizes and consequent spatial densities of the midget/parasol pair of ganglion cells in primates compared to the beta/alpha pair in cats.

ACKNOWLEDGMENTS

Supported in part by NIH grants EY02923, EY06098, and EY01730; the E. K. Bishop Foundation; the Chatlos Foundation; Research to Prevent Blindness, Inc.; and by NIH grant RR00166 to the Regional Primate Research Center at the University of Washington. We would like to thank William Calvin, Dennis Dacey, Harvey Karten, and Barry Lia for their comments on a draft of this paper, as well as Toni Haun for her numerous contributions to this study.

REFERENCES

Amthor FR, Takahashi ES, Oyster CW (1989) Morphologies of rabbit retinal ganglion cells with complex receptive fields. J Comp Neurol 280:97–121.

Behan M (1981) Identification and distribution of retinocollicular terminals in the cat. An electron microscopic autoradiographic analysis. J Comp Neurol 199:1–16.

Benevento LA, Standage GR (1983) The organization of projections of the retinorecipient and nonretinorecipient nuclei of the pretectal complex and layers of the superior colliculus to the lateral pulvinar and medial pulvinar in the macaque monkey. J Comp Neurol. 217:307–336.

Berman AL (1968) The Brain Stem of the Cat. Madison: The University of Wisconsin Press.

Boycott BB, Wässle H (1974) The morphological types of ganglion cells of the domestic cat's retina. J Physiol (Lond) 240:397–419.

Boycott, B.B., and H. Wässle (1991) Morphological classification of bipolar cells of the primate retina. Eur. J. Neurosci. 3:1069–1088.

Brandon, C (1991) Cholinergic amacrine neurons of the dogfish retina. Visual Neuroscience 6:553–562.

Brening RK, Rodieck RW (1986) Morphology of the cat ganglion cells that project to the superior colliculus. Invest Ophthalmol Vis Sci Suppl 27:223.

Buhl EH, Peichl L (1986) Morphology of rabbit retinal ganglion cells projecting to the medial terminal nucleus of the accessory optic system. J Comp Neurol 253:163–174.

Cajal, SR (1937) Recollections of My Life (translation by E. Horne Craigie). Philadelphia: The American Philosophical Society.

Chalupa LM, Williams RW, Henderson Z (1984) Binocular interaction in the fetal cat regulates the size of the ganglion cell population. Neuroscience 12:1139–1146.

Cooper HM, Magnin M (1987) Accessory optic system of an anthropoid primate, the gibbon (*Hylobates concolor*): Evidence of a direct retinal input to the medial terminal nucleus. J Comp Neurol 259:467–482.

Dacey DM (1989) Axon-bearing amacrine cells of the macaque monkey retina. J Comp Neurol 284:275–293.

Dacey DM (1990) The dopaminergic amacrine cell. J Comp Neurol 301:461–489.

Darwin C (1859) The Origin of Species. London: John Murray.

Darwin F (1896) The Life and Letters of Charles Darwin, Including an Autobiographical Chapter. New York: Appleton.

Ebbesson SOE (1970) On the organization of central visual pathways in vertebrates. Brain Behav Evol 3:178–194.

Ebbesson SOE (1972) A proposal for a common nomenclature for some optic nuclei in vertebrates and the evidence for a common origin of two such cell groups. Brain Behav Evol 6:75–91.

Farmer SG, Rodieck RW (1982) Ganglion cells of the cat accessory optic system: Morphology and retinal topography. J Comp Neurol 205:190–198.

Fredericks CA, Giolli RA, Blanks RHI, Sadun AA (1988) The human accessory optic system. Brain Res 454:116–122.

Goldsmith TH (1990) Optimization, constraint, and history in the evolution of eyes. Q Rev Biol 65:281–322.

Gregory KM, Giolli RA (1985) The dendritic architecture of the medial terminal nucleus of the accessory optic system in the rat, rabbit, and cat. Exp Brain Res 60:501–508.

Guillery RW, Geisert EE Jr, Polley EH, Mason CA (1980) An analysis of the retinal afferents to the cat's medial interlaminar nucleus and to its rostral thalamic extension, the "geniculate wing." J Comp Neurol 194:117–142.

Harwerth RS, Crawford MLJ, Smith EL III, Boltz RL (1981) Behavioral studies of stimulus deprivation amblyopia in monkeys. Vision Res 21:779–789.

Hayhow WR (1959) An experimental study of the accessory optic system in the cat. J Comp Neurol 113:218–313.

Hughes A, Wässle H (1976) The cat optic nerve: Fibre total count and diameter spectrum. J Comp Neurol 169:171–184.

Hutchins B, Weber JT (1985) The pretectal complex of the monkey: A reinvestigation of the morphology and retinal terminations. J Comp Neurol 232:425–442.

Illing R-B, Wässle H (1981) The retinal projection to the thalamus in the cat: A quantitative investigation and a comparison with the retinotectal pathway. J Comp Neurol 202:265–285.

Jacob F (1982) The Possible and the Actual. New York: Pantheon.

Kaas JH, Huerta MF, Weber JT, Harting JK (1978) Patterns of retinal terminations and laminar organization of the lateral geniculate nucleus of primates. J Comp Neurol 182:517–554.

Kaplan E, Shapley RM (1982) X and Y cells in the lateral geniculate nucleus of macaque monkeys. J Physiol (Lond) 330:125–143.

Kelly JP, Gilbert CD (1975) The projections of different morphological types of ganglion cells in the cat retina. J Comp Neurol 163:65−80.

Koch C, Poggio T, Torre V (1982) Retinal ganglion cells: a functional interpretation of dendritic morphology. Phil Trans Royal Soc B (Lond) 298:227−264.

Kolb H, Nelson R, Mariani A (1981) Amacrine cells, bipolar cells and ganglion cells of the cat retina: A Golgi study. Vision Res 21:1081−1114.

Koontz MA, Rodieck RW, Farmer SG (1985) The retinal projection to the cat pretectum. J Comp Neurol 236:42−59.

Leventhal AG, Keens J, Törk I (1980) The afferent ganglion cells and cortical projections of the retinal recipient zone (RRZ) of the cat's "pulvinar complex." J Comp Neurol 194:535−554.

Mariani AP (1990) Amacrine cells of the rhesus monkey retina. J Comp Neurol 301:382−400.

Moore RY (1983) Organization and function of a CNS circadian oscillator: The suprachiasmatic nucleus. Fed Proc 42:2783−2789.

Murakami DM, Miller JD, Fuller CA (1989) The retinohypothalamic tract in the cat: retinal ganglion cell morphology and pattern of projection. Brain Res 482:283−296.

Nathans J (1987) Molecular biology of visual pigments. Ann Rev Neurosci 10:163−194.

Nguyen-Legros J, Botteri C, Phuc LH, Vigny A, Gay M (1984) Morphology of primate's dopaminergic amacrine cells as revealed by TH-like immunoreactivity on retinal flat-mounts. Brain Res 295:145−153.

Paley W (1802) Natural Theology. Oxford: Vincent.

Partridge LD (1982) The good enough calculi of evolving control systems: Evolution is not engineering. Am J Physiol 242:R173−R177.

Perry VH, Cowey A (1984) Retinal ganglion cells that project to the superior colliculus and pretectum in the macaque monkey. Neuroscience 12:1125−1137.

Perry VH, Oehler R, Cowey A (1984) Retinal ganglion cells that project to the dorsal lateral geniculate nucleus in the macaque monkey. Neuroscience 12:1101−1123.

Potts AM, Hodges D, Shelman CB, Fritz KJ, Levy NS, Mangnall Y (1972a) Morphology of the primate optic nerve. I. Method and total fiber count. Invest Ophthalmol 11:980−988.

Rodieck RW (1973) The Vertebrate Retina: Principles of Structure and Function. San Francisco: W.H. Freeman and Company.

Rodieck RW (1979) Visual Pathways. Ann Rev Neurosci 2:193−225.

Rodieck RW (1988) The Primate Retina. In: Comparative Primate Biology: Volume IV, Neurosciences (Steklis HD, ed), pp 203−278. New York: Alan R. Liss.

Rodieck, RW (1991) Which cells code for color? In: From Pigments to Perception: Advances in understanding visual processes (Valberg A, Lee BB, eds), pp 83−93. New York: Plenum Press.

Rodieck RW, Binmoeller KF, Dineen JT (1985) Parasol and midget ganglion cells of the human retina. J Comp Neurol 233:115−132.

Rodieck RW, Brening RK (1983) Retinal ganglion cells: Properties, types, genera, pathways and trans-species comparisons. Brain Behav Evol 23:121− 164.

Rodieck RW, Watanabe M (1986) Morphologic diversity in the ganglion cell projection to different zones within the cat lateral geniculate nucleus. Neurosci Abst 12:1038.

Rodieck RW, Watanabe M (1988) Morphology of ganglion cells that project to the parvocellular laminae of the lateral geniculate nucleus, pretectum, and superior colliculus of primates. Neurosci Abst 14:1120.

Sanderson KJ (1971) The projection of the visual field to the lateral geniculate and medial interlaminar nuclei in the cat. J Comp Neurol 143:101–118.

Shapley RM, Kaplan E, Soodak R (1981) Spatial summation and contrast sensitivity of X and Y cells in the lateral geniculate nucleus of the macaque. Nature 292:543–545.

Simpson JI (1984) The accessory optic system. Ann Rev Neurosci 7:13–41.

Spear PD, McCall MA, Tumosa N (1989) W- and Y-cells in the C layers of the cat's lateral geniculate nucleus: Normal properties and effects of monocular deprivation. J. Neurophysiol. 61:58–73.

Szabo J, Cowan WM (1984) A stereotaxic atlas of the brain of the Cynomologus monkey (*Macaca fascicularis*). J Comp Neurol 222:265–300.

Wässle H, Illing R-B (1980) The retinal projection to the superior colliculus in the cat: A quantitative study with HRP. J Comp Neurol 190:333–356.

Wässle H, Grünert U, Röhrenbeck J, Boycott BB (1990) Retinal ganglion cell density and cortical magnification factor in the primate. Vision Res 30:1897–1990.

Watanabe M, Rodieck RW (1989) Parasol and midget ganglion cells of the primate retina. J Comp Neurol 289:434–454.

Weber JT, Giolli RA (1986) The medial terminal nucleus of the monkey: evidence for a 'complete' accessory optic system. Brain Res 365:164–168.

Westheimer, GW (1966) The Maxwellian view. Vision Res 6:669–682.

Williams RW, Bastiani MJ, Lia B, Chalupa LM (1986) Growth cones, dying axons, and developmental fluctuations in the fiber population of the cat's optic nerve. J Comp Neurol 246:32–69.

Winters WD, Kado RT, Adey WR (1969) A stereotaxic brain atlas for *Macaca nemestrina*. Berkeley: University of California Press.

The 1992 Helmerich Lecture: Introduction

Robert Shapley

One major function of the brain (besides estimating contrast!) is estimating the size of thing or of the distance of one thing from another. The dimensions of mental size or distance are not like size or distance in the three spatial dimensions of the "real" world, though these may enter into the mental calculation. People who make a strong impression are in some sense larger than and distant from the average as measured along cognitive axes. The presentation of the W. H. Helmerich III award of the Retina Research Foundation to Dr. Christina Enroth-Cugell is a good reason to consider the size of Christina in our mental coordinate systems and the dimensions of her character.

First, there is her scientific career. And, first and foremost, the famous 1966 paper in the *Journal of Physiology* with John Robson of Cambridge University. No honor contemporaries confer can match the influence of a great paper on generations of young scientists. The Enroth-Cugell and Robson paper is one of the landmarks of visual neuroscience. Its introduction of linear systems analysis to the mammalian retina was remarkable; its discovery of X and Y cells was memorable. Later on I will attempt to explain some of the mysterious attraction of X and Y cells, but here I will just assert that the concept of parallel processing in the visual system that Enroth-Cugell and Robson introduced in their 1966 paper is profound. Christina insists on giving John Robson full credit for the ideas in the paper. Nevertheless, her contributions to the research were essential. This was one of those fortunate cases of supralinear summation in science.

Christina's other scientific accomplishments have added to her magnitude along the scientific dimension. Among these is the proof of the importance of network interactions in retinal light adaptation. Her collaborative work with Brian Cleland, Peter Lennie, Gevene Hertz, Tom Harding, A. B. Bonds, John Troy, and me established the existence and the spatiotemporal character of network adaptation in the cat retina. This line of research was greatly influenced by another scientist from Cambridge, William Rushton.

Christina has also always been interested in the dynamics of response in cat retinal ganglion cells. Her doctoral dissertation on the flicker responses of cat retinal ganglion cells was her initial contribution in this field; subsequently she worked on the response dynamics of center and surround receptive field mechanisms and of different types of ganglion cells with many colleagues:

Cleland, Larry Pinto, Alan Freeman, Robert Linsenmeier, Hank Jakiela, Lennie, and me too. In her scientific work there are consistent qualities: quantitative precision of stimulus control and response measurements, as well as scrupulous attention to all methodological details.

The next cognitive dimension in which Christina Enroth-Cugell should be measured is that of nurturing collaborators and students and training young scientists. Many people have done their best work in collaboration with Christina. She demanded and still demands incredible productivity. How has she accomplished this? One factor has been the use of shameless flattery. Christina will often say, "You're a genius" or "all my genii," and this works wonders as a motivational tool. She has always been encouraging and has used positive reinforcement of all kinds, including compliments, cookies, and coffee. She has also set an example of dedicated hard work, always putting in extra effort in preparing talks and lectures and teaching her students how to clarify their own presentations and writing.

What makes Christina Enroth-Cugell so unusual in science is another dimension entirely, her nobility. We live in an era of common people. Even reigning monarchs and presidents are quite common nowadays, with characters of low amplitude and common aspirations. But Christina has a lot of class and is, by merit, raised to a kind of regal stature. One part of this is her extraordinary enjoyment of life, which contrasts starkly with her Scandinavian habit of "moaning and groaning," to use one of her pet phrases. Her enjoyment of life is expressed in her strong emotional attachment to people she loves. It is also evident in the relish with which she consumes good food and sherry. Another part of her class act is her sense of tradition and history in science and in her personal life. In scientific discourse this is expressed in her appreciation of her mentors, such as Granit and Forbes, Wald and Hartline, and William Rushton. In her honesty, energy, liveliness, intelligence, emotions, and sense of tradition, there is just more of her than there is of other people.

Then there is the dimension of ethics. Christina is puritanical about work. The goal is not sheer effort; the goal is to get the job done right. Coupled with this drive is an equally strong motivation toward honesty and integrity that she communicates to students and colleagues alike. In Christina's world, precision and accuracy are not merely desirable; they are morally necessary. Similarly, clarity of thought and precision of expression are her tests of character. Sloppiness of any kind is almost sinful. This attitude is one reason why Christina really has no respect for Authority. Authority must prove itself by clear thought and hard work like anyone else.

Perhaps the most important dimension of all is the most obvious: Christina is a Woman in Science. Morality, strength, nurturing behavior, elegance, and lack of respect for Authority may all be consequences of her being a woman among male scientists. One other consequence of her femininity may be the sexual undertone that pervades the famous 1966 paper on X and Y cells, and that may explain some of the paper's mysterious charm. The terms X and Y certainly suggest the sex chromosomes that carry genes for females and males, respectively. However, many of us know that the original names for the cells were I and D, supposedly standing for *interesting* and *dull*. However, this terminology may have been only a rationalization; really *I* and *D* were letters that spelled ID, suggesting that Freud was on the authors' minds. Scientists who have studied X and Y cells have also discerned that the X cells seem female, while the Y cells seem male. For instance, X cells prefer fine detail, are quite sensitive, have small size and spread, respond with high fidelity, and give a sustained response to stimulation. Y cells, however, respond to coarse and fine detail, have large bodies and branches, respond transiently and sometimes in a distorted manner to stimulation, and have stout, long axons.

Seriously, as a female scientist Christina Enroth-Cugell walked a lonely road for a long time, and she was one of the leaders of her generation of women in science. Perhaps this explains her drive to excel and her impatience with undeserved Authority. It is an honor to honor her.

9 The World of Retinal Ganglion Cells

Christina Enroth-Cugell

This chapter is intended as a tribute to those who started the field of sensory—and in particular visual—neurophysiology and did so much to further our understanding of retinal function. In addition I hope that some of the young people who are just beginning to study retinal neural networks are curious about the world of research surrounding retinal ganglion cells as it was almost seventy years ago. Reminders of a few of the early milestones along the road from 1926 to where we are today are also included. These pages are in no way intended to be an all-inclusive review of vertebrate retinal ganglion cells. The selection of topics is biased, because this story constitutes "a sentimental journey" for the author. Although the subject of this book is the role of contrast at different levels of the visual system, my own contribution will deal with that topic only to a very limited extent. Last, but certainly not least, these pages represent an inadequate but heartfelt attempt to express my gratitude to those who have been instrumental in my receiving the Helmerich Award.

EDGAR D. ADRIAN

Let me start with Adrian of The Physiological Laboratory in Cambridge and Yngve Zotterman, who came to Cambridge from Sweden to learn from Adrian. They initiated the era of single-cell neurophysiology by recording for the very first time the activity of a single nerve cell. They did it by isolating the activity of one axon originating in a stretch receptor. The work on stretch receptors was published in a series of three articles in 1926, the first one authored by Adrian alone (Adrian 1926; Adrian and Zotterman 1926a, 1926b). I read these papers as my very first lesson in neurophysiology forty-two years ago, and I must say that, on reading them once again, I am amazed at what these early masters accomplished with their brains and hands unaided—or should I say unhampered—by sophisticated recording equipment and computers. Moreover, the sometimes almost poetic quality of Adrian's language, together with the personal humility that his papers exude, makes the world look like a better place. So, as I proceed I will share a few passages with you to give you a feeling for what recording from sensory neurons was like in those days.

As you will see below, Adrian contributed several other "firsts" to physiology and at one time he discussed his work on the sensory systems with the father of all modern neurophysiology, Charles Sherrington (quoted from Granit 1966, p. 99). During this conversation Adrian pondered the nature of sensory neurons in general and commented, "The sensory messages are scarcely more complex than a succession of Morse dots," to which Sherrington responded, "How complex must not the central processes then be in order to explain the workings of our mind."

My guess is that the speakers on the first day of this meeting might say to themselves that the retinal message may look simple, but a lot has to happen before those Morse dots can be manufactured and sent on their way to the brain. The speakers during the second day will likely agree with Sherrington that central processes are very complicated. With regard to vision, at least, about ten years ago Horace Barlow (1983) seemed to agree with Sherrington, for he finished a talk entitled "Understanding Natural Vision" by pointing out that "We do not understand much of it."

Adrian and Zotterman's Work

A few years before Adrian and Zotterman started their experiments, a virtual revolution in electrophysiological experimentation had begun. It was fueled by pioneering technical advances on both sides of the Atlantic. At that time two different instruments were commonly used for recording electrical activity from muscle and nerve tissue: the mercury capillary electrometer and the string galvanometer. However, one of them, the capillary electrometer, had, to quote Adrian (1926, p. 50), "... fallen out of favor with the majority of physiologists because its records need analysis and because of its low sensitivity compared to the string galvanometer." The string galvanometer had its own serious drawbacks, however. Its problem was, quoting Adrian again, "... the limitation imposed by the inertia of the moving system. Owing to the mass of the string the record of its movement does not give a true picture of the change of the electromotive force applied to it, and the distortion, though of little account in the record of a muscle action current, is quite enough to obscure the true form of the much briefer responses of a nerve fiber" (Adrian 1926, p. 49).

But help was under way, for in this country Forbes and Thacher (1920) and Gasser and Newcomer (1921) were already using the vacuum tube amplifier in conjunction with recording instruments in physiological experiments, and in the following year, 1922, Erlanger and Gasser introduced the cathode ray oscilloscope. While these exciting developments occurred in the United States, in Cambridge Adrian was anxious to take advantage of them in his sensory nerve experiments, the goal of which was to record from single fibers. Forbes and his colleagues (1924)) had already recorded sensory signals from whole nerves by showing that, when a muscle is stretched, a compound action potential travels towards the spinal cord.

Adrian's major difficulty in his attempt to record from single axons was to achieve a recording system that was both sensitive and fast enough. In the first of the three 1926 papers (p. 49) he acknowledged that the cathode ray oscillograph was the recording instrument of choice, but he did not use it until a few years later. He wrote that the reason was "... the intensity of the illumination from the ray is far too small to allow photographs to be made from a single excursion, and similar excursions must be repeated many times over before the plate or the eye is affected." Therefore he chose to work with the reasonably distortion-free but insensitive capillary electrometer (Lucas 1912, p. 225) in conjunction with the valve amplifier. The nerve potential was applied to the input of the amplifier and its output was fed to the electrometer, where the nerve signal caused a vertical mercury pillar 0.03 mm in diameter to move up and down. The shadow of the moving pillar was cast on a glass photographic plate that was moved at a speed of 80 mm per second. In 1926 Adrian and Zotterman published the first records of action potential spikes obtained from any single neuron using this equipment.

How did they do it? They did it by selecting a suitable preparation and by employing their deft fingers and a big dose of patience. They used the sterno-cutaneous muscle of the frog, having established that this muscle always contains at least one muscle spindle, "... and as our results show there are usually three or four end-organs [in this muscle] which are stimulated by tension ..." (Adrian and Zotterman 1926a, pp. 151–152). They also determined that the nerve that supplies the muscle arises from the brachial nerve and contains only twelve to twenty-five axons. They connected this nerve to recording electrodes "with short lengths of moist carpet thread imbedded in gelatine" (Adrian and Zotterman 1926a, p. 152). To stimulate the end-organs they used weights that were "... attached to a thread from the muscle and allowed to hang over a light pulley" (same page).

There were no microelectrodes at that time. The first ones were introduced ten years later by Forbes and co-workers (Granit 1955, p. 4; Forbes et al. 1937). So some method had to be devised to permit the detection of electrical activity in only one axon of the whole A nerve that was connected to the electrodes. Adrian and Zotterman reasoned that, since the entire muscle contained only a small number of receptors, by cutting off a little piece of muscle at a time they might be lucky enough to eliminate one receptor at a time and eventually end up with only one functioning receptor in what was left of the muscle, and hence only one active axon in the nerve. And that is just what happened.

Figure 9.1 shows the results from one of their experiments. The time marker is seen at the top of the figure. The distance between two peaks represents 10 ms. To the best of my understanding, the black areas of each record represent the nervous activity. The weight was applied to the muscle 10 seconds prior to obtaining the top record, which shows the activity in the nerve when the muscle is intact. After obtaining this first record they removed a little strip of the muscle tissue, and after each successive strip was removed

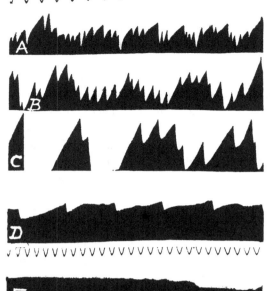

Figure 9.1 Neural responses generated in stretch receptors of the sternocutaneous muscle of the frog. The black part of each record represents nerve responses recorded from the whole nerve that supplies the muscle. Record D shows the action potentials from one individual sensory axon in that nerve. For details see text. (From Adrian and Zotterman 1926a)

they recorded the nerve activity again. In B one strip of the muscle has been removed, in C two strips, and in D a total of three strips has been removed.

As pieces were removed the total number of response peaks recorded over the total duration of each record also decreased, presumably because fewer and fewer receptors generated action potentials. In D the responses are regularly distributed "with a period of 0.030 sec." and "very nearly all of the same amplitude" (Adrian and Zotterman 1926a, p. 153). Finally, when one more strip of the muscle was removed, the response to stretch was completely abolished. Electrical stimulation of the muscle nerve, however, caused a muscle twitch (Adrian and Zotterman 1926a, p. 153), so the preparation was still viable.

About this result the authors wrote, "We have no direct proof that the regular responses shown in D are due to one nerve ending only, but the indirect evidence leaves very little doubt of it" (Adrian and Zotterman 1926a, p. 155). They scrutinized the validity of their indirect evidence in great detail and concluded that they had indeed recorded from an individual sensory fiber.

One of the important principles established by Adrian and Zotterman's results on the frog's stretch receptors was that, when the stimulus strength was increased, the impulses in an individual axon remained of the same amplitude, while the *frequency* of the impulse increased. That is, they established the all-or-none property of action potentials traveling in sensory axons and the principle of the gradation of impulse frequency with stimulus strength.

As far as I know, this was also the first time that a relationship between the level of sensation and impulse frequency in sensory nerves was proposed. Adrian and Zotterman pointed out that if, as they found, it is only the impulse frequency that varies with stimulus strength, the obvious fact that our sensations are graded is probably related to impulse frequency in the responding sensory neuron and to the number of neurons responding.

In other words, by 1926 Adrian and Zotterman had developed the very foundation of sensory neurophysiology: single sensory neurons produce all-or-none spikes, the frequency at which a sensory neuron fires impulses depends on the strength of the stimulus, and the grading of sensations is probably related to the firing frequency of sensory neurons.

As something to reflect upon when you next struggle to keep the list of references in one of your papers within bounds, here is the *total* list of references from the second of these three papers that together represent a turning point in the development of the physiology of senses (Adrian and Zotterman, 1926a).

REFERENCES.
1. Adrian. This Journ. 61. p. 49. 1926.
2. Erlanger and Gasser. Amer. Journ. Physiol. 70. p. 663. 1924.
3. Cooper and Adrian. this Journ. 58. p. 209. 1923; 59. p. 61. 1924.
4. Adrian and Forbes. Ibid. 56. p. 301. 1922.
5. Brücke. Ztsch. f. Biol. 76. p. 213. 1922.
6. Brevée and Dusser de Barenne. This Journ. 61. p. 81. 1926.

Adrian and Matthews

Very soon after Adrian brought electrophysiology into the era of single-neuron experimentation, he turned his attention to the visual system. His co-worker in the Cambridge laboratory was Rachel Matthews, and in 1927 they published the first recordings of retinal ganglion cell action potentials in a vertebrate—the conger eel. The potentials were not, however, from a single visual axon as they had hoped. Their plan was to place the whole optic nerve on gross electrodes and then use very small, sharply focused stimuli. In other words, they hoped to use an approach similar to the one Adrian and Zotterman had used so successfully in their experiments on the stretch receptors in muscle: restrict *stimulation* so that only one axon in the nerve became active. Here is what Adrian and Matthews said about their approach: "Since each fibre of the optic nerve must supply on the average an area at least 90 μ diam. on the retina (see p. 413) it would seem to be an easy matter to restrict the activity to a single nerve fibre" (Adrian and Matthews 1927a, p. 386). To achieve this goal they spent considerable effort obtaining the sharpest possi-

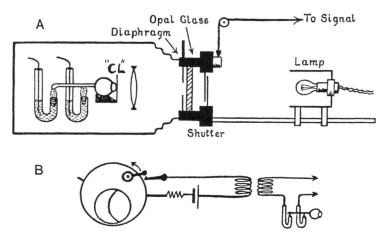

Fig. 1. A. Arrangement of apparatus for focussing an image of an illuminated disc on the retina.

    B. Detail of electric signal.

Figure 9.2. Experimental setup for recording from the whole optic nerve of the conger eel. The vertical line labeled "CL" is a microscope cover slip surrounded by fluid. (From Adrian and Matthews 1927a)

ble retinal image of very small stimuli. Adrian and Matthews' (1927a) experimental setup is shown in figure 9.2.

There is one particular detail in the upper part of this figure to which I want to draw attention lest somebody believe that contact lenses for protection of the cornea were first introduced to visual experimentation in the 1950s. The vertical line that I have marked "CL" is a microscope cover slip. According to the authors, it "was kept in optical contact with the cornea with fluid," an arrangement that certainly can be thought of as a satisfactory "home-made contact lens." An ophthalmoscope was used to refract the eye and, "with the refraction of the front surface of the cornea annulled by the cover glass" (Adrian and Matthews 1927a, p. 381), the eel's isolated eye was found to be several diopters hyperopic. The necessary correcting lenses were set up in a holder in front of the eye, and a sharp retinal image was thus formed on the retina. Adrian and Matthews also checked the quality of this image in other ways, and there can be little doubt that it was good.

In spite of their efforts, they did not succeed in activating only a single axon. Even a stimulus with a diameter of only 10 microns generated activity in several axons, as one must expect from what we now know about overlapping retinal ganglion cell receptive fields in vertebrates. But failure to activate a single axon in the optic nerve did not prevent Adrian and Matthews from making important contributions to the very beginning of visual electrophysiology. First, before them no one had recorded neural activity from a vertebrate optic nerve. Second, although their electrode picked up the activity from more than one axon at a time, the resolution of their multiaxon recording

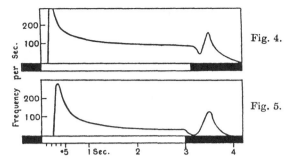

Fig. 4. Frequency of impulses per sec. during and after illumination. Duration of lighting shown below record. Exp. 16. Disc, diam. 36 mm. Illumination 830 metre candles.

Fig. 5. Ditto. Exp. 13. Disc, diam. 12·8 mm. Illumination 830 metre candles.

Figure 9.3 Recordings from the whole optic nerve of the conger eel. The white portion of the wide horizontal bar at the bottom of each record indicates the light stimulus. The luminance is the same in both panels, but the stimulus area is smaller in the bottom panel. Note that in both cases there is a burst of impulses when the light is turned off. (From Adrian and Matthews 1927a)

was sufficient for them to achieve a reasonably reliable estimate of the total number of spikes per unit time. And this enabled them to score another "first": they showed that some ganglion cells must respond with a burst of spikes at the offset of light.

In figure 9.3 you see the very first plot ever of the impulse frequency of vertebrate ganglion cells in response to the onset of light—and also the *increase* in firing that occurred when the light was turned off. Thus, there can be no doubt that off-bursts were produced by at least some of the ganglion cells from whose axons the electrodes recorded action potentials.

With their carefully controled optical quality of retinal images, Adrian and Matthews also investigated spatial interaction in the retina, and they have been credited with being the first to provide physiological evidence of spatial interaction in a vertebrate retina (See Granit 1947, p. 186; Hartline 1940; Barlow 1953; and Levick 1972, p. 532).

To conclude this description of Adrian's earliest contributions to electrophysiology, here is a quote from a talk he gave in 1953. The occasion was the inauguration of a new neurophysiology laboratory that had been created for Zotterman in Stockholm. Adrian began his talk by recalling what experimentation had been like in the early 1920s, and he made the following comment about the equipment that Gasser, Erlanger, Newcomer, and Forbes had introduced at that time: "The technique they were using was clearly not to be taken lightly; it contained all sorts of unfamiliar components, high tension batteries, condensers and resistances—electrical gear which now overflows our store cupboards but then had all to be made by hand in the laboratory" (Adrian 1953). I guess we have come a fair distance since then—at least as far as instrumentation is concerned.

H. KEFFER HARTLINE

The next big step, or rather steps, were taken by H. Keffer Hartline in this country. He provided the first description, in both invertebrates and in cold-blooded vertebrates, of how individual optic nerve fibers talk to the brain, and he also showed what they might tell the brain. He was one of the founders of present-day visual neurophysiology.

Work on Limulus

In 1931, inspired by the important contributions of Adrian and his co-workers in England, Hartline, together with C. H. Graham, began work on the visual system. In the summer of 1931, while at Woods Hole, they worked on the lateral eye of the horseshoe crab, the *Limulus*, which I understand is not a crab at all. They hoped to isolate, by dissection, a single axon from its optic nerve and record the activity in this isolated fiber. At the outset they used young specimens with clear eyes that yielded vigorous whole-nerve responses to light stimuli (Granit and Ratliff 1985, p. 270). But they were singularly unsuccessful in obtaining individual functioning axons.

Then, during one of the last days of their summer stay at Woods Hole, when their frustration was very high and they had only two old animals left, Hartline and Graham suddenly succeeded in isolating functional single axons and recording their all-or-none action potentials. During his many years of working on the *Limulus*, Hartline never understood why the experiments on young animals did not work. The first full paper about the signals in single optic nerve axons in the *Limulus* was published in 1932.

The Receptive Field

Before I move on to the vertebrate retina, let me briefly trace the history of a concept that will recur throughout this book: *the receptive field*. The term was coined by Sherrington (1906, p. 129) to describe "the whole collection of points of skin surface from which the scratch-reflex can be elicited ...." Our present use of this term differs from that original definition, because Sherrington's receptive field served more than one sensory neuron. Adrian (1932) was the first to use the term to refer to *one* sensory neuron. He called the area of the frog's skin innervated by a single afferent fiber a "receptive field" (quoted from Granit 1955, p. 58). With reference to vertebrate retinal ganglion cells the receptive field was first defined by Hartline (1938), as you will see below.

The Vertebrate Retina

To return to Hartline, he was also the first to record from a single retinal ganglion cell axon of the vertebrate eye, the eye of the frog. In this animal he did not attempt to dissect the optic nerve. Instead he excised the eye, removed the front part of it together with the corpus vitreum, and made a radial incision in the retina and the sclera from the edge of the eye cup almost to the nerve head so that the preparation could lie flat under a microilluminator. This enabled him to obtain sharply focused images of small light spots on the retina.

Hartline was not only a superb scientist; he also possessed extraordinary manual skills and manufactured his own instruments for microdissection. After the preparation was mounted he used his home-made scissors to cut off a small bundle of axons at the nerve head and then lifted the bundle onto the recording electrode. Then he dissected free a single axon from that bundle and did it so gently that the axon was still functional when he was through.

If you leaf through the papers that Hartline published between 1938 and the beginning of the 1940s, you will find that he must have isolated a very large number of frog axons over that period and that he described many, if not most, of the basic ganglion cell properties in vertebrates known to us today. Using his movable, well-focused stimuli of varying sizes, he determined that there is a specific region within which the stimulus must fall in order to obtain a response from the cell whose axon the electrode records from. In Hartline's own words, "This region will be termed the receptive field of the fiber. The location of the receptive field of a given fiber is fixed; its extent, however, depends upon the intensity and the size of the spot of light used to explore it and upon the condition of adaptation" (Hartline 1938, p. 410). Within this receptive field some cells responded to a light stimulus with a burst of spikes at ON and another burst at OFF. Other cells generated a spike burst only at ON, and yet a third kind responded with an initial high-frequency discharge followed by a steady firing at a lower rate as long as the light was on. These basic types of response patterns were not altered when stimulus conditions such as state of adaptation or stimulus strength or position were changed (Hartline 1938).

Hartline showed that sensitivity was at a maximum in the middle of the receptive field, that the magnitude of the discharge at light-off was a function of how long the light was on, and that two spatially separated stimuli interacted to determine the nature of the cell's response, and he also described how the frequency of discharge varied with stimulus strength. In other words, in this country Hartline did for retinal ganglion cell physiology what Adrian did in England for sensory neurophysiology—that is, he laid the foundation for our current knowledge.

Both his long-time co-worker and friend, Floyd Ratliff, and his friend of fifty years, Ragnar Granit, described Hartline as a rather quiet and very unassuming man who was slightly embarrassed by public acclaim. As an example of this, let me quote one of Granit's stories about Keffer Hartline. In 1967 he received the Nobel Prize (which he shared with Granit and George Wald). Shortly after the day that the selection of winners had been announced, Hartline got a phone call from a journalist who asked, "What exactly did you do when you heard that you had gotten the Prize?" Hartline answered, "I had my breakfast." The journalist, who sounded quite excited, then asked, "And what did you do *after* you had heard about the Nobel Prize?" Hartline replied, "I finished my breakfast."

RAGNAR GRANIT

The study of single *mammalian* retinal ganglion cells was ushered in by Ragnar Granit and his collaborators. He is usually associated with Sweden, and of course that is where he made most of his scientific contributions, but some of his important observations on the visual system were published while he was professor of physiology in Finland, where he was born and raised. In 1939 he accepted the post of director of one of the three Nobel Institutes for Research that were part of Karolinska Institutet in Stockholm, in part because of the ethnic political climate in Finland at that time.

The following is a simplified and slightly exaggerated description of how he decided to study neurophysiology. After finishing "gymnasium" (the equivalent of high school plus one or two years of undergraduate college) he wanted to become a psychologist, which, to quote Granit, is "a common weakness in young people," so he went to Germany to learn Gestalt psychology. There he decided that one cannot really make progress in psychology unless one knows how the human body works in health and sickness, so he went to medical school and, after obtaining his M.D. degree, he started to specialize in psychiatry. From that experience he decided that one needs to know how the central nervous system works in order to be useful in psychiatry, and that took him to Sherrington in England.

Granit was not only a student, but also an ardent admirer of Charles Sherrington, in whose Oxford laboratory he spent two extended periods in 1928 and 1932. He went there because of his interest in the neural mechanisms of the central nervous system in general and in the interplay of inhibition and excitation in particular. Another of Granit's heroes was Cajal, who, according to his own account, studied the histology of the retina only as a prelude to an attack on the histology of the rest of the central nervous system. The reason for this was that the retina, in Cajal's own words, "is a true nervous center" (Granit 1955, p. 38), and in his own writings Granit made it clear that it was Cajal's work that stimulated him to use the physiology of the retina in a similar way: as an introduction to the physiology of the central nervous system in general.

One of Granit's early ambitions was to demonstrate by electrophysiological experiments that retinal responses to light represent a balance between excitation and inhibition. Indeed he became the first to demonstrate inhibitory processes in the vertebrate retina in experiments he did with Therman in Granit's laboratory in Finland and published in 1935. They recorded from the frog's optic nerve in much the same way that Adrian and Matthews had done a few years earlier from the eel's optic nerve. That is, they measured activity from a sizable number of ganglion cell axons, but still from a small enough number that they could get an approximate count of the total number of

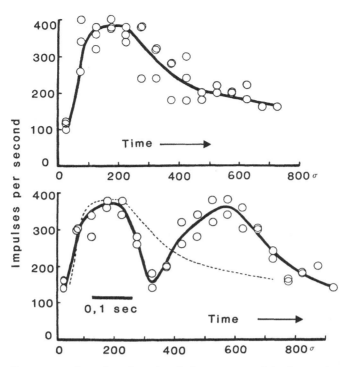

Figure 9.4 Recordings from the whole optic nerve of the frog to demonstrate retinal inhibition. For details see text. (From Granit and Therman 1935)

action potentials traveling past their electrode per unit time. The results from one such experiment are shown in figure 9.4.

In the upper half you see an optic nerve's response to the cessation of a light stimulus. The stimulus itself is not shown. Impulse frequency is plotted on the vertical axis and the time elapsed since the retinal illumination was turned off on the horizontal axis. In the lower half, the nerve first responds to the offset of a retinal light stimulus identical to the one used above. But this time the retina is reilluminated *during* the response to the first stimulus. The timing of the second stimulus is indicated by the short, heavy horizontal line. That flash clearly cut short—i.e., inhibited—spike production.

Single-Cell Recordings

After the move to Stockholm Granit concentrated on developing a technique for recording from single retinal ganglion cells. In this endeavor Gunnar Svaetichin, also from Finland, was of invaluable help. The major reason Granit was so eager to develop a technique for recording from individual mammalian ganglion cells was that he was looking for a tool—a tool better than the electroretinogram—with which to explore the neurophysiology of color vision. In addition, he wanted to study in more detail how excitation and inhibition together determine the response of ganglion cells, and thus the message that the eye sends to the brain.

Granit had an immense admiration for Hartline's technique of dissecting and recording from individual retinal ganglion cell axons in the frog. However, I suspect that he realized full well that Hartline's technique was not compatible with his own style. In the 1939 paper in which he described the experiments he performed with Svaetichin, Granit said that Hartline's technique "was too laborious for use in work which requires such a great number of observations" (p. 162), referring here to the measurements of numerous spectral sensitivity curves based on "threshold" responses from individual cells.

Instead of isolating axons by dissection, Granit and Svaetichin isolated action potentials with a small silver-in-glass electrode. After removal of the cornea and lens, it was lowered through the corpus vitreum until it made contact with the retinal surface. Figure 9.5 shows some of the very first recordings using this technique. These could well be two different isolated spikes, one large and one small, each originating in its own single neuron. Of course one would have to see these potentials on a faster sweep to be sure.

For more than ten years Granit never stated that the impulses came from a single ganglion cell. He talked about *retinal elements* or *units* and even mentioned that he might be recording from several cells with very well-synchronized activity. Not until William Rushton came to Granit's Stockholm laboratory in 1948 and demonstrated that the spikes came from "giant" retinal ganglion cells did Granit begin referring to the recordings as coming from

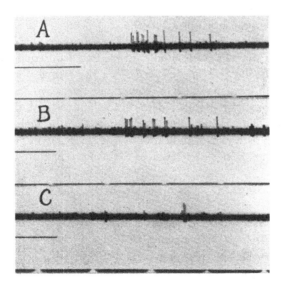

Figure 9.5 One of the first recordings of single-cell activity from a vertebrate (frog) retina using a microelectrode. All three records show off-responses to monochromatic flashes of light (6000 Å). Each short horizontal bar at the bottom of the figure represents 200 milliseconds. The duration of the stimulus is given in A to C by the thin horizontal line. (From Granit and Svaetichin 1939)

single retinal ganglion cells. I will comment later on a 1949 paper by Rushton based on experiments done in Stockholm. After 1950 Granit no longer worked on ganglion cells personally, and in 1952 the equipment in the "eye room" was dismantled, never again to resound to the delightful prop-prop-prop from hard-working ganglion cells.

Let me now say a few words about the foundation of knowledge about the *mammalian* retina, which Granit and his co-workers provided between 1941 and 1951. It included work on the cat, rabbit, guinea pig, rat, and mouse. Much of the fundamental insight gained from the work of Granit and his colleagues can be summarized as follows: whatever the retina tells the brain about the visual world around us, the message that leaves the retina in axons of mammalian retinal ganglion cells is the result of complicated interactions between excitatory and inhibitory processes within the retinal neural network. Before proceeding I should make it clear that the terms *excitatory* and *inhibitory*, as used here, simply imply any influence upon the ganglion cell that increases or decreases the cell's firing rate. Thus the term *excitatory input* does not specify whether an increase in firing rate is due to an increase in excitatory postsynaptic potentials, a decrease in inhibitory postsynaptic potentials, or some combination of both, across the ganglion cell membrane. The corresponding holds for the term *inhibitory input*.

Maintained Discharge

I must also mention the kind of retinal ganglion cell activity that was referred to in the 1940s primarily as *spontaneous activity of retinal elements* but is now mostly called *maintained activity*. Granit found that in any of his healthy mammalian preparations most retinal ganglion cells produced an irregular train of impulses when the retina was exposed to some uniform, steady, illumination or when it was left in complete darkness. The electrode rested on the surface of the retina but, since the front of the eye bulb had been removed, the eye had lost some of its rigidity. Moreover, sometimes the decerebration plus urethane anesthesia did not suppress all small eye movements. Thus there was a possibility that the maintained firing could have been due to a mechanical effect of the electrode upon the cell's spike-generating mechanism.

Granit was convinced this was not the case. He believed that the spontaneous firing was a physiological phenomenon that "was very useful in revealing inhibitory effects which would otherwise escape notice" by the next station in the central visual pathways (Granit 1947, p. 96). Since Granit wanted to use retinal ganglion cells to study inhibitory processes in the retina and he used extracellular recordings, the maintained discharge served as a background against which he could detect inhibitory inputs to the cell.

Several years later Kuffler, who also recorded from the retinal surface, reported that he also found spontaneous firing, and he cited several reasons why he believed it was not an artifact, but a normal phenomenon. He acknowledged that his findings were in general agreement with those of Granit (Kuffler 1953). Subsequently, when people began recording from axons of single retinal ganglion cells in the optic nerve or tract, it was found that with this technique too—i.e., in a situation in which the electrode could not possibly interfere with the generation of spikes—mammalian ganglion cells exhibit a maintained discharge.

Excitatory and Inhibitory Responses

In Granit's experiments, stimulating the retina with flashes of light produced *excitation*—i.e., a spike burst—only at onset of the stimulus in some cells, at offset in other cells, or both at onset and at offset in still other cells. In Granit's terminology, these were the retinal ON-elements, OFF-elements and ON-OFF elements. That ganglion cells receive *inhibitory* as well as excitatory signals was demonstrated in Granit's experiments in several ways. One expression of inhibition was the complete or partial suppression of the maintained discharge at the *onset* of a flash, without any burst at ON, but with a spike discharge at OFF (see for example, the records in figure 29, Granit 1955). Another situation in which inhibitory effects were obvious was when a light flash caused a peak of firing at onset and the cell continued to fire, but at some lower rate, while the stimulus remained on. In such cases the first effect of turning off the light was a pause and then a slow return to the prestimulus maintained discharge frequency, but no off-burst (see for example, the bottom record in figure 65a, Granit, 1947). These were given the terms *preexcitatory inhibitions* and *postexcitatory inhibitions* by Granit.

Using Granit's technique it was possible to record with relative ease from a large number of cells in succession during a single experiment on a live mammal that could be kept in good general condition for 12 to 20 hours. But this type of recording had one serious shortcoming compared to Hartline's excised frog-eye preparation. In the mammalian preparation, where the cornea and lens had been removed, the surface of corpus vitreum faced the stimulus beam, a situation that did not lend itself very well to producing sharp images on the retina. In Granit's lab the only stimuli used were therefore diffuse lights that covered virtually the entire retinal surface. Thus the outer limits of receptive fields were never determined, nor were differences in sensitivity or type of discharge pattern as a function of position explored.

By the beginning of the 1950s, at the end of the first decade of experiments, a first chapter on mammalian retinal ganglion cells had been written by Granit and co-workers. The highly variable discharge patterns observed were clearly the result of intricate interactions between excitation and inhibition. A detailed understanding of the *spatial organization* of this excitation-inhibition interplay remained to be provided by Kuffler in the United States and, to some extent, by Thomson in England. Kuffler worked on the cat, Thomson on the rabbit, and both left the animals' natural image-forming apparatus intact so that sharply focused images could be formed on the retinas. Kuffler made a hole in the sclera through which the electrode was advanced for recording from the retinal surface. Thomson, on the other hand, recorded from individual ganglion cell axons in the retrobulbar part of the optic nerve. As far as I know, he was the first one to record from single ganglion cell *axons* in a mammalian optic nerve or tract. Thomson died soon after his paper on retinal ganglion cells had been published in the *Journal of Physiology* in 1953, leaving Kuffler and his "eye boys," Hubel, Wiesel, and Barlow, to write much of the second chapter about mammalian retinal ganglion cells.

STEPHEN W. KUFFLER

Many members of today's neurobiology community are fortunate to have known Steve Kuffler well. I am lucky enough to have known him just a little bit, and, unless you completely lacked receptors for human qualities, it did not take many encounters to sense the kind of a man he was. Surely his human qualities were part of the reason why he was a scientist of great caliber and why so many outstanding researchers emerged from his laboratory.

Kuffler's impact on progress in neurobiology, including visual neurophysiology, cannot be overestimated. He did not start his work on the cat's retinal ganglion cells because he wanted to know what role they played in vision, and he personally did not continue to work on the retina after the mid-1950s. Kuffler, like Granit before him, believed that the vertebrate retina was well suited to studying many central nervous system processes in general. This I infer, for instance, from his talk at the 1952 Cold Spring Harbor Symposium on "The Neuron," in which he made the following introductory statement: "In this discussion emphasis will be laid on neuronal activity, probably representative of many parts of the central nervous system, rather than on problems of vision" (p. 281). This approach did not prevent him from making many invaluable contributions to visual physiology.

The 1952 and 1953 Papers

I will discuss only a few of Kuffler's contributions. When he explored the cat retina with spot stimuli, his results were similar to those Hartline (1938) had previously obtained in the frog. There was a retinal area, the receptive field, within which the stimulus had to fall in order to evoke a response, and Kuffler also stressed that, while the location of a receptive field was fixed, its extent depended upon stimulus conditions. If the stimulus was weak or of only moderate strength and was applied to the middle of the receptive field, then it always evoked a burst only at ON or at OFF; that is, the cell had an ON-center or an OFF-center. A stimulus applied far out in the periphery of the field generated a discharge at OFF in ON-center cells, at ON in OFF-center cells. In some intermediate zone the response consisted of a burst of spikes both at ON and at OFF.

These two types of cells, the ON-center and the OFF-center retinal ganglion cells, were the only two kinds that Kuffler encountered in the cat. He did not conclude that the cat possessed only two kinds of ganglion cells. On the contrary, one of the many developments that he, in his wisdom, predicted was expressed in the 1952 paper as follows: "It is almost certain that with more

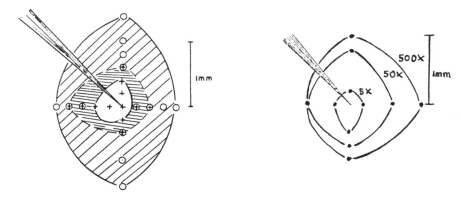

Figure 9.6 (Left) Map of receptive field of single cat retinal ganglion cell. Responses were elicited with a small spot of constant, moderate luminance and recorded intraocularly with a microelectrode. Against the photopic background used, these stimuli generated a spike burst only at the onset of the flash within the central region (crosses) of the receptive field, at offset only in the outlying parts (circles) of the receptive field, and both at onset and at offset when the stimulus was located in an intermediate area. That is, this is an ON-center cell. (Right) Sensitivity is at a maximum in the middle of the receptive field and falls off toward the periphery. The innermost line indicates the area beyond which the stimulus luminance had to be higher than 5 times the "threshold" luminance, which yielded a just-audible response to a short flash. Beyond the two other lines the stimulus had to be 50 and 500 times "threshold" as determined in the very middle of the field. Note that neither of these sketches shows a perfectly circular field and that in the right-hand sketch the sensitivity distribution is clearly asymmetric. (From Kuffler 1953)

refined methods a variety of ganglion cells of different behavior remains to be uncovered" (p. 292).

Figure 9.6 demonstrates several of Kuffler's findings in the form of two simple sketches. The one on the left illustrates schematically how the type of discharge varies with position when a receptive field is explored with a small spot of constant, moderate strength. I believe that this cartoon was first shown as a slide at the 1952 Cold Spring Harbor Symposium.

The right-hand sketch makes the point that sensitivity is at a maximum in the middle and falls off more or less smoothly with distance from the middle. These two sketches are, even now, 40 years later, some of the most frequently reproduced figures in basic neuroscience and vision texts, and deservedly so. The left-hand sketch in particular serves as a reminder of the shape of the receptive fields of Kuffler's cells. It is clear from figure 9.6 that they may be more "egg-shaped" than circularly symmetric. The degree to which they deviate from perfect circular symmetry has been discussed in several publications (e.g., Rodieck and Stone 1965a; Hammond 1974; Levick and Thibos 1982; Soodak et al. 1987). But modern-day mathematical modelers frequently assume circular symmetry, for this makes things simpler.

A word or two about terminology is in order before I proceed. In the two Kuffler papers, as well as in early papers by his co-workers, a ganglion cell's response was, by implication, equated with a stimulus-evoked *increase* in discharge frequency. As I have already mentioned, both Granit and Kuffler found

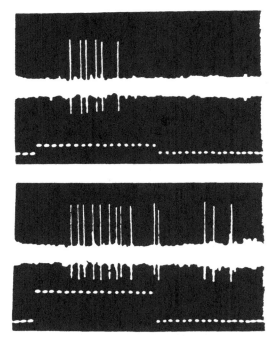

Figure 9.7 Responses from an ON-center cell elicited with a small flashing spot. The stimulus is located in the same place (in the middle) of the receptive field in both cases, but it is more luminous in the lower half of the figure. (From Kuffler 1952)

that cat retinal ganglion cells exhibited spontaneous activity that both of them considered a physiological phenomenon rather than a result of, say, electrode pressure. Hence it would seem more appropriate to think of any stimulus-evoked *change* in firing frequency as a response, be it an increase, a decrease, or some combination of the two. That is how the word is used here.

In Hartline's (1938) experiments on the frog the basic discharge pattern of a particular cell remained fixed irrespective of stimulus size, stimulus strength, etc., but this was not at all what Kuffler found in the cat. Instead he was impressed with what he referred to as the "fluidity" of a cell's response as stimulus conditions varied. One example of this fluidity is shown in figure 9.7, which is taken from figure 5 of Kuffler's 1952 paper.

Figure 9.7 shows the responses of an on-center cell when a relatively small stimulus (somewhat less than a degree in diameter) is flashed on and off in the very middle of the receptive field. In the upper panel the luminance of the spot is such that the cell responds with a weak on-discharge. In the lower panel the only change is an increase in the stimulus luminance, and now the cell responds with a stronger burst at ON and a discharge at OFF as well, although the latter is quite weak. This particular kind of "fluidity of response" was, if I read Kuffler right, at least part of the basis for the opinion he expressed in the following statement about the functional organization of receptive fields: "It must not be inferred, however, that the centers are quite uniform and receive no contribution which is characteristic of the surround" (Kuffler

1953, p. 62). As noted below, the behavior of the cell in figure 9.7 also agreed qualitatively with the subsequent difference-of-Gaussians model of Rodieck (1965).

Mutual Antagonism

Probably the most important legacy of the 1952 and 1953 papers for the understanding of ON- and OFF-center receptive fields is the concept that the signals from the center and those from the surround oppose each other. Kuffler's notion was that, when signals are simultaneously dispatched from different receptive field locations, they interact somewhere in the retinal neural circuitry in a manner that he himself expressed as follows: "Functionally the center and the surround regions are opposed, the one tending to suppress the other. The ganglion cell is subjected to multiple influences from its receptive field and its discharge will express the balance between these opposing and interacting influences" (1953, p. 62). To illustrate this, an experiment on an ON-center cell from Kuffler's 1953 paper is shown in figure 9.8.

In the uppermost panel one small spot was turned on and then off again in the middle of the receptive field, as indicated by the cartoon to the left. In the middle panel the central spot was not used. Instead a stimulus of twice the diameter of that in the uppermost panel and also more luminous was directed to the periphery. A moderately strong off-discharge resulted. In the bottom panel the two stimuli were applied simultaneously (in the same locations as before) and produced a weaker on-discharge than when the central spot alone was used. The off-discharge was weaker than when the peripheral stimulus alone was used. Because no maintained discharge was included in any of the records, one can not *see* the effect of inhibitory inputs on the ganglion cell when the flash goes ON in the uppermost panel or when the flash goes OFF in the middle panel. But in the text Kuffler explains that weakening of the discharges at ON and OFF occurred when both spots were applied simultaneously because the central stimulus did not only cause the cell to discharge at ON, but at offset it also "suppressed" the discharge generated by the peripheral spot at OFF. Correspondingly, the peripheral spot caused a discharge at offset, but when it went on it also "suppressed" the on-discharge set up by the central stimulus. In other words, the "functional antagonism" between the receptive field center and the periphery explained the results (Kuffler 1952, p. 286)

It is worth noting that Kuffler did not use the term "the inhibitory surround," an expression sometimes attributed to him by others who write on the interaction between the center and the surround in Kuffler cells. A forerunner of Kuffler's succinctly stated principle of mutual antagonism between a receptive field's center and its surround was Granit's often-repeated opinion that the ON- and the Off-systems antagonize each other. He was so impressed by this feature of the responses that he elicited with diffuse lights that the very last vision paper (1951) based on his own experiments bore the title "The antagonism between the on- and the off-systems in the cat's retina."

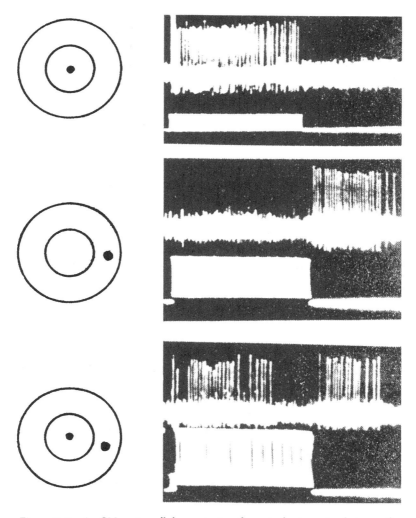

Figure 9.8 An ON-center cell demonstrating the mutual antagonism between the center and the surround. For details see text. (After Kuffler 1953)

I want to make one final comment on Kuffler's 1952 and 1953 papers by pointing out that you cannot read them without being impressed by his generosity and modesty, and therefore admire him even more. For example, he concluded his presentation at Cold Spring Harbor in the following gracious way: "That the retinal discharge is the result of inhibitory-excitatory influences has been discussed at length by Granit and his co-workers and these papers should be consulted (Donner and Willmer 1950; Granit 1947, 1950). By their different experimental procedures they have also shown the plasticity of discharge types. This paper merely stresses one new approach in the analytical study of these complex phenomena."

I will now leave the era of Granit and Kuffler and their co-workers, but not before stressing that what we have learned from them still constitutes a very large proportion of what we know today about vertebrate retinal ganglion cells with center-surround organized receptive fields. Of course, a fair amount of quantitative data has been added to our knowledge, and it is now fashionable to talk about receptive field properties in terms of models. That brings me to the third chapter of this brief saga about retinal ganglion cells, and it begins with Bob Rodieck.

R. W. RODIECK

Rodieck's experimental work with Jonathan Stone and the quantitative presentation of the model that emerged from that work unquestionably initiated the modern era of retinal ganglion cell study. It changed the manner in which many investigators of ganglion cells conducted their experiments and described their results.

Why Models?

Although both Granit and Kuffler chose to work on the mammalian retina because it is a readily accessible part of the central nervous system, there are other important reasons to study retinal ganglion cell behavior. One of these is to learn the role the retinal signal plays in how we see. To this end, one needs to know how ganglion cells respond, not only to one particular stimulus, such as a flashing spot or bar in some location within the receptive field, but also to arbitrary stimuli. If we know how a retinal ganglion cell's responsiveness (sensitivity or gain) varies as a function of position within the receptive field, and if the signals generated at different retinal positions combine linearly to set the magnitude of the cell's response, then we might be able to predict the cell's response to any arbitrary spatial pattern that falls on a part of the receptive field or covers the entire field, as most natural visual scenes do.

In the early 1960s Rodieck and Stone worked together in Peter Bishop's laboratory in Sydney, Australia. They used both moving spots of light and stationary flashing ones to determine the cells' responsiveness as Kuffler had done. One of the differences between their experiments and the previous ones of Kuffler was that Rodieck and Stone applied stimulus spots to more than one hundred locations within some of the receptive fields and judged the strength of the response at each location by listening to it. In addition, they used average response histograms as a quantitative measure of response magnitude (and time course). From these results they mapped the spatial distribution of responsiveness within the receptive fields of Kuffler cells. Initially they presented a qualitative model that explained the varying discharge patterns that they obtained at different locations (Rodieck and Stone 1965b, figure 8).

In the same year Rodieck (1965) published his quantitative version of the model in which the presumed properties of the receptive field were described in mathematical terms. This first quantitative model of mammalian receptive fields has come to be known as the *difference-of-Gaussians (DOG) model*.

Rodieck and Stone (1965b) suggested that one may view the receptive fields of Kuffler cells as having a *center response mechanism* and a *surround response mechanism*. Each mechanism may be visualized as a set of receptors and inter-neurons whose stimulus-evoked activities are independently pooled into a single output signal from the center mechanism and another output signal, of the opposite sign, from the surround mechanism.

The *sensitivity distribution* within each mechanism was represented by a Gaussian surface and, although the terms *center* and *surround* were retained, the assumption was that the two concentric Gaussian surfaces overlapped in the central portion of the receptive field. The center and surround signals were assumed to combine linearly to determine the rate at which the ganglion cell fires impulses. Figure 9.9 (based on Rodieck and Stone 1965a, 1965b) summarizes some of the main features of the DOG model. If you make a vertical cut through the midpoint of two concentric Gaussian surfaces, you get two Gaussian profiles. These are shown in the center of the figure. The center's

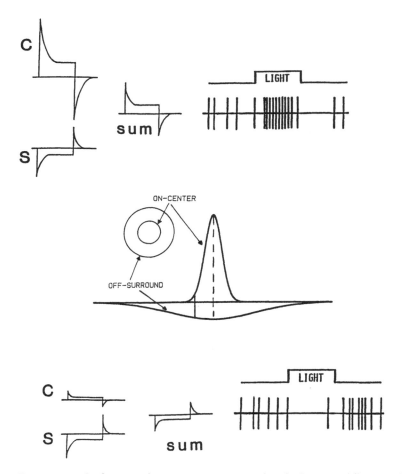

Figure 9.9 Qualitative, schematic representation of Rodieck's 1965 difference-of-Gaussians model, which is explained in full in text. (After Rodieck and Stone 1965)

profile is tall and narrow; the surround's is low and broad and has been drawn upside down to indicate that the two output signals are of different signs.

The time course of the output signals, according to Rodieck and Stone's suggestion, is sketched for the center and the surround (figure 9.9, C and S) assuming that the stimulus is a square pulse. For both of these hypothetical signals a deflection upwards implies that the response mechanism provides an excitatory drive to the ganglion cell, while a deflection downwards implies an inhibitory drive.

If a cell has an ON-center as is assumed in figure 9.9, then the center's output signal consists of a sudden rise at light onset, followed by an exponential-like decay (Rodieck and Stone 1965a. p. 588) to a plateau. At offset there is a sudden dip followed by an exponential-like rise. The surround signal follows an inverted time course. The amplitude of each signal is set by the responsiveness of the mechanism in question at the point at which the stimulus falls. As mentioned before, the outputs from the two mechanisms are assumed to combine linearly (as are signals within each mechanism). Therefore, according to the model, whether at any specific point within the receptive field a cell's response will be dominated by inputs from the center or from the surround will depend upon the difference between the responsiveness of the two mechanisms.

Figure 9.9 shows one stimulus being applied to the very middle of the receptive field, with a second one applied (at a different time) close to the "edge" of the center. For the central stimulus the presumed output signals from the center and the surround mechanisms, as well as the sum of these two, are shown above the sensitivity profiles, and for the peripheral stimulus the corresponding signals are shown below. In the middle of the receptive field the center's responsiveness is so high compared to the surround's that, when the outputs of the center and the surround are combined, the center "wins." This results in a discharge pattern with the characteristics shown: an excitatory burst of spikes at ON, an inhibitory pause at OFF. When the center and surround signals generated by the peripheral stimulus are combined, the surround "wins" and the "sum-signal" generates a very different response pattern: a short pause at ON and a weak discharge at OFF.

The above is a presentation in layman's language of some of the basic features of the difference-of-Gaussians model, and clearly Kuffler's concept of how the center and the surround oppose each other, as seen in figure 9.8, is an important feature of the model. Similarly Kuffler's result, shown in figure 9.7, can be understood in terms of the model: the stimulus in the upper panel generated an output signal from the very sensitive center mechanism but was too week to elicit one from the surround. The stronger stimulus in the lower panel of figure 9.7 was sufficient to stimulate the surround, too, which resulted in a weak off-burst.

Since Rodieck's 1965 model was first published, experiments have revealed some new information about the spatial organization of the receptive fields of mammalian retinal ganglion cells. It has become necessary to add new features to the original DOG model (e.g., Hochstein and Shapley 1976a,b) or to make modifications to accommodate new findings (e.g., Derrington and Lennie 1982). However, to many of us the DOG model has been and continues to be an invaluable aid for understanding signal processing in the neural network of center-surround organized receptive fields. Moreover, the fact that many of Kuffler's findings (as you have just seen) went into building the model once again points out how important he was to the study of the neural mechanisms of the mammalian retina.

PARALLEL PATHWAYS

The concept of parallel pathways from the retina to the cortex is presently a very popular topic in visual physiology (to be really up-to-date, one should talk about *parallel streams*), and some aspects of this topic will be dealt with later in this volume (see Chapter 11 by Peter Lennie). My justification for mentioning it here is that it started with retinal ganglion cells and is an important milestone along the road of retinal ganglion cell research from 1927 to 1992.

In the mid-1960s the cat was the most popular mammal for retinal ganglion cell experiments, but many other vertebrate species, mammals and nonmammals, had been or were also studied. Studies of these varied species taught us an important lesson: not all vertebrate retinal receptive fields are created equal. Not even all mammalian receptive fields are organized in the manner that Kuffler described.

Among nonmammals, since 1960 (Maturana et al.) the frog and since 1963 (Maturana and Frenk) the pigeon have been known to have ganglion cells with receptive fields that are organized very differently from that of the Kuffler cells. In 1963 (Barlow and Hill) the rabbit was shown to have ganglion cells with "funny receptive fields" that produced a response to a moving stimulus only if the motion was in a certain direction. To stationary flashing stimuli these cells responded with an on-off discharge, whatever the location of the spot within the field. Three years later (Michael 1966) the squirrel joined the club; it, too, was shown to have directionally selective ganglion cells. Then a footnote to the first of the two 1965 Rodieck and Stone papers hinted at what was to come with regard to cat retinal ganglion cells. They found one cell that did not behave as a proper ON- or OFF-center cell. However, it was not until the mid-1970s that several receptive fields other than the Kuffler type were described in the cat (for reviews see Rodieck 1979; Levick and Thibos 1983). Now we know that these non-Kuffler cells constitute approximately 35 percent of the cat's retinal ganglion cell population. Regrettably many of these developments were overlooked by investigators who worked on the cat retina in the late 1960s. They thought of the cat's retinal ganglion cells purely in terms of the types that Kuffler had described. It was believed that higher mammals had simpler retinas.

At this time Fergus Campbell in Cambridge had a young, bright student by the name of John Robson, and the two of them were convinced that sinusoidal grating patterns constituted a useful tool for investigating spatial properties of the human visual system. Their experiments, however, could not determine the extent to which the neural mechanisms for spatial vision resided in the retina. They were eager to find out, by animal experiments, how a retina that was presumed to be similar to that of man responded to gratings. Fergus Campbell had previously spent some months at Northwestern when the biomedical engineering program was in its very beginnings. He knew that I had a laboratory for recording from cat retinal ganglion cells, so in 1964 Fergus "shipped" John Robson—together with the world's first "grating machine" for use in single-cell experiments—to this side of the Atlantic. We recorded from Kuffler cells, hoping to learn how these ON- and OFF-center cells responded to gratings, and therefore what they might contribute to the cat's spatial vision.

It came as a surprise to us to find that both the ON-center and the OFF-center class could be divided into two functionally quite different kinds of cells. Because we did not know what the functional significance of these very different kinds was, we gave them the noncommittal names X and Y cells. There were several differences between the two groups, but the major one on which we (that is, John Robson) based the grouping was that X cells summed signals generated at different locations in the receptive field in an approximately linear fashion, Y cells in a very nonlinear way (Enroth-Cugell and Robson 1966).

Thus, by the mid-1970s it was clear that the cat's retina contains several classes of cell with quite different response properties: X cells, Y cells, and the various cells indicated above that are neither X nor Y. That retinal ganglion cells have different response properties implies that they extract different aspects of the optical image that falls on their receptive fields. That is, the cat retina had been shown to process information in parallel. It would soon become clear that this parallel processing extended beyond the retina all the way to the cortex. A substantial part of the work that led to this realization was done in Canberra, Australia, by Cleland, Dubin, Fukuda, Hoffmann, Levick, Stone, and others. In this country Sherman and co-workers made important contributions to this development.

The title of my chapter says that I will deal with retinal ganglion cells, so this is all that I will say about parallel pathways. However, I want to point out that not only are there parallel visual pathways, but unfortunately there are also parallel terminologies. I have only used one of these, which is not out of disrespect for the individuals who generated the other terminologies, but in order to minimize confusion. (For examples of these other terminologies, see Rodieck 1979; Thibos and Levick 1983; Rodieck and Brening 1983.)

AFTERTHOUGHTS

On these pages I have dealt only with the ancient and the not-quite-so-ancient history of the *physiology* of vertebrate retinal ganglion cells. There is a whole other side to the world of retinal ganglion cells, and that is their *morphology* and the relationship of morphology to physiological types. I would like to

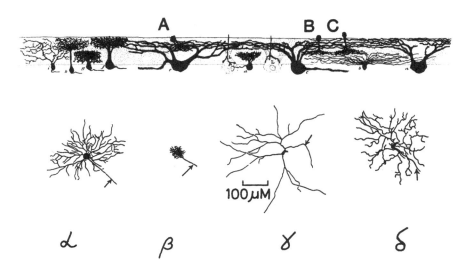

Figure 9.10 Ganglion cell layer of a dog retina (above; from Cajal 1892) and a cat retina (below; from Boycott and Wässle 1974). See text for a full description.

conclude with a few thoughts that come to mind as I think back to what has happened in visual neurophysiology over the past forty years.

For no less than one hundred years it has been known that mammalian ganglion cells, although a well-defined class of retinal neurons, certainly do not all look alike. This is obvious from a glance at figure 9.10. The upper part of the figure shows a vertical section through the ganglion cell layer of a dog retina, taken from Cajal's work published in 1892. The cells labeled A, B, and C are the only ones that are not ganglion cells. One need not consider any details to appreciate the morphological diversity among the ganglion cells of this particular mammal. It is also obvious that the soma sizes and axon diameters vary considerably, with a large soma giving rise to a thicker axon than a small soma. The differences in sizes and characters of the dendritic trees are also striking.

I find it rather curious that it took about eighty years after the publication of the picture of these dog ganglion cells before it was demonstrated that there is also a remarkable structural diversity among cat retinal ganglion cells and that there is a correlation between structure and function. Now, when one looks back, it is puzzling that suggestions failed to emerge earlier that in the cat the many differences in ganglion cell response properties—those of ON- and OFF-center cells, X and Y cells, and cells with several different properties unlike those of X or Y cells—might be related to ganglion cell morphology. Not until in 1974 were any exhaustive descriptions of the shapes of cat retinal ganglion cells and their relation to function published. Largely thanks to the fruitful interaction between the physiologists in Canberra (Cleland, Levick, and others) and two outstanding morphologists and their co-workers in Europe, Boycott and Wässle, we now understand the morphology of the cat's different functional cell classes (Cleland and Levick 1974; Boycott and Wässle 1974).

The lower half of fig. 9.10 shows four cells drawn from a flat-mount of the cat's retina (Boycott and Wässle 1974). The cell farthest to the left is of the anatomical alpha type, the cell next to it is of the anatomical beta type, and both of them are from the same retinal eccentricity (1.2 mm from the area centralis). The beta cell has a considerably smaller cell body and smaller spread of the dendritic tree. The alpha cell is physiologically a Y cell, and the beta cell corresponds to an X cell. The two cat cells farthest to the right belong to the class of functionally diverse cells that are neither X nor Y cells and are also morphologically diverse.

It is also surprising that different functional roles among the cat's retinal ganglion cells were not sought much earlier in view of what was known about transmission of sensory information in the somatic peripheral nervous system. As early as 1927 Erlanger suggested that information about *different sense modalities* is carried in fibers of different conduction velocities and hence different diameters (Granit 1955, pp. 45–46; see also Erlanger and Gasser 1938). Consider that in 1938 Bishop and O'Leary demonstrated that electrical stimulation of the cat's optic nerve generated two well-separated humps in the compound action potential recorded in the optic tract, and during the 1950s and 1960s it was established that the axons of the cat's retinal ganglion cells fall into groups of different conduction speeds (see the review by Thibos and Levick 1983). In spite of this knowledge, prior to 1971 (Cleland, Dubin, and Levick) little thought was given to the idea that retinal ganglion cell axons of different diameters and conduction velocities might transmit different "visual modalities"—i.e., that different aspects of the retinal image might travel in axons of different diameters.

My final "afterthought" is also tied to morphology. When William Rushton came to spend a year in Granit's laboratory in 1948 he was critical, as was his nature, of Granit's lack of serious attempts to establish exactly the structure from which the electrode picked up spikes. So Rushton decided to find out.

First of all he convinced himself that the Granit-Svaetichin type electrode did not record from clusters of synchronized cells. While recording spike potentials, he exerted pressure on the retina with a sharp electrode and noted that there was always a sudden and irreversible termination of firing, never "a step down to half size, etc." (Rushton 1949, p. 743). He also estimated how fast the spike amplitude declined when the electrode was moved away from the cell. In figure 9.11 you see Rushton holding the "rope," as he called it, of seven electrodes, each of which could be separately connected to the amplifier. During an experiment he first adjusted the position of the central electrode on the retina to record a spike at maximal amplitude. By knowing the distance between the midpoint of the central electrode and all the surrounding ones he determined that, at 0.1 mm in all directions from the optimal point, the amplitude of the same spike had fallen to only half of its maximal amplitude.

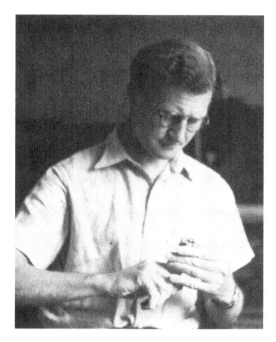

Figure 9.11 William Rushton in 1948 in Ragnar Granit's laboratory in Stockholm.

In several experiments in which the corpus vitreum was removed and the retina brightly lit, Rushton then recorded one or two well-isolated spikes, after which he drew a picture (using a low-power microscope) of the structures in the vicinity of the electrode tip. This drawing was later compared to a flat-mount of the retina. One such drawing is shown on the left side of figure 9.12.

Close to the bottom there is a vessel, and above and below it a few axons are drawn. The circle indicates the position of the tip of the electrode with which Rushton had recorded one very large, well-isolated spike as well as a second well-isolated spike half the size of the large one. Two large ganglion cells are drawn above the position of the electrode. On the basis of his knowledge of how far from a ganglion cell a spike can be recorded, Rushton noted that there were no other structures in the vicinity that could possibly have generated the two spikes. Rushton therefore concluded that the large spike came from the cell closest to the electrode, the smaller one from the cell farther away from the electrode. Although it was not drawn in this figure, Rushton points out in the text that the "giant cells" from which he recorded have "a wide-thrown ramification of branching filaments extending some 0.5 mm in all directions" (Rushton 1949).

On the right side of figure 9.12 you see one ON-alpha cell and one OFF-alpha cell taken from figure 12 of Wässle et al. 1981. Considering the similar sizes and relative positions of the members of the two cell pairs, including the fact that Rushton's cells (although not shown) have dendritic trees of much the same size as the two alpha cells, it seems likely to me that Rushton discovered Y cells forty-three years ago.

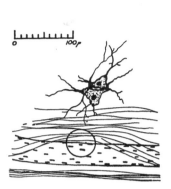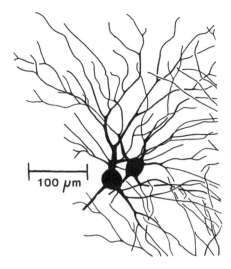

Figure 9.12   On the left side is figure 3 from Rushton 1949. Part of figure 12 from Wässle et al. 1981 is shown on the right. See text for an explanation.

As a "summary afterthought," it seems probable to me that we would have made faster progress in understanding how the retina works if physiology and morphology had started to walk hand in hand at an earlier stage.

Last of all, I want to stress once more that these pages do not by any stretch of the imagination include every important development with respect to our knowledge of retinal ganglion cells between the 1920s and the 1990s. For example, I have not mentioned contributions by Otto Creutzfeldt in Germany and those whom he trained, Maffei and his group in Italy, Horace Barlow's pioneering work on *what* it is that retinal ganglion cells signal and *how* they do it (e.g., Barlow and Levick 1969a, 1969b), or those who demonstrated the anatomical correlate of the functional ON- and OFF-center dichotomy (Nelson et al. 1978), nor have I touched upon many other aspects of the world of retinal ganglion cells. This has been a journey through time with only a few selected stops.

REFERENCES

Adrian ED (1926) The impulses produced by sensory nerve endings. Part 1. J Physiol 61:49–72.

Adrian ED (1935) The Mechanism of Nervous Action. Philadelphia: University of Pennsylvania Press.

Adrian ED (1953) Sensory messages and sensation. The response of the olfactory organ to different smells. Acta Physiol Scand 29:5–14.

Adrian ED, Matthews R (1927a) The action of light on the eye. Part I. The discharge of impulses in the optic nerve and its relation to the electric changes in the retina. J Physiol 63:378–414.

Adrian ED, Matthews R (1927b) The action of light on the eye. Part II. The processes involved in retinal excitation. J Physiol 64:279–301.

Adrian ED, Matthews R (1928) The action of light on the eye. Part III. The interactions of retinal neurones. J Physiol 65:273–298.

Adrian ED, Zotterman Y (1926a) The impulses produced by sensory nerve endings. Part II. The response of a single end-organ. J Physiol 61:151–171.

Adrian ED, Zotterman Y (1926b) The impulses produced by sensory nerve endings. Part III. Impulses set up by touch and pressure. J Physiol 61:465–483.

Barlow HB (1953) Summation and inhibition in the frog's retina. J Physiol 119:69–88.

Barlow HB (1983) Understanding natural vision. In: Braddock OJ, Sleigh AC, eds. Physical and Biological Processing of Images, Vol. 11, pp 2–14. Berlin: Springer.

Barlow HB, Hill RM (1963) Selective sensitivity to direction of movement in ganglion cells of the rabbit retina. Science 139:412–414.

Bishop GH, O'Leary JL (1938) Potential records from the optic cortex of the cat. J Neurophysiol 1:391–404.

Boycott BB, Wässle H (1974) The morphological types of ganglion cells of the domestic cat's retina. J Physiol 240:397–419.

Cajal SR (1893) La retine des vertebres. La Cellule 9:17–257. (Translated by Maguire D and Rodieck RW.) In The Vertebrate Retina. San Francisco: Freeman, 1973.

Cleland BG, Dubin MW, Levick WR (1971) Sustained and transient neurones in the cat's retina and lateral geniculate nucleus. J Physiol 217:473–496.

Cleland BG, Levick WR (1974) Brisk and sluggish concentrically organized ganglion cells in the cat's retina. J Physiol 240:424–456.

Derrington AM, Lennie P (1982) The influence of temporal frequency and adaptation level on receptive field organization of retinal ganglion cells in cat. J Physiol 333:343–366.

Enroth-Cugell C, Robson JG (1966) The contrast sensitivity of retinal ganglion cells of the cat. J Physiol 187:517–552.

Enroth-Cugell C, Robson JG (1984) Functional characteristics and diversity of cat retinal ganglion cells. Invest Ophthalmol 25:250–267.

Erlanger J (1927) The interpretation of the action potentials in cutaneous and muscle nerve. Am J Physiol 82:644–55.

Erlanger J, Gasser H (1937) Electrical signs of nervous activity. Philadelphia: University of Pennsylvania Press.

Forbes A, Campbell CJ, Williams, HB (1924) Electrical records of afferent nerve impulses from muscular receptors. Am J Physiol 69:283–303.

Forbes A, Renshaw B, Rempel B (1937) Units of electrical activity in the cerebral cortex. Am J Physiol 119:309–310.

Forbes A, Thacher C (1920) Amplification of action currents with the electron tube in recording with the string galvanometer. Am J Physiol 52:409–471.

Gasser HS, Erlanger J (1922) A study of the action currents of nerve with the cathode ray oscillograph. Am J Physiol 62:496–524.

Gasser HS, Newcomer HS (1921) Physiological action currents in the phrenic nerve. An application of the thermionic vacuum tube to nerve physiology. Am J Physiol 57:1–26.

Granit R (1947) Sensory mechanisms of the retina. London: Oxford University Press.

Granit R (1951) The antagonism between the on- and off-systems in the cat's retina. L'annee Psychol 50:129–134.

Granit R (1955) Receptors and Sensory Perception. New Haven: Yale University Press.

Granit R (1966) Charles Scott Sherrington, an Appraisal. London: Thomas Nelson.

Granit R, Ratliff F (1985) Haldan Keffer Hartline: 1903–1983. Biographical memoirs of fellows of the Royal Society. 31:236–292.

Granit R, Svaetichin G (1939) Principles and technique of the electrophysiological analysis of colour reception with the aid of microelectrodes. Upsala Läkareförenings förhandlingar. Ny följd, Bd. XLV. 1–4. Upsala: Almqvist & Wiksells Boktryckeri-A.-B.

Granit R, Therman PO (1935) Excitation and inhibition in the retina and in the optic nerve. J Physiol 83:359–381.

Hammond P (1974) Cat retinal ganglion cells: size and shape of receptive field centres. J Physiol 242:99–118.

Hartline HK (1938) The response of single optic nerve fibers of the vertebrate eye to illumination of the retina. Am J Physiol 121:400–415.

Hartline HK (1940) The effects of spatial summation in the retina on the excitation of the fibers of the optic nerve. Am J Physiol 121:700–711.

Hartline HK, Graham CH (1932) Nerve impulses from single receptors in the eye. J Cell Comp Physiol 1:277–295.

Hochstein S, Shapley RM (1976a) Quantitative analysis of retinal ganglion cell classifications. J Physiol 262:237–264.

Hochstein S, Shapley RM (1976b) Linear and nonlinear spatial subunits in Y cat retinal ganglion cells. J Physiol 262:265–284 .

Kuffler SW (1952) Neurons in the retina: organization, inhibition, and excitation problems. Cold Spring Harbor Symposia on Quantitative Biology Volume XVII: The Neuron. Cold Spring Harbor, LI: Long Island Biological Association.

Kuffler SW (1953) Discharge patterns and functional organization of mammalian retina. J Neurophysiol 16:37–68.

Levick WR (1972) Receptive fields of retinal ganglion cells. In: Fuortes MGF, ed. Handbook of Sensory Physiology. Vol. VII/2 Physiology of Photoreceptor Organs, pp 531–566. Berlin: Springer-Verlag

Levick WR, Thibos LN (1982) Analysis of orientation bias in cat retina. J Physiol 329:243–261.

Levick WR, Thibos LN (1983) Receptive fields of cat ganglion cells: classification and construction. IN: Progress in Retinal Research (Osborne N, Chader G, eds), pp 267–314.

Lucas K (1912) On a mechanical method of correcting photographic records obtained from the capillary electrometer. J. Physiol 44:225–242.

Maturana H, Frenk S (1963) Directional movement and horizontal edge detectors in the pigeon retina. Science 142:977–979.

Maturana H, Lettvin JY, McCulloch WS, Pitts WH (1960) Anatomy and physiology of vision in the frog (Rana pipiens). J Gen Physiol 43:129–175.

Michael CR (1966) Receptive fields of directionally selective units in the optic nerve of the ground squirrel. Science 152:1092–1094.

Nelson R, Famiglietti, Jr EV, Kolb H (1978) Intracellular staining reveals different levels of stratification for on- and off-center ganglion cells in cat retina. J Neurophysiol 41:472–483.

Rodieck RW (1965) Quantitative analysis of cat retinal ganglion cell response to visual stimuli. Vision Res 5:583–601.

Rodieck RW (1979) Visual pathways. Ann Rev Neurosci 2:193–225.

Rodieck RW, Brening RK (1983) Retinal ganglion cells: properties, types, genera, pathways and trans-species comparisons. Brain Behav Evol 23:121–164.

Rodieck RW, Stone J (1965a) Response of cat retinal ganglion cells to moving visual patterns. J Neurophysiol 28:819–832.

Rodieck RW, Stone J (1965b) Analysis of receptive fields of cat retinal ganglion cells. J Neurophysiol 28:833–849.

Rushton WAH (1949) The structure responsible for action potential spikes in the cat's retina. Nature 164:743–744.

Sherrington, C (1906) The integrative action of the nervous system. New Haven: Yale University Press.

Soodak RE, Shapely RM, Kaplan E (1987) Linear mechanism of orientation tuning in the retina and lateral geniculate nucleus of the cat. J Neurophysiol 58:267–275.

Thomson LC (1953) The localization of function in the rabbit retina. J Physiol 119:191–209.

Wässle H, Peichl L, Boycott BB (1981a) Morphology and topography of on- and off-alpha cells in the cat retina. Proc R Soc Lond B 212:157–175.

III Central Visual Pathways

Contrast sensitivity may begin within and depend upon the retina, but it affects the function of all central visual processing. This is evident in the chapters under this heading.

Ehud Kaplan, Pratik Mukherjee, and Robert Shapley have studied information processing in the lateral geniculate nucleus (LGN) with grating stimuli and have observed state-dependent spatiotemporal filtering by LGN neurons. The function of parallel pathways and their relation to contrast sensitivity is taken up by Peter Lennie in his chapter, next. A. B. Bonds then presents his view on the mechanism of the cortical contrast gain control—a cortical mechanism observed in the primary visual cortex of the cat. This mechanism is responsible for regulating cortical responsiveness contingent on local contrast in the image. At the end of this section, Karen and Russell De Valois present the results of their research about lines labeled for pattern and color within the human visual pathway.

10 Information Filtering in the Lateral Geniculate Nucleus

Ehud Kaplan, Pratik Mukherjee, and
Robert Shapley

The mammalian lateral geniculate nucleus (LGN), strategically interposed between the retina and the visual cortex, has been the focus of intensive investigations for many years. Here we wish to focus on two aspects of LGN function: *stimulus*-dependent and *state*-dependent information filtering. We will forge a link between the recent biophysical findings from in vitro studies and the physiological results we and others have obtained in vivo. Several excellent reviews of LGN structure and function exist in the literature (for example, Singer 1977; Sherman and Koch 1986; Casagrande and Norton 1991). Therefore, we will not attempt another comprehensive review, but rather report some results from our ongoing investigation of LGN function, which exploits the simultaneous recording from a single retinal ganglion cell and its LGN target. We will begin with a brief synopsis of some of the relevant findings regarding information filtering in the LGN.

SOME ANATOMY, PHYSIOLOGY, AND BIOPHYSICS

The LGN is the thalamic relay station for visual information into the higher centers of the brain. In addition to the input from the retina, the LGN receives massive projections from layer VI of the visual cortex, from the brain stem, and from other brain structures. It is estimated that 80 to 90 percent of the synapses on LGN relay cells convey nonretinal inputs to the LGN (Sherman and Koch 1986). Anatomically, two major cell types can be distinguished: principal relay cells and interneurons (Guillery 1966). Elaborate synaptic complexes, called glomeruli (Szentágothai 1973) dot the landscape and provide ample opportunity for interactions among the various inputs and local elements of the LGN. The signals from the two eyes are segregated into separate layers, and in many old-world primates there are six layers, three from each eye. The function of the multiple representation of the world in the various layers has still not been completely determined. The essential elements in the LGN circuitry are shown in the simplified diagram in figure 10.1.

Recent work, mostly in vitro, has added much to our knowledge of the neurotransmitters that are active in the LGN and has established the importance of acetylcholine, GABA (both A and B receptor types), norepinephrine,

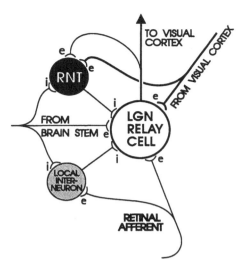

Figure 10.1 The essential elements of the LGN circuitry. Excitatory synapses are marked with an *e*, inhibitory ones with an *i*.

serotonin, and glutamate, with glutamate receptors of both the NMDA (voltage-sensitive) and non-NMDA (voltage-insensitive) types playing an important role (Sillito et al. 1990a,b; Kwon et al. 1991).

The segregation of the ocular inputs; the multiplicity of layer; the variety of cell types, connections, and neurotransmitters; and especially the massive nonretinal inputs from the visual cortex and from the brain stem, all suggest that the LGN could significantly modify the flow of visual signals from the retina to the visual cortex and serve as a gate, a filter, or both. However, most of the studies undertaken to establish just what this transformation might be have shown only minor differences between the organization of receptive fields in the retina and that seen in the LGN. This is because most attempts to get at the LGN transformation have compared populations of retinal receptive fields with populations of LGN receptive fields. A much more powerful approach is the direct comparison of a single retinal afferent with the function or properties of its LGN target cell. This is made possible by the fact that in the thalamus it is easy to record afferent activity in the form of slow synaptic (S) potentials, which are also called pre-potentials (Bishop et al. 1958; Hubel and Wiesel 1961; Cleland et al. 1971; Lee et al. 1983; Kaplan and Shapley 1984). It has now been firmly established that (1) every action potential in a retinal afferent fiber elicits an S potential in the LGN (Cleland et al. 1971) (2) all S potentials observed in the LGN are due to the activity of retinal ganglion cells (Kaplan and Shapley 1984), and (3) most LGN principal cells receive the bulk of their excitatory input from a single retinal ganglion cell (Cleland et al. 1971). These observations make it possible to compare quantitatively the input and output of a particular LGN neuron by monitoring both its S potentials and its action potentials.

LGN TRANSFORMATIONS OF RETINAL MESSAGES

The most obvious difference between the retinal and LGN discharges is the significantly lower firing rate of LGN neurons. On average, for every ten retinal spikes only approximately four LGN spikes are relayed to the cortex. This is true for both spontaneous activity and driven responses (Kaplan et al. 1987).

Another prominent difference between receptive fields in the retina and in the LGN was reported by Hubel and Wiesel (1961), who compared the strength of surround inhibition in the retina with that measured in the LGN and found that the LGN surround was substantially stronger. Lee et al. (1983) reported similar results in the monkey. This type of spatial filtering is more pronounced at low temporal frequencies, high contrasts, or deep anesthesia (Kaplan et al. 1987; Kaplan and Shapley unpublished observations). In addition to this modification of the spatial organization of the receptive field, it was observed by Coenen and Vendrick (1972) that the arousal level of the animal modified the relay of retinal activity to the cortex: the ratio of LGN spikes to retinal spikes increased upon arousal. We shall return to this topic later.

An intriguing response observed in the LGN and not in the retina can be recorded from the so-called lagged cells, which respond to steps with a pronounced delay and an anomalous discharge at stimulus offset (Mastronarde 1987a,b; Saul and Humphrey 1990). Recently the possibility has been raised that the lagged cells do not constitute a distinct anatomical group, but rather each cell can become lagged (or nonlagged) under the right circumstances, such as brainstem stimulation (Uhlrich et al. 1990, but compare Humphrey and Saul 1991). The function of such responses will become clearer once this issue is resolved.

Significant insight into the function of the LGN was gained when Llinás and Jahnsen (1982) discovered that thalamic neurons, including those in the LGN, employ calcium channels of a peculiar type (T channels). These channels are inactive at normal resting potential, but are deinactivated when the cell is hyperpolarized (Jahnsen and Llinás 1984) and will produce the so-called low-threshold calcium spike when the hyperpolarized cell is then stimulated. The voltage sensitivity of the T channels provides a potent mechanism for dynamic tuning of thalamic neurons, which can be transformed from a tonic, relaylike behavior when the T channels are inactivated into a phasic, band-pass-filtering mode when the channels are active. The two activity modes are illustrated in figure 10.2, taken from Jahnsen and Llinás (1984).

It would seem that much of the biophysics, neurochemistry, and connectivity of the LGN are devoted to the regulation of the membrane potential of relay cells which, in turn, controls their dynamic response to the retinal input. In fact, it has recently been shown that the steady-state conductance of the T channels is not a step function of membrane potential, but rather varies gradually with the membrane potential of the cells, providing an exquisite tuning mechanism for the filtering action of the LGN. This is illustrated in figure 10.3, redrawn from Coulter et al. 1989.

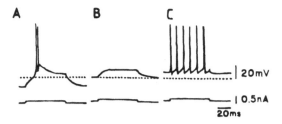

Figure 10.2 The response of thalamic cells to depolarizing current injections applied at three different membrane potentials, from the most hyperpolarized (A) to the most depolarized (C). A typical burst of conventional (Na) action potentials is seen riding the low-threshold calcium spike at A, whereas a sustained discharge results from stimulation at C. (Reproduced with permission from Jahnsen and Llinás 1984)

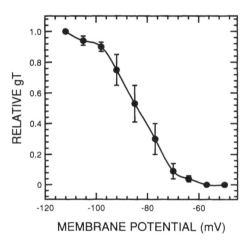

Figure 10.3 The dependence of the steady-state inactivation of the T current in rat thalamo-cortical relay neurons. Note that the available Ca conductance varies gradually, rather than abruptly, as a function of membrane potential. The range of membrane potential in vivo probably never goes more negative than − 75 mV. Error bars represent 1 SEM. (Replotted with permission from Coulter et al. 1989)

The Effect of Stimulus Contrast on Retina-LGN Transmission

Because contrast is a crucial aspect of any visual stimulus, we compared the responses to contrast of retinal ganglion cells with those of their LGN targets. The result was somewhat surprising: increased contrast impaired the steady-state transmission of visual signals from the retina to the cortex. This can be seen in figure 10.4 from Kaplan et al. (1987), which shows the amplitude of responses of a monkey retinal ganglion cell and its LGN target cell in response to a drifting grating. At low contrasts the retina and LGN produced similar responses, but as contrast increased the retinal ganglion cell increased its response more than the LGN neuron did. The transmission ratio, therefore, declined with contrast. This compression of the response range is not simply

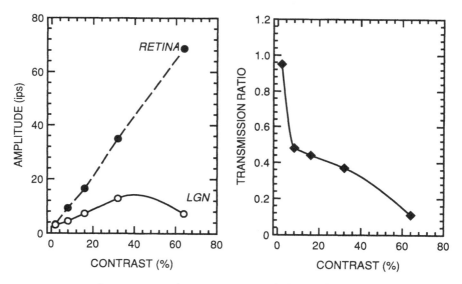

Figure 10.4 (Left) Transmission from retina to LGN declines with contrast. Shown are responses from a monkey retinal ganglion cell and its LGN (parvocellular) target. The stimulus was a black and white grating, 0.8 c/deg, drifting on the face of a CRT (100 cd/m² at 1 Hz. (Right) The transmission ratio (LGN response/S potential response) as a function of contrast. The behavior shown in this figure was typical of both monkey and cat LGN cells. (Reproduced with permission from Kaplan et al. 1987)

due to saturation of LGN neurons at lower contrasts, since we have shown (Kaplan et al. 1987, figure 9) that transmission ratios increase with LGN response if one keeps the stimulus contrast constant and varies other stimulus parameters, such as the temporal or spatial frequency.

The attenuation of retina-to-LGN transmission is a form of automatic gain control, a mechanism whose purpose could be to protect cortical neurons from saturation. If cortical summation were linear, then the contrast gain of cortical cells (the slope of their response vs. contrast function) would be proportional to the number of LGN neurons that synapse on each of the cortical neurons. That number is estimated by Tanaka (1983) to be between ten and thirty neurons, and the resulting high contrast gain would rob the cortex of any useful dynamic range of contrast. In addition to the LGN compression described here, inhibitory mechanisms in the cortex itself probably contribute to further compression of the LGN input.

The cellular mechanism subserving this form of contrast transmission control is unknown, but it is reasonable to assume that it represents an inhibitory response that increases with contrast and that, perhaps, has to exceed a threshold. Such inhibition could be mediated by either the reticular nucleus of the thalamus (RNT, see Ahlsén et al. 1985) or by local GABA-ergic interneurons in the LGN itself. Indeed, Koch (1985) proposed that shunting inhibition would develop once the retinal firing reaches a certain frequency. This could be due to the activity of the relatively fast $GABA_A$ receptors. However, recent work (see Crunelli and Leresche 1991) demonstrated that the slower $GABA_B$

receptors function in the LGN as well, and thus more subtle forms of gain control could be possible even during low retinal activity.

Although it is reasonable to attribute the contrast-induced decline in transmission ratio to inhibition, we should point out that this idea may be at odds with the observation cited above, that transmission ratios increase with LGN response. Therefore, other mechanisms might be involved. For example, it is possible that the transmission gain adjustment is accomplished via the excitatory corticofugal feedback, which could regulate the membrane potential of the relay cells. Since NMDA type glutamate receptors have been implicated in retina/LGN transmission (Kwon et al. 1991), reduced excitation from the cortex would lower the membrane potential, decrease the size of the EPSPs from the retina, and lower the fraction of S potentials that elicit LGN spikes. Further research is needed to establish firmly the biophysical mechanism of transmission control by contrast.

STATE-DEPENDENT INFLUENCES ON INFORMATION TRANSMISSION THROUGH THE LGN

Spontaneous Changes in Retina-LGN Transmission

It has long been known that the activity of the lateral geniculate nucleus is affected by changes in arousal during the sleep-wake cycle (McIlwain 1972; Singer 1977; Livingstone and Hubel 1981). The maintained discharge of cat LGN relay cells is higher during waking states and during rapid eye movement (REM) sleep than during slow-wave sleep, which is characterized by high-amplitude low-frequency synchronized activity in the electroencephalogram (EEG). Recordings from monkey LGN indicate that visual responses are reduced in sleep states as compared to waking states and are also more phasic, tending to respond preferentially to the onset of stimulation and suppress the sustained components (Singer 1977). During low arousal states, cat LGN neurons tend to fire characteristic "bursts" of action potentials, a firing pattern that is not observed during waking states (McIlwain 1972). In the monkey these bursts have been called *grouped discharges* (Singer 1977).

The agent of these state-dependent effects is the brain stem projection to the LGN. It has been shown that electrical stimulation of midbrain reticular structures during EEG-synchronized states increases the maintained discharge and the visually driven responses of LGN cells in the cat and monkey, thus mimicking the effect of arousal. In the cat a particularly effective area for regulating LGN function is the parabrachial nucleus (Hu et al. 1989), which sends a largely cholinergic projection to thalamic relay cells and to interneurons (Uhlrich et al. 1988).

Using quasi-intracellular recording methods in the LGNs of unanesthetized cats, Coenen and Vendrik (1972) reported significant variability in the proportion of retinal EPSPs that generate action potentials. This fraction is close to 1.0 during waking states, as characterized by desynchronized EEGs, but it falls to less than 0.5 during EEG-synchronized states. Hence the responsiveness of the LGN to its retinal input appears to vary considerably, depending on the behavioral state of the animal. This is illustrated in figure 10.5, which shows results obtained in our laboratory from simultaneous recording of the maintained discharge of S potentials and spikes from an ON-center Y cell, recorded in the LGN of a cat anesthetized with urethane and paralyzed with Flaxedil. Part A shows over 40 minutes without any modulation of the visual input. The physiological state of the animal (heart rate, blood pressure, CO_2 level in the blood) was constant throughout the recording session. Nevertheless, during this period both retinal input and LGN output varied, but the variations in the LGN discharge were significantly higher than those seen in the retinal discharge, so that the ratio between the firing rates of the LGN and the retina, shown in part B, varied widely. In part C the power spectrum of these fluctuations in LGN transmission demonstrates that most of the variability occurs on a very slow time scale, with periods in the range of 100 to more than 1000 seconds. The details of this power spectrum can be expected to change considerably for various cells, animals, or levels of anesthesia. The exact source of these variations is not yet firmly established, although they are likely to involve the projections from the brain stem.

Recent intracellular recordings from cat LGN relay cells in vivo have implicated the low-threshold Ca^{2+} spikes of Llinás and Jahnsen (1982) as the mechanism for the burst discharges recorded extracellularly during states of low arousal (Lu et al. 1990; Sherman et al. 1991). Bursts can be reliably identified from extracellular LGN spike trains as clusters of action potentials with interspike intervals (ISIs) less than or equal to 4 msec. The studies report that bursts occur when the cell is at relatively hyperpolarized resting membrane potentials, which is consistent with the in vitro findings for low-threshold Ca^{2+} spikes, and that this bursting activity declines when the cell's resting potential rises or during electrical stimulation of the parabrachial nucleus. This is consistent with another in vivo intracellular study of the cat LGN which showed that the membrane potential of relay cells is hyperpolarized during slow-wave sleep states relative to the potential during waking states (Hirsch et al. 1983).

A burst discharge, followed by tonic (nonburst) spikes from the extracellularly recorded response of an OFF-center Y cell to the dark portions of a drifting sinusoidal grating, is shown in figure 10.6. The three spikes in the burst occur with ISIs of less than 4 msec. We have observed that bursts always precede tonic spikes in the response to the onset of a visual stimulus, as also reported by Lu et al. (1990). The arrow labeled B in figure 10.6 indicates an S potential triggering a tonic spike with a latency of less than 1 msec. Virtually all LGN spikes occur within 1 to 3 msec of an S potential (Levick et al, 1972; Lee et al. 1983). However, the situation is different for spikes fired in a burst. They do not show the inflection, like the one at arrow B, that is typical of tonic spikes. Instead we observe that each burst is consistently preceded by an S potential, with a latency of 3 to 10 msec between the S potential and the first spike of the burst. An example is shown at arrow A in figure 10.6, where the S potential precedes the burst by about 4 msec. We routinely observe that S potentials trigger burst discharges after a delay of between 3 and 10 msec.

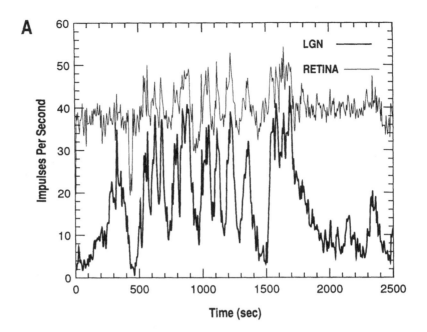

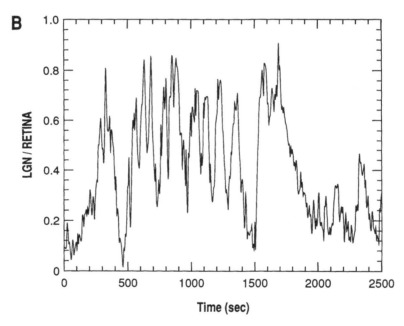

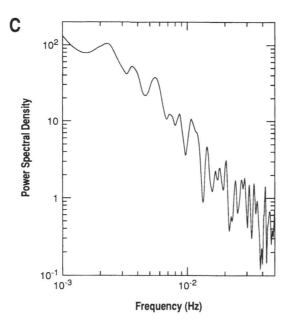

Figure 10.5 Spontaneous changes in the responsiveness of an ON-center Y cell to its S potential input. The recording is from the LGN of a cat anesthetized with urethane and paralyzed with Flaxedil. (A) Variation in the maintained discharge rate of the S potential (thin, upper line) and its LGN target neuron (thick, lower line) during 2500 s of continuous recording. Each data point represents the average firing rate for a period of 6 s. (B) Variations in transmission ratio (LGN rate/S potential rate) in A for each 6-second period. (C) Smoothed power spectrum of the temporal fluctuations in transmission ratio shown in B.

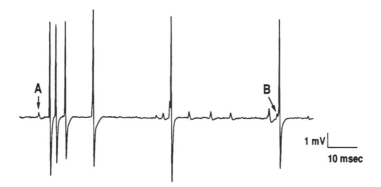

Figure 10.6 LGN spikes and S potentials recorded from an OFF-center Y cell in cat LGN in response to the dark portion of a sine wave grating (28 percent contrast, 1 c/deg) drifting at 2 Hz. The first three spikes form a burst discharge, with interspike intervals less than 4 msec. Note also the variability in the peak-to-peak amplitude of these three spikes. Arrow A indicates the S potential triggering the burst of spikes. Arrow B indicates an S potential triggering a tonic spike.

This longer latency for burst discharges is consistent with the idea that these bursts are generated from more hyperpolarized resting membrane potentials and hence require more time to reach firing threshold. We wish to emphasize that our data suggest that the bursts are not an interruption of the information flow from the retina to the visual cortex, but rather constitute a distinct mode of transmission.

The dynamics of the T type Ca^{2+} channel can be expected to influence the temporal response characteristics of relay cells when they are at hyperpolarized resting membrane potentials (Sherman and Koch 1986). Quantitative kinetic data from rat thalamus indicate that the T channel inactivates over a time course of tens of msec and requires more than 100 msec to recover completely from inactivation (Coulter et al. 1989). Hence relay cells generating bursts should respond poorly to high frequencies of stimulation, as there would not be sufficient time during the stimulation period to deinactivate the T channel and generate the Ca^{2+} spikes upon which action potential bursts depend. This is confirmed by the recent study of McCormick and Feeser (1990), who measured responses of relay cells in slices of guinea pig LGN to electrical stimulation of the optic tract. In hyperpolarized cells the responses to stimulation rates higher than 15 Hz were greatly attenuated. This high-frequency attenuation was not present in more depolarized cells firing only tonic spikes. Since the phasic nature of the burst response would attenuate low frequencies as well, McCormick and Feeser predicted that the optimal stimulation bandwidth for hyperpolarized cells in vivo would be 7 to 14 Hz.

Experimental results consistent with the prediction of McCormick and Feeser are shown in figure 10.7, where the temporal frequency (TF) responses of a cat ON-center Y cell and those of its retinal input are illustrated at two different levels of arousal. In part A, the LGN shows a band-pass TF response relative to its retinal input, with peak transmission between 2 and 8 Hz. In part B, an ISI histogram of the spikes recorded during the TF response measurement show that a significant percentage (12 percent) occur at less than 4 msec, which is characteristic of burst discharges. An EEG record taken during the maintained discharge of the neuron following the TF measurement is shown in part C, along with its power spectrum. Prominent slow-wave activity is present that is reflected as a peak near 1 Hz in the power spectrum. The fraction of S potentials that generated spikes during this period of the maintained discharge was only 0.3. Both these measures indicate that the animal was in a low arousal state, which is in agreement with the results of Coenen and Vendrik (1972).

The situation shown in parts A–C of figure 10.7 contrasts with the results shown in parts D–F, which were obtained from the same relay cell 65 minutes later. The TF response of the LGN cell is now relatively flat compared to its retinal input, with less attenuation than observed earlier at both low and high TFs. The ISI histogram shows much less bursting activity during these responses, as only 3 percent of the ISIs were less than 4 msec. The EEG taken during the maintained discharge of the cell just prior to the TF measurement shows that the high-amplitude, low-frequency waves that were present before

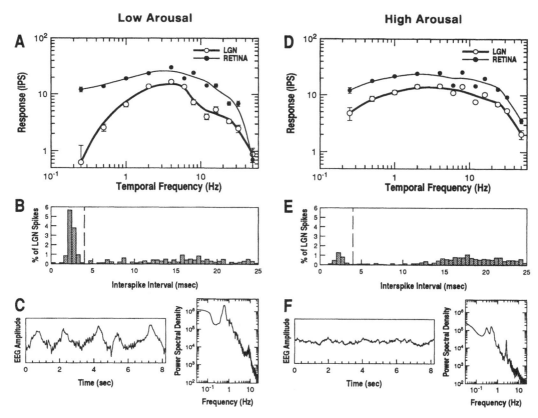

Figure 10.7 Temporal frequency responses of an ON-center Y cell from a cat LGN and its S potential input during states of low arousal (A–C) and high arousal (D–F). (A) First harmonic (Fourier fundamental) amplitudes of the response to a sinusoidal grating of 40 percent contrast and 1.2 c/degree, drifting at temporal frequencies (TFJ between 0.25 Hz and 50 Hz. The error bars represent ±1 SEM. The two 1ines are drawn through smoothed versions of the data points for the LGN and for the retina to indicate the trends in the data. (B) Histogram of the interspike intervals between 0 and 25 msec collected during the TF responses of the LGN in (A). ISls less than 4 msec are to the left of the dashed line. (C) An 8-s sample of the EEG recorded over area 17 during the maintained discharge of the cell after the TF trial in (A). The bandwidth for the EEG recording was 0.1 to 300 Hz. The power spectrum shown is the smoothed average spectral density of 15 EEG samples of 16 s each. (D) The TF responses, taken 65 min after the trial in (A), to an identical stimulus. (E) Histogram of interspike intervals between 0 and 25 msec collected during the TF responses in D. (F) An 8-s sample of the EEG that was recorded prior to the TF trial in D. The power spectrum shown represents the smoothed average spectral density of 15 EEG samples of 16 s each.

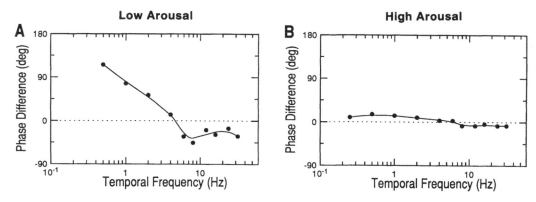

Figure 10.8 The phase difference between the (sinusoidal) LGN response and the retinal responses shown in figure 10.7 Note the pronounced phase lead followed by a phase lag in (A) and the almost constant phase difference between the LGN and the retina in (B).

are now largely absent. The fraction of S potentials that elicited LGN spikes during this period increased from 0.3 to 0.8. All these measures correlate with a higher arousal state.

The phase difference between the responses of the LGN and the retina changed significantly with the state of arousal. It was nearly constant at all temporal frequencies when the animal was in a high arousal state (figure 10.8B), but decreased continuously with temporal frequency at the low arousal state (figure 10.8A). Thus the phase of the LGN response led the retinal response phase at low temporal frequencies and lagged behind it at high temporal frequencies. The band-pass nature of the LGN temporal filter is thus seen to reflect the operation of a differentiator (phase lead) at low frequencies and an integrator (phase lag) at high frequencies. These are intimately related to the rise and decay of the calcium current carried by the T channel.

It should be emphasized that the two conditions shown in figure 10.7 do not represent discrete types of LGN activity. Rather the properties of the LGN response change in a continuous manner as the arousal level of the animal rises and falls. This reflects, at least in part, the gradual change in the level of deinactivation of the T type Ca^{2+} channel as the resting membrane potential of the LGN neuron shifts in response to nonretinal (probably brain stem) influences. This dependence was illustrated above in figure 10.3 from Coulter et al. (1989).

The band-pass temporal transfer function of LGN relay cells measured during prominent bursting activity agrees with the in vitro results of McCormick and Feeser (1990). However, our in vivo results show peak transmission at 2 to 8 Hz, a somewhat lower frequency range than their prediction of 7 to 14 Hz. This may reflect a species-specific difference in the inactivation kinetics of the T channel, as it has been reported that low-threshold Ca^{2+} spikes last twice as long in the cat as in the rat, and presumably in the guinea pig as well (McCormick et al. 1991). To illustrate the effect of changes in the LGN temporal transfer function in the time domain, in figure 10.9 we show responses of an ON-center X cell to a small flashing spot centered on its recep-

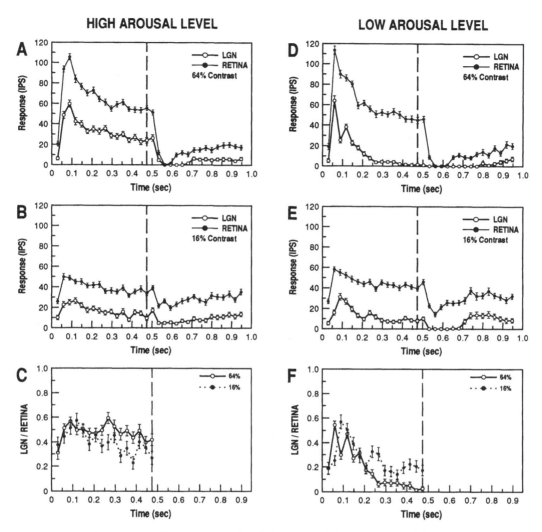

Figure 10.9 Step responses of an ON-center X cell from cat LGN and those of its S potential input during high (A–C) and low (D–F) arousal. (A) PSTHs of spikes and S potentials to 64 presentations of a central contrast-reversing spot, 1 deg in diameter, of 64 percent contrast modulated with a period of 1 s. The dashed line separates the ON step of the stimulus on the left from the OFF step on the right. Error bars represent 1 SEM. The LGN maintained discharge at this time was half the S potential maintained rate. (B) Same as A, but with a 16 percent contrast. (C) The ratio of the LGN and retinal PSTH responses to modulation of 64 percent contrast (solid line) and to 16 percent contrast (dotted line). The values during the OFF responses to the stimulus are not shown because the responses were too small for the ratio to be meaningful. (D) PSTHs of spikes and S potentials to the same stimulus protocol as in (A), taken 37 min later. The LGN maintained discharge at this time was one-tenth the S potential maintained rate. (E) PSTHs of spikes and S potentials to the same stimulus protocol as in B, taken 37 min later. (F) The ratio of the LGN and retinal PSTH responses to 64 percent contrast (solid line) and to 16 percent contrast (dotted line). Both low arousal and high contrast make the LGN response more transient.

tive field while the animal was in two different behavioral states. The spot was temporally modulated with a square wave at two contrasts (64 percent and 16 percent) with a period of 1 second. During the spontaneous discharge prior to the stimulation, the fraction of S potentials eliciting spikes was 0.5. As the solid line in part C shows, this proportion remained relatively constant at around 0.5 during the ON response of the cell to the stimulus. However, 37 minutes later the LGN maintained discharge had fallen to one-tenth the S potential rate, suggesting a lower arousal level. A repeat of the same measurement (in part D) shows that the LGN now responds much more phasically to its retinal input. The solid line in part F illustrates the point that the LGN relays its retinal input faithfully near the onset of the ON step of the stimulus, but that its response drops close to zero by the end of the ON step. As expected, temporal frequency responses (not shown) measured under these two different behavioral states confirmed that the LGN temporal transfer function had become more band-pass, with significantly stronger low-frequency attenuation in the state illustrated by the right-hand side of figure 10.9. The results for 16 percent contrast under these two conditions do not show as strong an effect as those for 64 percent contrast. Thus, during low arousal the degree of tuning of the LGN temporal transfer function may be contrast-dependent, with higher contrasts producing sharper tuning. This is an example of interaction between the state-dependent and stimulus-dependent aspects of LGN filtering.

Experimentally Induced Changes in Retina-LGN Transmission

Barbiturates are known to be powerful agents for depressing arousal and promoting synchronized low-frequency activity in the EEG. It has also been shown that barbiturates are potent antagonists of the excitatory effect of acetylcholine on thalamic relay cells, thereby blocking the effect of ascending cholinergic brain stem projections to the thalamus (Pape and Eysel 1988). In addition, the well-known enhancement of GABA-ergic inhibition by barbiturates will increase the effectiveness of local interneurons and interneurons of the reticular nucleus on relay cells. Hence one would expect LGN activity under barbiturate anesthesia to be bursty and its temporal transfer function to be band-pass. This has been anecdotally observed by many in the field, and it is confirmed by the results in figure 10.10, which shows the TF responses of an ON-center X cell before (A) and 2 minutes after (C) the injection of a 4 mg/kg IV dose of the barbiturate thiamylal (Surital). The ISI histograms of the LGN spikes collected during the TF trials are shown in parts B and D. The histograms show clearly that the barbiturate was very effective in promoting bursting activity in the LGN, presumably by hyperpolarizing the LGN relay cell. The magnitude and time course of this barbiturate effect is dose-dependent and variable among cells and among animals but, for doses in the range of 4 to 7 mg/kg, the strongest effects are seen 2 to 15 minutes after the injection. Electrical stimulation of the parabrachial nucleus should elicit the opposite transformation in LGN relay cells, with a suppression of the

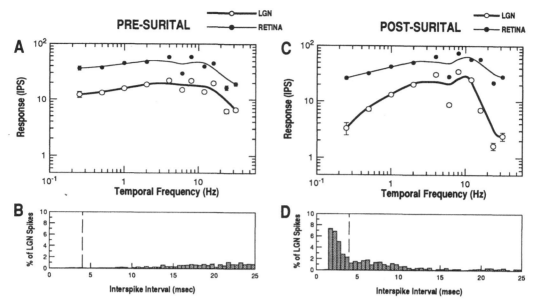

Figure 10.10 Temporal frequency responses of an ON-center X cell from cat LGN and its S potential input before and after an IV injection of a barbiturate (Surital). (A) First harmonic amplitudes of the response to sinusoidal gratings, of 40 percent contrast and 2.4 c/degree, drifting at TFs between 0.25 Hz and 32 Hz. The error bars represent 1 SEM. The two lines are drawn through smoothed versions of the data points for the LGN and for the retina, and are meant to convey the trend in the data. (B) Histogram of the interspike intervals between 0 and 25 msec collected during the TF responses in (A). Intervals less than 4 msec are to the left of the dashed line. (C) Responses of the cell to the identical stimulus as in (A), beginning 2 min after a bolus IV administration of 4 mg/kg Surital. (D) Histogram of the interspike intervals between 0 and 25 msec collected during TF responses in (C).

bursting response and a decrease in the temporal tuning of the cell. Given the anticholinergic property of barbiturates, however, one would predict that parabrachial stimulation would be less effective under barbiturate anesthesia than under other forms of anesthesia.

SUMMARY

We have shown several examples of the ways in which the LGN selects the information it passes on to the cortex, and have linked them to recently discovered biophysical mechanisms. The brief bursts of spikes that LGN relay neurons fire in the hyperpolarized state of low arousal could serve to alert the cortex to new stimuli that require attention, and the dynamics of the LGN under these conditions permit only stimuli from a restricted parameter range to be transmitted.

It is thus clear that it is grossly inaccurate to describe the LGN as a mere "relay nucleus," and it is also clear that this nucleus is capable not merely of gating the information arriving from the retina, but also of filtering it with a variety of mechanisms. The multitude of neurotransmitters and neuromodulators, synaptic arrangements, and ionic channels provides a very rich environment for the fine-tuning of the level and type of information that is relayed from the retina to the cortex. The involvement of NMDA-type glutamate receptors, with their voltage sensitivity and reported involvement in neuronal plasticity, is especially intriguing and challenging. Elucidating the ways in which the brain orchestrates the various players of this strategic structure will require further in vitro and in vivo studies, as well as computational modeling approaches to aid researchers in sorting out the complex circuit combinations.

ACKNOWLEDGMENTS

This work was supported by NIH grants EY 4888 (E. K.), EY 1472 (R. M. S.), and EY 1428. We thank Y. Holland for her help in preparing the manuscript.

REFERENCES

Ahlsén G, Lindström S, Lo F-S (1985) Interaction between inhibitory pathways to principal cells in the lateral geniculate nucleus of the cat. Exp Brain Res 58:134–143.

Bishop, PO, Burke W, Davis R (1958) Synapse discharge by single fibre in mammalian visual system. Nature 182:728–730.

Casagrande VA, Norton TT (1991) Lateral geniculate nucleus: a review of its physiology and function. In: Vision and Visual Dysfunction: The Neural Basis of Visual Function, Vol. 4. Leventhal AG, ed. Macmillan, 41–84.

Cleland BG, Dubin MW, Levick WR (1971) Sustained and transient neurones in the cat's retina and lateral geniculate nucleus. J Physiol (Lond) 217:473–496.

Coenen AML, Vendrik AJH (1972) Determination of the transfer ratio of cat's geniculate neurons through quasi-intracellular recordings and the relation with the level of alertness. Exp Brain Res 14:227–242.

Coulter DA, Huguenard JR, Prince DA (1989) Calcium currents in rat thalamocortical relay neurones: kinetic properties of the transient, low-threshold current. J Physiol (Lond) 414:587–604.

Crunelli V, Leresche N (1991) A role for GABA$_B$ receptors in excitation and inhibition of thalamocortical cells. Trends Neurosci 14:16–21.

Guillery RW (1966) A study of Golgi preparations from the dorsal lateral geniculate nucleus of the adult cat. J Comp Neurol 128:21–50.

Hirsch JC, Fourment A, Marc ME (1983) Sleep-related variations of membrane potential in the lateral geniculate body relay neurons of the cat. Brain Res 259: 308–312.

Hu B, Steriade M, Deschênes M (1989) The effects of brainstem peribrachial stimulation on neurons of the lateral geniculate nucleus. Neuroscience 31:13–24.

Hubel DH, Wiesel TN (1961) Integrative action in the cat's lateral geniculate body. J Physiol (Lond) 155:385–398.

Humphrey AL, Saul AB (1991) Stimulation of the brainstem reticular formation does not abolish the lagged/non-lagged cell distinction in the cat LGN. Soc Neurosci Abstr 17:282.5.

Jahnsen H, Llinás R (1984) Electrophysiological properties of guinea-pig thalamic neurones: an in vitro study. J Physiol (Lond) 349:205–226.

Kaplan E, Purpura K, Shapley RM (1987) Contrast affects the transmission of visual information through the mammalian lateral geniculate nucleus. J Physiol (Lond) 391:267−288.

Kaplan E, Shapley R (1984) The origin of the S (slow) potential in the mammalian lateral geniculate nucleus. Exp Brain Res 55:111−116.

Koch C (1985) Understanding the intrinsic circuitry of the cat's lateral geniculate nucleus: electrical properties of the spine-triad arrangement. Proc R Soc Lond B 225:365−390.

Kwon YH, Esguerra M, Sur M (1991) NMDA and Non-NMDA receptors mediate visual responses of neurons in the cat's lateral geniculate nucleus. J Neurophysiol 66: 414−428.

Lee BB, Virsu V, Creutzfeldt OD (1983) Linear signal transmission from prepotentials to cells in the macaque lateral geniculate nucleus. Exp Brain Res 52:50−56.

Levick WR, Cleland BG, Dubin MW (1972) Lateral geniculate nucleus of cat: retinal inputs and physiology. Invest Ophthalmol Vis Sci 11:302−311.

Livingstone MS, Hubel DH (1981) Effects of sleep and arousal on the processing of visual information in the cat. Nature 291:554−561.

Llinás R, Jahnsen H (1982) Electrophysiology of mammalian thalamic neurones in vitro. Nature 297:406−408.

Lu S-M, Guido W, Sherman SM (1990) Low threshold calcium spikes in LGN cells during responses to visual stimuli. Soc Neurosci Abstr 16:72.3.

Mastronarde DN (1987a) Two classes of single-input X-cells in cat lateral geniculate nucleus I. Receptive-field properties and classification of cells. J Neurophysiol 57:357−380.

Mastronarde DN (1987b) Two classes of single-input X-cells in cat lateral geniculate nucleus II. Retinal inputs and the generation of receptive-field properties. J Neurophysiol 57:381−413.

McCormick DA, Feeser HR (1990) Functional implications of burst firing and single spike activity in lateral geniculate relay neurons. Neuroscience 39:103−113.

McCormick DA, Huguenard J, Strowbridge B (1991) Determination of state dependent processing in thalamus by single neuron properties and neuromodulators. In: Single Neuron Computation (McKenna T, Davis J, Zornetzer SF, eds). Academic Press.

McIlwain JT (1972) Nonretinal influences on the lateral geniculate nucleus. Invest Ophthalmol Vis Sci 11:311−322.

Pape H-C, Eysel UT (1988) Cholinergic excitation and inhibition in the visual thalamus of the cat—influences of cortical inactivation and barbiturate anesthesia. Brain Res 440:79−86.

Saul AB, Humphrey AL (1990) Spatial and temporal response properties of lagged and non-lagged cells in cat lateral geniculate nucleus. J Neurophysiol 64:206−224.

Sherman SM, Koch C (1986) The control of retinogeniculate transmission in the mammalian lateral geniculate nucleus. Exp Brain Res 63:1−20.

Sherman SM, Lu S-M, Guido W (1991) Visually evoked burst discharges in cat LGN cells: spatial and temporal tuning. Soc Neurosci Abstr 17:249.10.

Sillito AM, Murphy PC, Salt TE, Moody CI (1990a) Dependence of retinogeniculate transmission in cat on NMDA receptors. J Neurophysiol 63:347−355.

Sillito AM, Murphy PC, Salt TE (1990b) The contribution of the non-N-methyl-D-aspartate group of excitatory amino acid receptors to retinogeniculate transmission in the cat. Neuroscience 34:273−280.

Singer W (1977) Control of thalamic transmission by corticofugal and ascending reticular pathways in the visual system. Physiol Rev 57:386−420.

Szentágothai J (1973) Neuronal and synaptic architecture of the lateral geniculate body. In: Handbook of Sensory Physiology (Jung R, ed) Vol 7 part 3B, pp 141–176. Berlin: Springer.

Tanaka K (1983) Cross-correlation analysis of geniculostriate neuronal relationships in cats. J Neurophysiol 49:1303–1318.

Uhlrich DJ, Cucchiaro JB, Sherman SM (1988) The projection of individual axons from the parabrachial region of the brain stem to the dorsal lateral geniculate nucleus in the cat. J Neurosci 8:4565–4575.

Uhlrich DJ, Tamamaki N, Sherman SM (1990) Brainstem control of response modes in neurons of the cat's lateral geniculate nucleus. Proc Natl Acad Sci USA 87:2560–2563.

11 Roles of M and P Pathways

Peter Lennie

Most of the major discoveries of physiological mechanisms underlying perception result from our looking for something in particular. We have some theory about mechanism—albeit a vaguely formulated theory, often developed in the course of seeking an explanation of perceptual phenomena—and we go looking for that mechanism with the microelectrode. Notable discoveries of this sort include the substrates of lateral inhibition, light and dark adaptation, chromatically opponent mechanisms, and trichromacy.

Our understanding of the most widely examined parallel visual pathways —the so-called M and P pathways in primates[1] and the possibly homologous X and Y pathways in the cat—has not developed in the usual way. We have a wealth of anatomical and physiological information about the organization of these pathways, but that has been accumulated almost entirely unprovoked by the need to explain perceptual phenomena. I can think of no case in which perceptual observations impelled anyone who did not already know about M and P pathways to postulate mechanisms with the properties we associate with these pathways. If perceptual observations and experiments have not led visual scientists to postulate pathways of the kind we now know exist, we ought to fear that one or other pathway has only a subtle influence on perception or that we have been looking at the wrong kinds of perceptual tasks in trying to find roles for the pathways

In this chapter I examine various ideas about the roles of M and P pathways. I begin by summarizing the properties of the two pathways below the cortex; I then consider some general benefits of parallel organization before going on to weigh evidence on how the pathways contribute to seeing.

GENERAL PROPERTIES OF M AND P PATHWAYS

The M and P pathways appear to be distinct from an early stage (they are driven by substantially distinct populations of bipolar cells), and in the macaque monkey remain wholly segregated at least as far as striate cortex. Table 11.1 summarizes the major physiological and anatomical differences between M and P cells.

Table 11.1. Attributes of M and P cells in the macaque

Attribute	M cells	P cells
Percent of ganglion cells	10	80
Distribution on retina	Densest in fovea?	Densest in fovea
Conduction velocity	~ 15 m/sec	~ 6 m/sec
Central projection		
Ganglion cells	LGN (ventral layers)	LGN (dorsal layers)
LGN cells	V1 (layer 4Cα)	V1 (layers 4Cβ, 4A)
Chromatic opponency	Almost none	Well-developed (two types: L vs. M; S vs. L + M)
Rod input	Yes	Sometimes
Contrast sensitivity	Higher (>60)	Lower (<20)
Spatial resolution	Lower	Higher (single-cone center in fovea)
Temporal resolution	Higher (60 Hz?)	High (30 Hz?)
Periphery effects	Some	None?

Most suggestions about the perceptual significance of parallel pathways draw inspiration from the known anatomical and physiological properties of the M and P systems or their associated streams in the cortex. For example, P cells are widely thought to be the substrate of color vision because only P cells express clear chromatic opponency. However, one should not place too much weight on this kind of argument for two reasons: first, it depends on the properties of the pathways being adequately characterized. We actually understand very little about the properties of most neurons in the visual pathway. For example, we know remarkably little about the complex, nonlinear cells that are so prevalent in striate and extrastriate cortex—and I think it is hazardous to infer their perceptual roles from the properties revealed by studies with simple visual stimuli. Second, even when dealing with well-characterized neurons like M and P cells in the primate, we can be quite easily misled. For example, an inference often drawn from the observation that the contrast sensitivities of M cells are substantially higher than the contrast sensitivities of P cells is that stimuli of low contrast excite only the M pathway. This is definitely suspect. Evidence from several sources that I shall touch upon shortly shows that chromatic discriminations must depend on the P pathway; yet, when we measure the detectability of a change in chromaticity, we find that under fairly standard conditions a single P cell is about sevenfold less sensitive than the human observer. The moral is that we cannot know what significance to attach to differences in sensitivity until we know how signals within a pathway are combined in giving rise to a perceptual decision. The broader lesson is that the physiological properties of cells may be a poor guide to their perceptual roles.

THE ADVANTAGES OF PARALLEL, MODULAR ORGANIZATION

Computer scientists are fond of parallel architectures because they permit (at least in principle) a computational load to be divided among multiple mechanisms acting concurrently, with the result that the problem is solved faster. Two forms of parallelism distinguished in computational work have potential biological counterparts, one less interesting than the other. The duller form is spatial parallelism, which is represented by the sampling of the image by a single class of ganglion cell—for example, the P cell, of which there are over a million in each eye. Essentially the same operation is undertaken concurrently for every point in the image. The benefits of this kind of image sampling are easily seen when we contrast it with the sampling undertaken by a television camera, which uses a serial scan to capture the whole image.

For our present purposes, the interesting form of parallelism is that which breaks a complex problem into different component tasks that are solved concurrently and to some degree independently. There is a pervasive belief, traceable to work on computational vision (Barrow and Tenenbaum 1978; Marr 1982), that modular organization is fundamental to efficient perceptual analysis, and it has become central to most recent discussions of how the visual system works (e.g., Livingstone and Hubel 1987). The multiple visual cortical areas identified in higher mammals are widely presumed to reflect specialization for different analyses. Is the parallel organization that is found lower in the visual pathway a special adaptation to facilitate this?

Parallel pathways fed by fibers from distinct classes of ganglion cells are common in almost all species that have been examined, both at the level of major fiber tracts (e.g., tectal vs. thalamic) and at the level of subdivisions within major tracts (for reviews see Lennie 1980; Rodieck 1988). In the tectal pathway—the most important in lower animals—cells often have elaborate receptive fields and are highly selective for circumscribed classes of visual stimuli. This is undoubtedly useful when the visual demands on an animal are limited, for perceptual decisions can be made at the periphery and conveyed in mechanisms of very low bandwidth. For example, the notional bug detector in the frog's retina analyzes a great deal of information but sends a simple signal for action. However, the selectivity of the bug detector is purchased by discarding information, and it leaves the animal ill equipped for detecting new classes of objects. To deal with new objects it has to develop a new detector with different properties, and so it gradually accumulates a variety of special mechanisms. The very sharp selectivity of the specialized detectors leaves them poorly equipped for any substantial role in the kind of modular analysis envisaged above; the detectors simply throw away too much information about the image.

M and P cells in the monkey, and X and Y cells in the cat appear to be much better candidates for providing inputs for a higher-level modular analysis. They have (broadly) linear, isotropic receptive fields that filter the image modestly and discard relatively little information (other than about level of illumination). Cells with such comparatively simple receptive fields exist principally (perhaps only) in the thalamic pathway. The predominance of this pathway in mammals, most especially in primates and carnivores (in macaques it carries 90 percent of the fibers that leave the retina) does not appear to make the higher mammals see better than other vertebrates; there are many species—notably birds—that clearly see as well as or better than we do in the sense of having better resolution or sensitivity. Rather, evolution of this pathway has brought about a "change in what can be done with what is seen, rather than in what can be seen" (Masterton and Glendenning, 1978).

While we can be reasonably confident that M and P cells have evolved to support the kinds of perceptual analysis of which only higher mammals are capable, nothing that we know about the requirements for modular analysis suggests why we might need two distinct pathways, either of which might be able to do the job on its own.

SUGGESTED ROLES OF M AND P CELLS

The significance of the parallel pathways has long been recognized, for the lamination of the LGN has almost universally been taken to indicate the segregation of sensory elements with different functions (Walls 1953). It is therefore not surprising that there is a long history of attempts to account for the different classes of cells and that early ones focused on the importance of lamination.

Binocular Vision

In primates, which have the most frontal eyes, the LGN has pronounced lamination. Inputs from the two eyes are interleaved and in precise retinotopic register. This encourages the inference that the different classes of cells have some special role in binocular vision. Since *Tarsius* and *Tupaia* have laminated LGNs and completely crossed pathways, the distinct cell classes implied by lamination probably have no particular significance for binocular vision. However, the frontal arrangement of the eyes in most primates and the cat, although permitting the alignment of specialized retinal regions near the optic axes, restricts the overall size of the visual field and places a premium on the animal's capacity for shifting gaze (through eye and/or head movements). This requirement may be important in the evolution of the M and P pathways. I will return to it later.

Photopic vs. Scotopic Vision

The oldest theory is attributed by Walls to Henschen (1931), and asserts that the parvocellular laminae receive inputs from cones and support the chromatic aspects of vision, while the magnocellular laminae support the perception of brightness (both scotopic and photopic). Walls provides a good deal of evidence that in its strong form this is probably wrong—there are well-

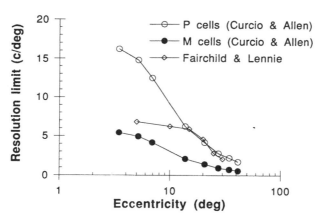

Figure 11.1 Variation of spatial resolving power with eccentricity. Open diamonds, human resolution limit for identifying a grating in scotopic vision (from Lennie and Fairchild 1992); circles, sampling limit for the mosaics of P ganglion cells (open circles) and M ganglion cells (filled circles) estimated from the ganglion cell counts of Curcio and Allen (1990), assuming that the proportions of M and P cells are the same as in the macaque monkey, that the sampling mosaic is triangular, and that an ON-center/OFF-center pair of cells provides a single sampling element.

developed parvocellular and magnocellular divisions in nocturnal primates such as *Galago* and *Aotus*—but there is some reason to ask whether the magnocellular pathway is especially adapted for scotopic vision (or conversely, whether the parvocellular pathway is peculiarly ill equipped to support it).[2] Clark (1943) found that, after maintaining monkeys in red light for a month, there was pronounced atrophy of the magnocellular layers of the LGN, but not of the parvocellular layers. Recent work by Purpura, Kaplan, and Shapley, (1988) which has shown that P cells but not M cells are very insensitive at low levels of illumination, revives the question of how P cells are involved in rod vision. There is clear evidence for rod input to some P cells (Wiesel and Hubel 1966; Virsu and Lee 1983; Lennie and Krauskopf unpublished observations), but what sort of vision can this support?

Mark Fairchild and I (1993) tried to find out. We measured scotopic acuity for identifying interference fringes formed directly on the retina at a range of eccentricities from 5 deg to 30 deg and compared the measured acuities with those calculated for the mosaics of M and P ganglion cells in the human retina on the assumption that the proportions of the two classes are the same in humans and macaques. Figure 11.1 shows the results of the comparison. At all eccentricities the mosaic of M cells is too coarse to support the observed acuity. Therefore, scotopic visual acuity must depend to a significant extent on the P pathway.

Color Vision

An early idea about the organization of the LGN linked it to color vision. Clark (1941) suggested that the lamination reflected the segregation of three pathways, each of which carried one of the signals for normal trichromatic vision. Whatever the code, the trichromacy of vision requires that each local region of the retina give rise to an independent signal for each chromatic dimension. Since ganglion cells are believed to be univariant, we might suppose that each point on the retina is sampled by as many different cell types as there are dimensions to be represented—three.

Walls (1953) very soundly disposed of the notion that LGN lamination and color vision were simply linked by showing that whether an animal was trichromatic or dichromatic was unrelated to the number of laminae in its LGN. However, a modern variant of Clark's idea deserves more scrutiny. This assigns two chromatically opponent channels ("red-green" and "yellow-blue") to the parvocellular laminae (making no distinction between the two laminae) and an achromatic channel to the magnocellular ones. There are several things wrong with this idea. First, the mosaic of M cells samples the image too coarsely for these cells to be the substrate of the high-resolution mechanism of achromatic vision (see below). Second, the organization of the P system is not what one would expect of a mechanism specialized for color vision: the "red-green" cells, which constitute perhaps 90 percent of the population of P cells, sample the image much more densely than would be needed to support acuity for colored objects. Moreover, the center-surround organization of their receptive fields ensures that their chromatic characteristics depend upon the spatial properties of the stimulus that excites them. The most comprehensive interpretation of these observations is that the "red-green" cells do double duty, carrying a multiplexed signal that can be decoded later by comparing the signals from two or more cells (Lennie and D'Zmura 1988).

The parvocellular system alone seems to be equipped to carry all the information we need to support the three dimensions of color vision. Lesions of the P pathway make chromatic discriminations impossible; lesions of the M pathway leave color contrast sensitivity unaffected (Merigan 1989; Schiller, Logothetis, and Charles 1990b). There is some reason to believe that M cells are responsible for the $V(\lambda)$ spectral sensitivity function (Lee, Pokorny, Smith, Martin, and Valberg 1990), but I believe that the mechanism responsible for $V(\lambda)$ is quite distinct from the one that supports achromatic form vision and that provides the third dimension of color in normal life. I know of no evidence that implicates the M system in color discriminations.

Spatiotemporal Aspects of Vision

One thing we know firmly from anatomical work is the distribution of the M and P cells on the retina beyond the fovea. This allows us to estimate what visual acuities the two pathways might sustain. Figure 11.2 shows that the limit to normal visual acuity must be set by P cells, as the sampling density of the mosaic of M cells is too coarse to sustain the observed performance at both scotopic and photopic levels of illumination.

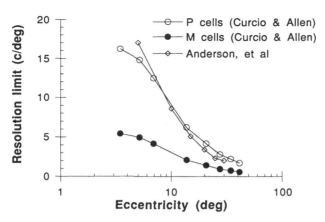

Figure 11.2 Variation of spatial resolving power with eccentricity. Open diamonds, human resolution limit for identifying a grating in photopic vision (from Anderson, et al. 1991); circles, sampling limit for the mosaics of P ganglion cells (open cirdes) and M ganglion cells (filled circles), estimated from the ganglion cell counts of Curcio and Allen, (1990), assuming that the proportions of M and P cells are the same as in the macaque monkey, that the sampling mosaic is triangular, and that an ON-center/OFF-center pair of cells provides a single sampling element.

Ibotenic acid lesions confined to the parvocellular layers of the LGN (Merigan, Katz, and Maunsell 1991) or exposure to neurotoxins that damage P cells selectively (Merigan and Eskin 1986) leave macaques with much-reduced visual acuity and leave their contrast sensitivity much reduced, except for stimuli of low spatial and high temporal frequency. Lesions of the M pathway in the LGN (leaving intact the P pathway and others that reach the cortex through the superior colliculus) affect contrast sensitivity only for stimuli of low spatial frequency and high temporal frequency (Merigan and Maunsell 1990; Merigan, Byrne, and Maunsell 1991; Schiller, Logothetis, and Charles 1990a). Even these signs of M pathway activity are confined to low contrasts: lesions of the M pathway do not impair flicker resolution of high-contrast stimuli (Merigan and Maunsell 1990).

There is an interesting parallel between this circumscribed involvement of the M pathway in spatiotemporal contrast thresholds and the suggestion made by Tolhurst (1973) and Kulikowski and Tolhurst (1973) that the spatio-temporal contrast sensitivity of the normal observer reflects contributions of two classes of mechanisms: one (called the *sustained channel*) that is, preferentially sensitive to medium and high spatial frequencies, and another (the *transient channel*) that is most sensitive to low spatial frequencies. The sensitivity of the transient channel is thought to exceed that of the sustained channel only when stimuli flicker. The important point in the present context is that the distinction drawn by Tolhurst was based on the appearance of gratings at threshold: when detection is presumed to be mediated by the transient mechanism the observer is aware of temporal variation, but not the spatial structure; when the sustained mechanism determines threshold the spatial structure is evident, but not the temporal variation.

Lennie: Roles of M and P Pathways

Complex Visual Discriminations

Work that has looked at the effects of M or P pathway lesions on more complex visual discriminations (Schiller et al. 1990a, 1990b; Lynch, Silveira, Perry, and Merigan 1992) provides little further evidence of the perceptual importance of the M pathway in normal vision: fine stereopsis is disrupted by lesions of the P system, but not by lesions of the M system; motion perception is affected by M lesions only when stimuli are fast moving and of low contrast and therefore probably not detectable through P cells. M lesions seem to bring about no general weakening of the capacity to discriminate speed and direction of movement. Nonetheless, monkeys that have been poisoned with acrylamide and appear to have no functioning P systems at all show few outward signs of visual abnormality when they are casually observed (W. H. Merigan, personal communication). When pushed, the isolated M system must be capable of supporting coarse form discrimination. That is not to say that in the normal animal it does the same thing.

Conclusions

By providing plentiful evidence for the importance of P cells, though revealing no solid role for M cells, the work just reviewed sharpens some of the issues, but leaves us still unclear about why the visual system is organized the way it is. Our conscious vision is not dominated by objects that give rise to low contrast, high temporal frequency, and low spatial frequency signals of the kind to which the M pathway seem relatively most sensitive. Indeed, the only normal circumstances under which we might come close to giving the M system some advantage over the P system are those in which we move our eyes or some object moves fleetingly. Are M cells especially important in just this context, or is their normal role too subtle or too far removed from anything we have so far contemplated to be revealed by the kinds of psychophysical experiments undertaken to explore it?

ANOTHER POSSIBLE ROLE OF M CELLS: ALERTING AND DIRECTING GAZE

Monkeys and cats have the capacity to direct attention visually and to make eye movements that capture and, if necessary, pursue, an object of interest. Visual capture (by voluntary saccades) and pursuit are recently evolved capabilities possessed only by animals, such as primates and cats, that have frontal eyes and some central specialization of the retina. Moreover, the eye movements are under attentional control and are disrupted by lesions of the striate cortex (Mohler and Wurtz 1977; Segraves, Goldberg, Deng, Bruce, Ungerleider, and Mishkin 1987).

In this last section I want to explore the possibility that M cells might have a special role in this. I am not suggesting that the M pathway controls the allocation of attention or that it is in any way tied to either the "sustained" or the "transient" components of attention recently distinguished by Nakayama and Mackeben (1989). Rather, the idea is that M cells provide a conduit through which visually significant objects can rapidly attract attention and subsequent foveation.

In the laboratory voluntary saccades are generally fast, especially when they are made to targets isolated in the visual field. The latency of a normal saccade is typically around 200 msec—significantly faster than other visual reaction times—and it may, under special circumstances, be as short as 100 msec (Becker 1991). The average error of the primary saccade to a target is about 10 percent and this is usually corrected by one or more secondary saccades. In a richer visual environment saccades can be quite different. If an observer is presented with two targets that are separated by up to 10 to 20 deg but quite distinct perceptually and is instructed to select one target or to foveate the targets in turn, the saccade is made to some point between the two—the "global" effect (Findlay 1982). This tendency to make a saccade to the center of gravity of a complex display is much reduced for long-latency saccades that result either from the observer's striving for accuracy (Ottes, van Gisbergen, and Eggermont 1985) or from his being prevented from making a saccade until some time after the appearance of the target (Coëffé and O'Regan, 1987).

The improvement in accuracy is purchased at considerable expense—latencies may be increased by several hundred msec—an observation that led Jacobs (1987) to suggest that the center-of-gravity tendencies reflect a useful adaptation: the primary saccade sends the eye as rapidly as possible to somewhere near the middle of an interesting target complex, and a secondary saccade brings the target to the fovea. For the conditions examined by Jacobs, this sequence of movements captures a target more efficiently than does a single, slower, saccade. Might the M pathway provide the signal that permits the detection and speedy but coarse localization of a peripheral objects as a precursor to a saccadic movement? In the following paragraphs I examine some evidence that bears on this possibility.

Signals from M cells arrive in the cortex sooner than do those from P cells. The difference between the conduction velocities of M and P pathways is of the order of 4 msec from the retina to the cortex (slightly less for Y cells vs. X cells in the cat) and is probably too small to be significant on its own. However, M cells have inherently higher contrast sensitivity than do P cells—greater than would be expected from a simple summation of signals from the number of P cells that cover the same region of the retina.[3] This greater contrast sensitivity is likely to result in the latency of a reliable visual response (that is, the time after the onset of the visual stimulus at which the discharge of a neuron reliably exceeds its previous rate), being a good deal shorter for an M cell than for a P cell (less so for a Y cell vs. an X cell), because a stimulus of given contrast will generally evoke a much greater response from the M cell. Observations made by Troy and Lennie (1987) on the cat suggest that, for a fivefold difference in sensitivity between two cells (which is typical of the difference between that of M and P cells) and a stimulus of contrast near the threshold of the less sensitive cell, the response of the more sensitive one will be detected 40 msec sooner.

M cells express a "shift effect," a discharge evoked by a shift in the spatial position of a grating pattern that occupies an annular region between about 20 and 50 deg from the center of the receptive field (Krüger 1977). Large rectified responses can be evoked by a shift of one bar width (ca. 0.25 deg) once or twice a second. The shift effect is very clear in M cells (as in the Y cells of the cat), but is weak in P cells (Krüger, 1977).[4] It appears to be the expression of a nonlinearity that is well-characterized in cat (Hochstein and Shapley, 1976), but to which only a little attention has been given in primate (Kaplan and Shapley, 1982). M cells are therefore sensitive to change of local contrast in a substantial region around the classical receptive field.

M cells may be relatively sparse in the fovea. Silveira and Perry (1990) have measured the density of M cells at eccentricities of 4.5 deg and higher, but we have no direct observations on their density nearer the fovea. However, one line of evidence (Ogden and Miller 1966), which shows that the fast component of the compound action potential recorded in the optic nerve cannot be elicited by stimulation of the foveal margin of the optic disk, suggests that M cells must be relatively sparse in and near the fovea (or have much smaller axons). This is not strong evidence, but it is consistent with the idea that the function of the M pathway is to underpin the capture of visual stimuli.

What sorts of evidence would strengthen this case? We would like most of all to know how lesions of the magnocellular pathway affect the speed and accuracy of saccadic and pursuit eye movements. We already know that M cells project (indirectly, but relatively heavily) to cortical areas that are implicated in the control of pursuit eye movements (Newsome, Wurtz, Dürsteler, and Mikami 1985), but we have no solid evidence how damage confined to the subcortical M pathway affects eye movements. Page, King, Merigan, and Maunsell (1993) examined eye movements in monkeys that had lesions confined to the magnocellular LGN, and they found little effect, but the visual stimuli used in the experiments—small bright, red spots—were ill suited to exploring the role of M cells. It would be useful to know how the contrast and spatial frequency of targets affect the accuracy and latency of eye movements. It would also be valuable to know more precisely how the spatial characteristics of large, complex targets affect the latency and precision of saccades.

CONCLUSIONS

The best evidence we have indicates that the P pathway is overwhelmingly important for the conscious analysis of the image. This is not to say that the M pathway can play no role in concsicous vision, for when the M system is left isolated by destruction of the P ganglion cells, monkeys are evidently not blind. Nonetheless, under normal circumstances the need for the M pathway seems so slight that we should look in a different domain for its major function. The argument made here is that the M pathway is peculiarly well adapted to supporting the rapid gaze shifting that is so important for animals with frontal eyes. We do not normally see with the M pathway, but the M pathway is very important for seeing.

ACKNOWLEDGMENTS

This work was supported by NIH grants EY04440 and EY01319.

NOTES

1. Here I am using the nomenclature that in recent years has become widely adopted: the M pathway originates in a distinct class of large ganglion cells (the *parasol* cells of Polyak, 1941) and the P_α cells of Perry, Öhler, and Cowey, 1984) and projects to the magnocellular division of the lateral geniculate nucleus (LGN). The P pathway originates in the class of ganglion cells in and near the fovea that correspond to the *midget* ganglion cells or P_β cells, and projects exclusively to the parvocellular layers of the LGN.

2. Specialization for photopic and scotopic vision cannot be the reason for the evolution of X and Y cells in the cat: both cell types are overwhelmingly driven by rods under most circumstances, but both also receive inputs from cones (Enroth-Cugell, Hertz, and Lennie 1977).

3. The center of an M cell's receptive field covers a region that would include about nine P cell centers (giving an expected threefold improvement in sensitivity over a P cell) yet, for some reason that we do not yet understand, the M cell is perhaps five times more sensitive.

4. One should not infer from this kind of experiment that the mechanism exists only far from the receptive field; the experiments are designed to minimize the activation of mechanisms in the classical receptive field. In the cat the greatest weight comes from the near inner edge of the annulus, and the mechanism is probably strongest near the center of the receptive field.

REFERENCES

Anderson, S. J., Mullen, K. T., and Hess, R. F. (1991). Human peripheral spatial resolution for achromatic and chromatic stimuli: limits imposed by optical and retinal factors. J. Physiol. 442, 47–64.

Barrow, H. G., and Tenenbaum, J. M. (1978). Recovering intrinsic scene characteristics from images. In A. R. Hanson & E. M. Riseman (Eds.), Computer Vision Systems. New York: Academic Press.

Becker, W. (1991). Saccades. In R. H. S. Carpenter (Ed.), Vision and Visual Dysfunction (pp. 95–137). Boca Raton: CRC Press.

Clark, W. E. L. G. (1941). The laminar organization and cell content of the lateral geniculate body in the monkey. J. Anat., 75, 419–433.

Clark, W. E. L. G. (1943). The anatomy of cortical vision. Transactions of the Ophthalmic Society, U.K., 62, 229–245.

Coëffé, C., and O'Regan, J. K. (1987). Reducing the influence of non-target stimuli on saccade accuracy: predictability and latency effects. Vision Res., 27, 227–240.

Curcio, C. A., and Allen, K. A. (1990). Topography of ganglion cells in human retina. J. Comp. Neurol. 300, 5–25.

Enroth-Cugell, C., Hertz, B. G., and Lennie, P. (1977). Cone signals in the cat's retina. J. Physiol., 269, 273–296.

Findlay, J. (1982). Global visual processing for saccadic eye movements. Vision Res., 22, 1033–1045.

Henschen, S. E. (1931). Ueber spezifische Lichtsinn- und Farbensinnzellen im Gehirn. Acta Psychiat. Neur., 6, 347–358.

Hochstein, S., and Shapley, R. M. (1976). Linear and nonlinear spatial subunits in Y cat retinal ganglion cells. J. Physiol., 262, 265–284.

Jacobs, A. M. (1987). On localization and saccadic programming. Vision Res., 27, 1953–1966.

Kaplan, E., and Shapley, R. M. (1982). X and Y cells in the lateral geniculate nucleus of the macaque monkey. J. Physiol., 330, 125–144.

Krüger, J. (1977). The shift-effect in the lateral geniculate body of the rhesus monkey. Exp. Brain Res., 29, 387–392.

Kulikowski, J. J., and Tolhurst, D. J. (1973). Psychophysical evidence for sustained and transient detectors in human vision. J. Physiol., 232, 149–162.

Lee, B. B., Pokorny, J., Smith, V. C., Martin, P. R., and Valberg, A. (1990). Luminance and chromatic modulation sensitivity of macaque ganglion cells and human observers. J. Opt. Soc. Am. A, 7, 2223–2236.

Lennie, P. (1980). Parallel visual pathways: a review. Vision Res., 20, 561–594.

Lennie, P., and D'Zmura, M. (1988). Mechanisms of color vision. CRC Crit. Rev. Neurobiol., 3, 333–400.

Lennie, P., and Fairchild, M. D. (1993). Ganglion cell pathways for rod vision. Vision Res., in press.

Livingstone, M. S., and Hubel, D. H. (1987). Psychophysical evidence for separate channels for the perception of form, color, movement, and depth. J. Neurosci., 7, 3416–3468.

Lynch, J. J., Silveira, L. C. L., Perry, V. H., and Merigan, W. H. (1992). Visual effects of damage to P ganglion cells in macaques. Vis. Neurosci. 8, 575–583.

Marr, D. (1982). Vision: A Computational Investigation into the Human Representation and Processing of Visual Information. San Francisco: W. H. Freeman.

Masterton, B. R., and Glendenning, K. K. (1978). Phylogeny of the vertebrate sensory systems. In B. R. Masterton (Eds.), Sensory Integration (pp. 1–38). New York: Plenum.

Merigan, W. H. (1989). Chromatic and achromatic vision of macaques: role of the P pathway. J. Neurosci., 9, 776–783.

Merigan, W. H., Byrne, C., and Maunsell, J. H. R. (1991). Does primate motion perception depend on the magnocellular pathway? J. Neurosci., 11, 3422–3429.

Merigan, W. H., and Eskin, T. A. (1986). Spatio-temporal vision of macaques with severe loss of Pβ retinal ganglion cells. Vision Res., 26, 1751–1761.

Merigan, W. H., Katz, L. M., and Maunsell, J. H. R. (1991). The effects of parvocellular lateral geniculate lesions on the acuity and contrast sensitivity of macaque monkeys. J. Neurosci., 11, 994–1001.

Merigan, W. H., and Maunsell, J. H. R. (1990). Macaque vision after magnocellular lateral geniculate lesions. Vis. Neurosci., 5, 347–352.

Mohler, C. W., and Wurtz, R. H. (1977). Role of striate cortex and superior colliculus in visual guidance of saccadic eye movements in monkeys. J. Neurophysiol., 40, 74–94.

Nakayama, K., and Mackeben, M. (1989). Sustained and transient components of focal visual attention. Vision Res., 29, 1631–1647.

Newsome, W. T., Wurtz, R. H., Dürsteler, M. R., and Mikami, A. (1985). Deflcits in visual motion processing following ibotenic acid lesions of the middle temporal visual area. J. Neurosci., 5, 825−840.

Ogden, T. E., and Miller, R. F. (1966). Studies of the optic nerve of the rhesus monkey: nerve fiber spectrum and physiological properties. Vision Res., 6, 405−506.

Ottes, F. P., van Gisbergen, J. A. M., and Eggermont, J. J. (1985). Latency dependence of colour-based target vs. nontarget discrimination by the saccadic system. Vision Res., 25, 849−862.

Page, W. K., King, W. M., Merigan, W., and Maunsell, J. (1993). Pursuit deficits revealed by step-ramp tracking errors in monkeys with LGN lesions. Vision Res., in press

Perry, V. H., Oehler, R., and Cowey, A. (1984). Retinal ganglion cells that project to the dorsal lateral geniculate nucleus in the macaque monkey. Neuroscience, 12, 1101−1123.

Polyak, S. L. (1941). The Retina. Chicago: University of Chicago Press.

Purpura, K., Kaplan, E., and Shapley, R. M. (1988). Background light and the contrast gain of primate P and M retinal ganglion cells. Proc. Natl. Acad. Sci. U.S.A., 85, 4534−4537.

Rodieck, R. W. (1988). The primate retina. In Comparative Primate Biology (pp. 203−278). Alan R. Liss.

Schiller, P. H., Logothetis, N. K., and Charles, E. R. (1990a). Functions of the color-opponent and broad-band channels of the visual system. Nature, 343, 68−70.

Schiller, P. H., Logothetis, N. K. and Charles, E. R. (1990b). Role of the color-opponent and broad-band channels in vision. Vis. Neurosci., 5, 321−346.

Segraves, M. A., Goldberg, M. E., Deng, S., Bruce, C. J., Ungerleider, L. G., and Mishkin, M. (1987). The role of striate cortex in the guidance of eye movements in the monkey. J. Neurosci., 7, 3040−3058.

Silveira, L. C. L., and Perry, V. H. (1990). The topography of magnocellular projecting ganglion cells (M-ganglion cells) in the primate retina. Neuroscience, 40, 217−237.

Tolhurst, D. J. (1973). Separate channels for the analysis of the shape and the movement of a moving visual stimulus. J. Physiol., 231, 385−402.

Troy, J. B., and Lennie, P. (1987). Detection latencies of X and Y type cells of the cat's dorsal lateral geniculate nucleus. Exp. Brain Res., 65, 703−706.

Virsu, V. and Lee, B. B. (1983). Light adaptation in cells of macaque lateral geniculate nudeus and its relation to human light adaptation. J. Neurophysiol., 50, 864−877.

Walls, G. L. (1953). The lateral geniculate nucleus and visual histophysiology. In J. M. D. Olmsted, S. F. Cook, H. B. Jones, & J. L. Kirk (Eds.), University of California Publications in Physiology (pp. 1−100). London: Cambridge University Press.

Wiesel, T., and Hubel, D. H. (1966). Spatial and chromatic interactions in the lateral geniculate body of the rhesus monkey. J. Neurophysiol., 29, 1115−1156.

12 The Encoding of Cortical Contrast Gain Control

A. B. Bonds

CORTICAL RESPONSE TO DIFFERENT CONTRASTS

In the many studies of the relationship of the response amplitude of cortical cells to stimuli of differing contrast, the one dominant finding is nonlinearity. Maffei and Fiorentini (1973) were the first to describe cat cortical cells as having a clear contrast threshold. They characterized the response amplitude of simple cells as linear with log contrast, with saturation at high contrasts. Complex cells behaved similarly, but saturated at lower levels. This general model is consistent, with some variation, throughout the literature. Both Tolhurst, Movshon, and Thompson (1981) and Dean (1981) confirmed a distinct threshold for cat cortical cells but describe the suprathreshold response as linear with contrast, with saturation beginning about 1 log unit above the threshold contrast.

In a detailed study of 247 cells from cat and monkey visual cortices, Albrecht and Hamilton (1982) concluded that the most appropriate mathematical description of the cortical response-vs.-contrast (RVC) relationship is a hyperbolic ratio function, which satisfactorily fit about 70 percent of that population. While this function does not have a hard threshold, it embodies a region of linearity with log contrast (usually over about a log unit of contrast) and saturation. Three other mathematical functions (linear, log, and power) were found to have much less general applicability across the same population.

As will be shown below, the RVC relationship may not result from a single process; hence, fitting with a single function may be inappropriate. The linearity with contrast that was proposed earlier was not strictly incorrect, but the conclusion may have been misleading due to limitations of methodology. Albrecht and Hamilton pointed out that logarithmic and linear fits are virtually indistiguishable over ranges of less than a log unit, and Tolhurst, Movshon, and Thompson (1981) and Dean (1981) limited their measurements to contrasts no greater than 25 percent which is about one log unit above threshold.

CONTRAST MEDIATION OF RESPONSE NONLINEARITIES

The nonlinearity of the cortical RVC function results in two apparent paradoxes: (1) Even a quasilinear relationship between input and output is limited to about a log unit, and most cells saturate or even supersaturate (suffer response decline; see, for example, figure 12.7A at higher contrasts. Our behavioral capability to distinguish contrasts, however, extends to well over two log units. This can be explained to some extent by the observation that the effective range of contrasts signaled varies from cell to cell, with some cells responsive to low contrasts and others with higher thresholds but less saturation at higher contrasts (Albrecht and Hamilton 1982, figure 5). (2) Response saturation at higher firing rates would predict that the well-known cortical tuning characteristics for spatial frequency and orientation (e.g., Maffei and Fiorentini 1973; Henry, Bishop, Tupper, and Dreher 1973) would vary significantly depending on contrast. Specifically, operation in a region of saturation would afford broader tuning since the response would increase less rapidly at high levels (Robson 1975).

While this prediction would wreak havoc with models of visual processing as a more or less linear mechanism dependent on fixed filter characteristics (e.g., De Valois and De Valois 1988), fortunately it does not come to pass. Spatial frequency band-pass measured either via a method of thresholds (yielding contrast sensitivity) or by response amplitude is remarkably constant (Movshon, Thompson, and Tolhurst, 1978). Both orientation and spatial frequency tuning have subsequently been shown to be independent of stimulus contrast (Sclar and Freeman 1982; Albrecht and Hamilton 1982). Examination of RVC curves from nonoptimal stimulus configurations shows that this comes about because the primary suprathreshold nonlinearities (compression and saturation) are mediated by contrast and not by response amplitude. This result has also been extended to eye dominance (Li and Creutzfeldt 1984).

The dependence of cortical response amplitude nonlinearities on contrast has a profound consequence on understanding the operation of the visual cortex. Since compression or saturation in the RVC function can occur at widely differing response levels, this means that the control of response gain (firing rate vs. input amplitude) cannot arise within the cell itself or from more central mechanisms driven by the cell, but rather must arise from other cells contributing their information through a parallel network. All of the fundamental properties of the cortical cell must therefore be considered as a sum of lateral network activities, rather than as the result of strictly serial processes.

DOES THE VISUAL CORTEX REALLY MODIFY CONTRAST TRANSFER PROPERTIES SIGNIFICANTLY?

Within the context of this caveat let us consider the serial impact of cortical processing on contrast information by comparing RVC curves measured at the input stage (from lateral geniculate nucleus (LGN) neurons) and the output stage (from cortical neurons). In this way the nonlinearities introduced by

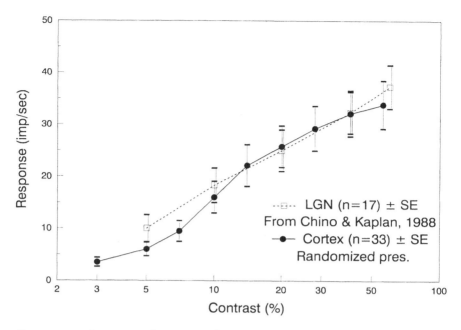

Figure 12.1 Comparison of response vs. log contrast (RVC) curves averaged across populations of LGN cells (open squares, dashed line) and cortical (filled circles, solid line) cells. The LGN response is first harmonic at the frequency of stimulation, and the cortical response (with 17 simple, 16 complex cells) is DC component. Bars indicate the standard error of the mean; bars are offset for LGN responses. Cortical responses were measured in the usual way, with contrasts presented in randomized order.

the cortical cells themselves can be clarified. Figure 12.1 (dotted line, open squares) shows an RVC curve averaged across 17 cat LGN cells (Chino and Kaplan 1988). Response is expressed in absolute impulses/sec at the fundamental frequency of stimulation, with error bars denoting the standard error of the mean. Overlaid on this is a similar average (solid line, filled circles) across 33 cat cortical cells (17 simple, 16 complex) taken from the database of Bonds (1991). This curve is likewise based on absolute response amplitude, with bars denoting standard error and, in the fashion of all similar studies, contrasts presented in random order (see below). Both simple and complex cell responses were calculated from average (DC) firing levels. This might be criticized because it is customary to express simple cell responses in terms of power at the stimulus fundamental frequency, as was done for the LGN responses. However, a comparison of fundamental response components from LGN and simple cells alone yields nearly identical results.

At least three points may be drawn from this figure: (1) Within a broad range of contrasts (10 to 60 percent) there is virtually no difference in the average firing rate of LGN cells and cortical cells. Thus despite significant convergence of LGN signals onto cortical cells, estimated at around 10 to 30 (Tanaka 1985), net cortical output amplitude is nearly unchanged. This suggests high selectivity in terms of what the cortex deems fit to pass on, and it also suggests that an average firing rate of 10 to 40 spikes/sec is functionally optimal for these signaling pathways. (2) The standard error of these two curves is remarkably similar. Even though the firing rates of different cortical cells at different contrasts are usually characterized as varying extremely broadly, there is in fact not much more populational variation than is found in the input stream. (3) There is a marked difference between the two curves at contrasts below 10 percent, with cortical cells appearing to be much less responsive. In view of LGN convergence and the resulting opportunity for probability summation this seems counterintuitive, since it would appear that cortical cells are losing low-contrast information even though they are, if anything, slightly more responsive to medium-contrast (14 to 40 percent) information.

CORTICAL CONTRAST GAIN IS VARIABLE

One would not expect cortical cells to reject low-contrast information that might be critical to survival. Hints at what might be happening first arose in the observation that "the responsiveness of cortical cells to a constant stimulus can vary over time" (Henry et al. 1973). This suggestion inspired nearly universal acceptance of the multiple histogram stimulation paradigm for cortical cells, in which the temporal sequence of presentation of different stimulus parameters is randomly interleaved. The resulting spread of variability across all stimulus conditions significantly enhanced the reliability of quantitative comparative studies, but tended to mask an important cortical response property. At least some component of response variability has been shown to be deterministic and dependent on stimulation. Repeated presentations of high-contrast stimuli yield slow decays (over seconds) in response amplitude (Vautin and Berkley 1978). The dependence of response reduction on stimulus contrast was quantified by Ohzawa, Sclar, and Freeman (1985), who presented several series of contrasts, each narrowly grouped about some mean value. When that mean value was increased the resulting RVC curves shifted rightward, indicating gain reduction that was equivalent to logarithmic contrast attenuation. The work of Vautin and Berkley and Ohzawa et al. was modeled on examples of psychophysical adaptation resulting from exposures of long duration to high contrast (e.g., Blakemore and Campbell 1969). In that context, results were sought only after extended periods of adaptation (seconds to minutes), with the implication that contrast adaptation is both slow and insensitive and therefore less important to day-to-day vision.

To see if adaptation could take place within a shorter time frame, cat cortical cells were presented with series of grating exposures in which contrast increased stepwise, then decreased in a sequential order (Bonds 1991). In a typical experiment, exposures to each contrast level were 3 seconds long and were followed by an immediate step to the next higher or lower contrast. The only zero-contrast stimulation was after completion of a series. With a typical range of nine contrast levels, the entire measurement cycle required 54 seconds to ascend in 0.15 log steps from 3 percent to a peak contrast of

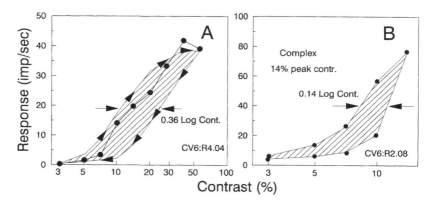

Figure 12.2 (A) Cortical RVC curves showing ordered and sequential contrast presentation. The filled circles (solid line) represent the RVC relationship when contrasts are presented in randomized order. The shaded area represents the response envelope from contrast presentation in ascending order (upper bound, up arrows), then descending (lower bound, down arrows) order. Each contrast level was presented for three seconds, and the full cycle was repeated 10 times. The horizontal arrows represent half the maximum response, at which level the dynamic hysteresis is equivalent to 0.36 log units of contrast. (B) Dynamic response hysteresis at low contrast levels. Each datum represents a 3 contrast presentation, with a peak contrast of only 14 percent.

56 percent and return to 3 percent. Each cycle was repeated ten times for measurement reliability.

This procedure was applied to a total of 36 cells (17 simple, 19 complex) in the cat visual cortex. For comparison with other RVC studies, curves were also measured with these cells using the more standard randomized contrast presentation procedure. Typical results from the randomized presentation (Figure 12.2A, filled circles) show the now-familiar pattern of threshold, a linear-with log contrast segment and saturation. Results from sequential presentation are more complex. The shaded area of figure 12.2A denotes the envelope of the response, with the upper boundary representing the response to increasing contrasts and the lower boundary the response to decreasing contrasts. The most prominent feature of this curve is the significant dynamic response hysteresis: at a given contrast level, the response is always greater when that level is preceded by a lower contrast than when it is preceded by a higher contrast. A figure of merit for the degree of hysteresis was derived by observing the shift in log contrast required to generate a response of half the maximum amplitude (horizontal arrows) for the rising and falling legs of the curve. Across 36 cells, this averaged 0.36 (± 0.15 log SD) log units, with a minimum of 0.1 log unit and a maximum greater than 1 log unit. No such adaptation was found in four LGN cells that were similarly tested, implying that contrast adaptation first arises in the cortex.

Another feature of the hysteresis curve of figure 12.2A is the suggestion that response saturation is a dynamic property. Nearly all cells showed a flattening of the curve as higher contrasts were reached on the ascending leg. In nearly every case, the first contrast decrement after the peak contrast yielded a response significantly lower than that found at the same contrast level on the ascending leg. This would not be expected if saturation resulted from response compression, in which case the trajectory would simply be retraced. Instead, gain reduction resulting from exposure to higher contrasts appears to linger even after reduction of the contrast.

Under the above-mentioned measuring conditions, dynamic response hysteresis may simply be considered as another expression of the cortical contrast adaptation described earlier, which results from long periods of stimulation with high contrasts. Acknowledging the possibility that contrast adaptation could be significant in natural behavioral vision, the next step was to assess lower limits of sensitivity and speed. The sensitivity of the gain-setting system to low levels of contrast was explored by testing seven cells with sequences of five contrasts peaking at 14 percent. In four cases, hysteresis averaging 0.12 log contrast was seen (figure 12.2B), although three cells showed negligible adaptation under these circumstances. Cells with high contrast sensitivity demonstrated modest hysteresis even for exposures to near-threshold contrasts. A peak contrast of 5 percent (shown for 3 seconds) yielded a response differential of nearly 50 percent at a 3 percent test contrast. This same cell showed a slight (but repeatable) response reduction at 1 percent contrast after exposure to a peak contrast of 3 percent for 3 seconds. In many cases contrasts that are barely suprathreshold are thus sufficient to alter the gain of a cell.

The impact of gain control on normal behavioral vision is also dependent on the speed of its activation, but measurements of the rate of gain change are difficult. Some response histogram waveforms show consistent amplitude loss over a few seconds of stimulation (Albrecht, Farrar, and Hamilton 1984). Other histograms can be flat or even show a slight rise over time despite clear adaptation of average response amplitude (Bonds 1991). This suggests the possibility that, in the classical pattern of any well-designed automatic gain control, gain reduction takes place quite rapidly, but its effects linger for some time.

A direct measurement of the rate at which adaptation occurred using a probe stimulus of varying stimulus onset asynchrony (e.g., Enroth-Cugell and Shapley 1973) proved impossible because of the complicated temporal format of cortical responses to brief stimuli. However, it was possible to show that the gain-setting process can occur over very brief periods of time by presentation of very brief adaptation stimuli. In these experiments (figure 12.3) a pedestal stimulus (drifting grating, 14 percent contrast) of two seconds' duration was used to establish a baseline firing rate. Adaptation resulted from the introduction of a temporary increase in contrast (to 28 percent) starting 0.5 second after the appearance of the pedestal. The adapting stimulus duration ranged from 50 msec to 750 msec. Adaptation was measured by taking the ratio of spikes generated during the first and last 500 msec of the 2-second pedestal period. Because of the inherently transient nature of the cortical response (probably reflecting adaptation by the pedestal stimulus itself), this ratio was 0.81 without any adapting stimulus. Even a 50-msec adapting stimu-

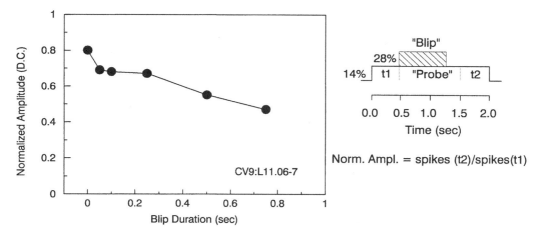

Figure 12.3 Speed of gain modification. A pedestal of 14 percent contrast is presented to this complex cell, which elevates its firing nearly uniformly in time. Half a second later, the contrast is incremented to 28 percent for a variable length of time (50 to 750 msec). A ratio is taken of the number of spikes during the first and last 500 msec of the pedestal period (2 s altogether). This ratio is reduced slightly for a 50-msec increment and by nearly half for a 750-msec increment.

lus reduced this figure slightly, and the decline was more or less linear with adapt duration to 750 msec, where the ratio was reduced by about 50 percent. Exposure to even brief increases in contrast can thus reduce the firing rate of the cell noticeably and for some period of time.

As in the case of the nonlinearities found in the statically measured response vs. contrast function, the dynamic nonlinearities were also dependent on stimulus contrast rather than the response level of the recorded cell. Two experiments were performed to test explicitly the dependence of hysteresis on contrast. Emulating the paradigm of Sclar and Freeman (1982), hysteresis curves were measured for different peak response levels in the same cell. These levels were defined by selecting different grating orientations for the tests. At each orientation the same set of contrasts was delivered. Over a range of peak amplitudes from 40 to 70 imp/sec generated at five different orientations, the magnitude of the hysteresis remained essentially constant, ranging from 0.25 to 0.28 log unit. Figure 12.4A shows the similarity between three such curves normalized to the same peak amplitude.

A second approach tested for the existence of hysteresis under conditions of constant contrast by modifying response amplitude through sequential presentations of differing orientations. A control hysteresis curve was first measured under normal conditions (by varying contrast; cross-hatched area in figure 12.4B). Next, response amplitude was varied over the same total range and time frame by varying orientation, while contrast was fixed (shaded area, figure 12.4B). Hysteresis is reduced by about 30 percent although not eliminated, when induced with fixed contrast. This was the smallest loss found; in three other similar experiments, losses exceeding 60 percent were found. Both

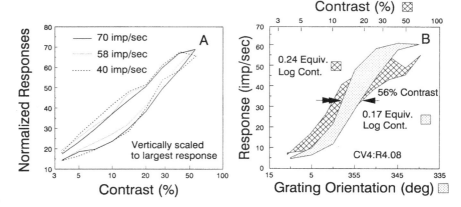

Figure 12.4 Evidence of contrast mediation of gain control. (A) Hysteresis measured at three different orientations, with peak firing rates of 40, 58, and 70 imp/sec. Firing rate is modified by changing the stimulus orientation (at a fixed contrast). Response curves are normalized to the same height and demonstrate essentially the same trajectories; hysteresis is constant at 0.25 to 0.28 log unit despite the variation of the peak firing rate. (B) Hysteresis induced by contrast variation (line shading) is compared with hysteresis induced by orientation variation at fixed contrast (dot shading). In the latter case hysteresis is reduced, though not eliminated.

experiments thus indicate that contrast, rather than response level, is of primary importance in setting the operating level of cortical cells.

A REEXAMINATION OF CORTICAL CONTRAST TRANSFER PROPERTIES

The speed and sensitivity of the cortical gain control demonstrated by the above experiments implies that virtually any suprathreshold stimulus can dynamically adapt a cell from its resting state. For this reason much of the nonlinearity measured in cortical RVC curves is likely to depend on measuring conditions. Equipped with this knowledge, a reexamination of the average relationship between the system input (LGN RVC curve) and output (cortical RVC curve) seems worthwhile. Ideally one would measure cortical responsiveness by presenting contrast levels in isolation, with sufficient time for recovery to adaptation interspersed, but this is impractical due to the time required. Moreover, in real-world visual situations there is a high likelihood that low contrast levels will be (temporally) associated with low contrast levels and high with high. For this reason, the comparison will be made by averaging the responses to the rising edge of the sequential contrast presentations described above (figure 12.5A).

At low contrasts (below 7 percent) the cortical response levels are essentially identical with those from the LGN. This would suggest that there is some physical limitation on responsiveness with so little information present. At moderate contrasts (10 to 28 percent) cortical responsiveness actually exceeds that from the LGN, but it is sharply less at contrasts above 28

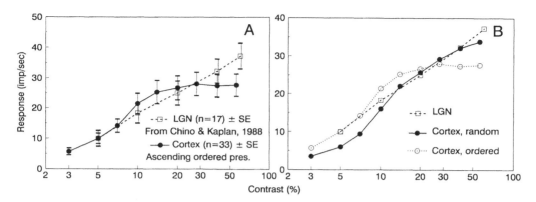

Figure 12.5 Comparison of LGN and cortical RVC curves as in figure 12.1, with the exception that cortical responses were measured by presenting the contrasts in a sequentially increasing order. (B) Combination of curves from figures 12.1 and 12.2A. LGN response is represented by open squares, dashed line; cortical response (randomized presentation) by filled circles, solid line; cortical response (ordered presentation) by open circles, dotted line.

percent. Enhancement of responsiveness at moderate contrasts is reasonable, but a transfer ratio of less than one at high levels seems less than optimal. One interpretation of this result is that, in a given contrast context, the absolute contrast (signaled by the absolute response level from LGN) is less important than higher sensitivity to incremental changes in contrast. The rapid ascent to and subsequent stabilization at a firing rate of about 25 imp/sec as contrast is increased suggests that this level is optimal for signaling both incremental and decremental changes in contrast. The positioning of this level midway within the average firing range (10 to 40 imp/sec) may be more than coincidental.

For a complete comparison, the combination of all three curves (LGN, cortex (random presentation) and cortex (ordered presentation)) is shown in figure 12.5B. The cortical curves cross one another. For random contrast presentations, on average lower contrasts are approached from much higher contrasts (hence responsiveness is lower than with ordered presentations), and higher contrasts are approached from much lower contrasts (hence responsiveness is higher than with ordered presentations). In this sample, the average contrast sensitivity increased 36 percent from 28.8 to 39.3, with sequential rather than randomized presentations, indicating that contrast sensitivity can be significantly underestimated when mixed contrasts are presented. With the exception of the very highest contrast, the transfer ratio of the cortex can be at least unity under different conditions of adaptation, although (as is pointed out above) a unity transfer ratio may not be ideal for information processing, especially at higher contrasts.

Cortical Gain Control and Inhibition

Cortical gain control always results in the reduction of responsiveness from the unadapted condition. It must result from inhibition. No stimulus-driven gain modification is seen in the afferent input stream from the LGN, so it must take place in cortical cells. The compressive nonlinearities seen in both the cortical RVC curves and the gain control are primarily contrast-driven, not response-driven, so the mediating signals must arise from other neurons in the network and be transferred via inhibition.

Intracortical inhibition has also been implicated in controlling the spatial filter properties (orientation and spatial frequency) unique to cortical cells. So-called cross-orientation inhibition results in reduction of a driven response when a grating or bar with a nonoptimal orientation is presented (Morrone, Burr, and Maffei 1982; Bonds 1989). A similar reduction in firing rate can occur when a grating of optimal orientation but nonoptimal spatial frequency is superimposed (De Valois and Tootell 1983; Bauman and Bonds 1991). Both of these mechanisms serve as a kind of lateral inhibition in the appropriate domain, enhancing the selectivity of the cortical neuron for the optimal stimulus. One might model contrast adaptation, which enhances sensitivity to changes in contrast at higher contrast levels, as a sort of lateral inhibition as well, only manifested across time rather than space. The question naturally arises as to whether the inhibition associated with spatial selectivity stems from the same mechanism and pathways that support contrast adaptation (a "universal inhibition theory").

Neurochemical Mediation of Inhibition

One of the most prevalent inhibitory neurotransmitters in the visual cortex is GABA (Shaw 1986). When cortical cells are exposed to microiontophoresis of the GABA antagonist bicuculline (or n-methyl-bicuculline), orientation selectivity is reported to be significantly reduced or eliminated (Sillito 1975, 1979), suggesting that the inhibition that mediates spatial selectivity is GABA-based. However, even though application of either GABA or bicuculline changes firing rate markedly, it does not change contrast adaptation behavior (DeBruyn and Bonds 1986; Vidyasagar 1990), suggesting that this effect is controlled via a different neurochemical pathway. On the basis of this evidence, spatially specific inhibition and contrast adaptation appear to be supported by two different mechanisms.

Cortical Spike Sequences

Further evidence for the independence of spatial inhibition and contrast adaptation arises from a totally different method of analysis. The distribution of individual impulses in a cortical spike train cannot be modeled by any continuous function. Instead, spikes are for the most part grouped in bursts with interspike intervals of 10 msec or less, with a burst followed by a refractory period of about 15 to 20 msec (Cattaneo, Morrone, and Maffeil 1981). Burst behavior in a spike sequence can be characterized by two parameters: (1) the number of bursts, or bursts per second (BPS), and (2) the duration of the

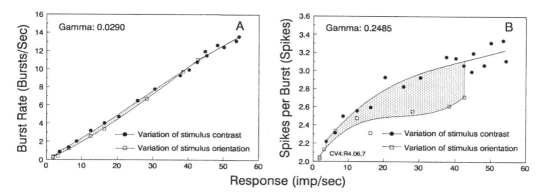

Figure 12.6 Burst statistic dependence on firing level. (A) The burst rate (bursts/sec) is plotted against firing level. The difference between the curves in which orientation is varied and contrast is varied is small (gamma = 0.029). (B) The burst length (spike/burst) likewise varies with firing rate, but in a way that is dependent on stimulation. At a given firing level, bursts are markedly shortened when firing rate is determined by orientation (open squares) rather than by contrast (filled circles). The difference between the curves (gamma, represented by the shaded area) is 0.2485.

bursts, or spikes per burst (SPB). Both parameters are strongly correlated with overall firing rate, but when that confounding variable is removed there is some difference in their behavior depending on what sort of stimulus generated the response.

Cat cortical spike sequences were analyzed for burst groupings using the simple rule that spikes with interspike intervals of 8 msec or less belonged in bursts (DeBusk, Bonds, and DeBruyn 1992). Several more sophisticated adaptive algorithms yielded essentially identical results. Comparisons were made between two types of experiments in which spike rate was changed either by changing contrast (at a fixed stimulus orientation) or by changing orientation (at a fixed stimulus contrast). Under all conditions, burst frequency (BPS) depended solely on average firing rate (figure 12.6A). To quantify the differences between contrast-parametric and orientation-parametric experiments, third-order polynomials were fit to curves generated under both conditions, and the (shaded) area between the curves was integrated over the range of measured firing rates. This parameter, called *gamma*, equaled about 0.03 for BPS in this case. At similar firing rates, burst length (SPB) is markedly shorter when firing rate is defined by varying orientation (open squares, figure 12.6B) rather than contrast (filled circles). In this example, gamma (about 0.25) is nearly ten times that found for BPS. In similar experiments across a population of 31 simple cells and 28 complex cells, gamma for BPS averaged 0.0114 and gamma for SPB averaged 0.1471, underscoring the sensitivity of burst length to stimulus orientation.

This result demonstrates a clear violation of the principle of univariance. The structure of the spike sequence at a given average firing rate can vary substantially on the basis of how the firing rate was generated. Presentation of nonoptimal orientations at higher contrasts yields spike bursts that are shorter than those generated by lower contrasts at the optimal orientation. This result, in combination with the finding that GABA causes response reduction at nonoptimal orientations, leads to the hypothesis that GABA inhibition acts to reduce firing by shortening bursts. At least in the cat somatosensory cortex, microiontophoretic injection of GABA has just that effect, and injection of bicuculline lengthens the bursts (Dykes et al. 1984).

Modulation of burst length has an impact on both signal transmission and cortical spatial filter properties. Because of postsynaptic temporal integration, concentrated bursts of spikes with short interspike intervals will be much more effective in generating depolarization than the same number of spikes distributed more evenly over longer intervals. The shortening of bursts resulting from nonoptimal orientations could thus effectively narrow the orientation tuning of a given cell at the level of the postsynaptic cell (Cattaneo et al. 1981). Burst length modulation can also be viewed as dynamic variation of the strength of coupling between nerve cells that is independent of firing rate.

Bursts and Contrast Transmission

While orientation manipulations result in inhibition that acts to change burst length, contrast manipulations appear to maintain a fixed relationship between firing rate and burst length. These results support the notion that there are at least two distinct forms of cortical. inhibition, with unique physiological bases differentiated by the burst organization. The existence of two types of inhibition is also consistent with the results discussed above, in which spatially dependent inhibition was GABA sensitive and contrast-dependent inhibition was not. The hypothesis that the two forms of inhibition are independent can be further tested by examining the behavior of spike bursts in the presence of explicit contrast-dependent inhibition. The model would predict that, in experiments involving response hysteresis, in which only contrast is changed, burst duration would depend only on absolute firing rate.

Burst analysis was applied to seven cells tested for response hysteresis; representative results are summarized in figure 12.7. When hysteresis measures involve high contrasts and response saturation (part A), BPS remains a constant function of firing rate, but the SPB trajectory (filled circles, part B) is mixed. SPB rises with spike rate on the presentation of ascending contrast, but with saturation it drops dramatically and remains depressed over the remainder of the contrast presentations. This would suggest that the same mechanism that shortens bursts at nonoptimal orientations also influences contrast gain control, which is at odds with the model of two independent inhibitory processes proposed above. However, a second manipulation on the same cell helps to reconcile the results. In this experiment (part C) the peak contrast was limited to 14 percent which avoided any evidence of response saturation but still yielded significant response hysteresis. The SPB trajectory is exactly iden-

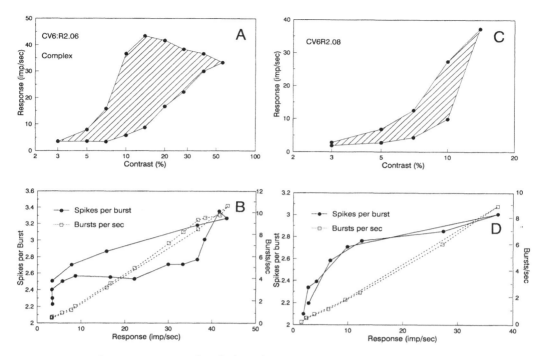

Figure 12.7 Burst length dependence on response hysteresis. (A, C) Response curves to sequentially ascending and descending contrasts, 3 s per datum. In (C) the peak contrast is 14 percent (see also figure 7.2B). (B, D) Corresponding plots of spikes/burst (open squares) and bursts/sec (filled circles) vs. firing rate. Bursts per second is simply proportional to firing rate in both plots. In (B), spikes/burst are noticeably depressed by exposure to contrasts that yield saturation, and this depression appears to linger throughout all descending contrasts. In (D), spikes/burst follow identical trajectories for both ascending and descending contrasts; no evidence of saturation or burst shortening is apparent.

tical for both ascending and descending contrasts (part D), indicating that in this case the burst-shortening mechanism was not activated.

We can thus conclude that in the limited case of gain control that is invoked under conditions of moderate contrast not involving saturation, gain can be reduced without evidence of the inhibitory mechanism that shortens bursts. Equally interesting is the evidence showing that response saturation is a nonlinearity that results from burst shortening, which is the same inhibitory mechanism that helps to define spatial filter properties. Note in figure 12.B that in the region of supersaturation (contrasts above 14 percent) the decrease in burst length is far greater than the decrease in number of bursts. Saturation could arise via inhibitory linkages from cells that have spatial tuning that is different from that of the recorded cell. These cells could then act as "lateral inhibitors" in the appropriate domain (orientation or spatial frequency) to sharpen the spatial selectivity of the recorded cell. Presentation of low-contrast stimuli that are optimal for the recorded cell (and thus nonoptimal for the inhibitory cells) would not activate the inhibitors, but higher contrasts would result in their recruitment, which could then result in saturation via burst shortening.

CONCLUSIONS

Unlike cells at earlier stages in the visual pathway, cells in the visual cortex demonstrate response nonlinearities that are dynamically controlled by contrast. The control mechanism is both sensitive and rapid, enabling it to operate under most natural viewing conditions. Its purpose appears to be the enhancement of incremental contrast information at the expense of information on absolute contrast. The loss of absolute contrast information in the cortex would seem no more problematic than the loss of absolute luminance information that is seen in the retina (Shapley and Enroth-Cugell 1984). One question that remains is why response attenuation is necessary. The gain control might serve to enhance contrast discrimination to the advantage of individual cells by holding their average firing level within a physiologically optimal range. If this were the case, the gain control should depend on the firing rate of the cell itself, but instead it is contrast-set. The independent adaptation of individual cells toward some optimum firing level would in fact be self-defeating, since uniform firing across all cells would tend to eliminate visual features. Uniform gain control across the cellular population would preserve the activity spectrum generated by the contrasts of the visual image, but would maintain a fairly constant total output from the cortex. This may be necessary to prevent input overload on subsequent structures due to convergence.

The results presented above are consistent with the idea that the unique patterns of cortical responses are defined by two kinds of inhibitory mechanisms. One mechanism is activated by nonoptimal spatial configurations (orientation and spatial frequency) and is characterized by shortening of bursts in the cortical spike train. It appears to be influenced by GABA. The other mechanism results in contrast-mediated response attenuation and is most likely responsible for nonlinearities seen at moderate contrasts. The neurotransmitter is unknown. Profound nonlinearities (saturation and supersaturation) from spatially optimal stimulation at higher contrasts appear to result from a combination of the two mechanisms, implying that in such cases the GABA-mediated burst-shortening mechanism is recruited only at higher contrasts.

ACKNOWLEDGMENTS

This work was performed with the help of Lisa Bauman, Ed DeBruyn, and Brian DeBusk. John Robson provided enriching conversation on stimulation by sequential contrasts and the global nature of gain control. Supported by NIH (RO1 EY03778) and a Vision Core Grant to Vanderbilt University.

REFERENCES

Albrecht DG, Hamilton, DB (1982) Striate cortex of monkey and cat: Contrast response functions. J Neurophysiol 48:217–237.

Albrecht DG, Farrar SB, Hamilton DB (1984) Spatial contrast adaptation characteristics of neurones recorded in the cat's visual cortex. J Physiol 347:713–739.

Bauman LA, Bonds AB (1991) Inhibitory refinement of spatial frequency selectivity in single cells of the cat striate cortex. Vision Res 31:933–944.

Blakemore CB, Campbell FW (1969) On the existence of neurones in the human visual system selectively sensitive to the orientation and size of reitna images. J Physiol 203:237–260.

Bonds AB (1989) The role of inhibition in the specification of orientation selectivity of cells in the cat striate cortex. Vis Neurosci 2:41–55.

Bonds AB (1991) Temporal dynamics of contrast gain in single cells of the cat striate cortex. Vis Neurosci 6:239–255.

Cattaneo A, Maffei L, Morrone, C (1981) Two firing patterns in the discharge of complex cells encoding different attributes of the visual stimulus. Exp Brain Res 43:115–118.

Chino YM, Kaplan E (1988) Abnormal orientation bias of LGN neurons in strabismic cats. Invest Ophthal Vis Sci 29:644–648.

Dean AF (1981) The relationship between response amplitude and contrast for cat striate cortical neurones. J Physiol 318:413–427.

DeBruyn EJ, Bonds AB (1986) Contrast adaptation in cat visual cortex is not mediated by GABA. Brain Res 383:339–342.

DeBusk, BC, Bonds, AB, DeBruyn, EJ (1992) Spike clustering in cat cortical cells supports independent coding of spatial and contrast information. Invest Ophthalmol Vis Sci (Suppl.) 33:1255.

De Valois KK, De Valois RL (1988) *Spatial Vision*. New York: Oxford Press.

De Valois KK, Tootell RBH (1983) Spatial-frequency-specific inhibition in cat striate cortical cells. J Physiol 336:359–376.

Dykes RW, Landry P, Metherate R, Hicks TP (1984) Functional role of GABA in cat primary somatosensory cortex: Shaping receptive fields of cortical neurons. J Neurophysiol 52:1066–1093.

Enroth-Cugell C, Shapley RM (1973) Adaptation and dynamics of cat retina ganglion cells. J Physiol 233:271–309.

Henry G, Bishop PO, Tupper RM, Dreher B (1973) Orientation specificity of cells in cat striate cortex. Vision Res 13:1771–1779.

Li CY, Creutzfeldt OD (1984) The representation of contrast and other stimulus parameters by single neurons in area 17 of the cat. Pflügers Archiv 401:304–314.

Maffei L, Fiorentini A (1973) The visual cortex as a spatial frequency analyzer. Vision Res 13:1255–1267.

Morrone MC, Burr DC, Maffei L (1982) Functional implications of crossorientation inhibition of cortical visual cells. Proc Roy Soc London B 216:335–354.

Movshon JA, Thompson ID, Tolhurst DJ (1978) Spatial summation in the receptive fields of simple cells in the cat's striate cortex. J Physiol 283:53–77.

Ohzawa I, Sclar G, Freeman RD (1985) Contrast gain control in the cat's visual system. J Neurophysiol 54:651–667.

Robson JG (1975) Receptive Fields: Neural representation of the spatial and intensive attributes of the visual image. In: Carterette EC, Friedman MF, ed. Handbook of Perception V: Seeing, pp 81–116. New York: Academic Press.

Sclar G, Freeman RD (1982) Orientation selectivity in the cat's striate cortex is invariant with stimulus contrast. Exp Brain Res 46:457–461.

Shapley RM, Enroth-Cugell C (1984) Visual adaptation and retinal gain controls. Prog Retinal Res 3:236–346.

Shaw C (1986) Laminar distribution of receptors in monkey (*Macaca fascicularis*) geniculostriate systems. J Comp Neurol 248:301–312.

Sillito AM (1975) The contribution of inhibitory mechanisms to the receptive field properties of neurones in the striate cortex of the cat. J Physiol 250:305–329.

Sillito AM (1979) Inhibitory mechanisms influencing complex cell orientation selectivity and their modification at high resting discharge levels. J Physiol 289:33–53.

Tanaka K (1985) Organization of geniculate inputs to visual cortical cells in the cat. Vision Res 25:357–364.

Tolhurst DJ, Movshon JA, Thompson ID (1981) The dependence of response amplitude and variance of cat visual cortical neurones on stimulus contrast. Exp Brain Res 41:414–419.

Tsumoto T, Eckart W, Creutzfeldt OD (1979) Modification of orientation sensitivity of cat visual cortex neurons by removal of GABA-mediated inhibition. Exp Brain Res 34:351–363.

Vautin RG, Berkley MA (1978) Responses of single cells in cat visual cortex to prolonged stimulus movement: Neural correlates of visual aftereffects. J Neurophysiol 40:1051–1065.

Vidyasagar TR (1990) Pattern adaptation in cat visual cortex is a co-operative phenomenon. Neuroscience 36:175–179.

13 Spatial Channels and Labeled Lines

Karen K. De Valois and Russell L. De Valois

The visual system allows an observer to gain information about the presence and character of objects at a distance. We wish to address one aspect of this process, which is related to how, at the level of the striate cortex, the visual system encodes information about the identity of objects.

An early step in vision must be that of identifying characteristics related to the presence of visual objects as opposed to irrelevant information. The response of the visual system to this problem takes into account the fact that most objects do not emit light, but rather reflect some portion of the incident illumination. Contrast $(L_{max} - L_{min}/2L_{mean})$ is a measure that refers to the relative amounts of light coming from different parts of a complex scene. The contrast formed by an object viewed against a background is invariant with illumination level, even though the absolute amount of light reflected by both object and background varies with light level. Contrast thus represents characteristics of the object and its background, not the relatively uninteresting character of the illuminant. It is often stated that the visual system converts its response from one dependent upon intensity to one dependent upon contrast at the earliest opportunity. Intensity information as such is indeed largely lost within the retina but, by the level of V1, the information that is conserved is not that of overall pattern contrast, but rather of amplitude within different two-dimensional spatial frequency bands. This fact, in combination with the nonflat spatial contrast sensitivity function, raises some interesting questions that we wish to explore further below.

The contrast at which a visual pattern will first become detectable can be predicted from a knowledge of the observer's contrast sensitivity function and the Fourier amplitude spectrum of the pattern (Campbell and Robson 1968). It is the amplitude of the individual Fourier components, not the contrast of the pattern as a whole, that determines whether the pattern will be seen (Graham and Nachmias 1971). These and related observations led to the suggestion that the visual system does not directly encode pattern contrast per se, but rather decomposes a complex pattern into its individual two-dimensional spatial frequency components, responding to each according to its amplitude (see De Valois and De Valois 1988 for a review of relevant data). Physiological recordings from individual neurons in the primary visual cortex, V1, confirm

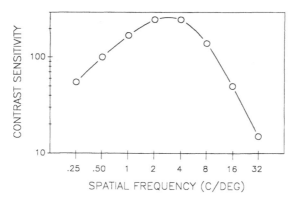

Figure 13.1 A typical spatial contrast sensitivity function for luminance-varying patterns. Contrast sensitivity (the reciprocal of threshold contrast) is plotted as a function of spatial frequency.

that each can be described in terms of its selectivity for two-dimensional spatial frequency.

The effective amplitude of a given frequency component—and thus ultimately the effective pattern contrast—is the product of the pattern amplitude at a particular spatial frequency and the observer's contrast sensitivity at the same frequency. Consider what would happen if an observer with the contrast sensitivity function shown in figure 13.1 were to view a very simple object, such as a plaid made up of two differently oriented components, one a sinusoidal grating of 0.5 c/deg and 5 percent contrast, the other a grating of 4 c/deg and 5 percent contrast. The first would be 5 times threshold contrast, since contrast sensitivity at 0.5 c/deg (for this observer) is 100. The contrast of the 4 c/deg component, however, would be 12.5 times its detection threshold, given a contrast sensitivity of 250 at that spatial frequency. At these relatively low physical contrasts, the *apparent* contrasts of the two components would be different (Georgeson and Sullivan 1975; Cannon 1979), with the component of higher frequency appearing to have the greater contrast.

If the same pattern were moved so that its distance from the observer was quadrupled, the retinal spatial frequencies of its two component gratings would be 2 and 8 c/deg, respectively, but the physical contrasts of the components would be largely unaffected. (Here we ignore the effects of increased attenuation by the eye's optics, which would simply exaggerate the effect we are discussing.) The lower-frequency component would now be 12.5 times its detection threshold contrast, while the higher would be only 2.5 times its threshold. Although the object itself would have changed only in position, not in character, its representation, at least through the V1 level, would be drastically modified. Yet if the ultimate task of the visual system is to construct (or reconstruct) an accurate representation of the visual world, important object invariances must be extracted without significant degradation.

These observations raise our second question, namely, how does the visual system allow the observer to determine what the object is? In other words, how is identifying information about the object encoded? The question of how information is encoded and transmitted from the peripheral sensory apparatus to the ultimate perceptual level is an old one. One widely accepted model assumes that individual neurons in the visual pathway act as labeled lines. The intellectual history of this idea can be traced to Johannes Mueller's prescient formulation (1826) of the Doctrine of Specific Nerve Energies. Mueller was interested in the question of how information about the quality of a stimulus could be transmitted through a sensory nerve. His conclusion, which has since become accepted dogma, was that information about stimulus quality is implicit in the identity of the responding nerve and is, in fact, independent of the particular event that produced the response. Thus, the message conveyed by excitation of the optic nerve is always that a visual event occurred, irrespective of the fact that the actual stimulus could have been physical pressure, for example, as in mechanically induced phosphenes.

This solution to the problem of how to convey stimulus quality is both elegant and flawed—elegant because of its simplicity and flawed because of its limitations. Since excitation of the optic nerve is almost always due to the occurrence of a visual event, signaling its quality by the mere identity of the responding nerve is efficient. No complex processing with its concomitantly large anatomical investment is required. The simplicity of the solution, however, also produces its limitations. Without sophisticated analyzing machinery, the processing required to discriminate between and differentially signal the presence of multiple classes of stimuli is not possible. Thus we "see" mechanical pressure and electrical currents when they are applied to the eye.

Mueller's concern, appropriate to the state of knowledge in the early nineteenth century, was with whole nerves. Although we are obviously able to observe and analyze sensory systems on a finer scale today, much of our thinking is still guided by the fundamental principle he was first to enunciate clearly. The basic idea is that the information transmitted by a given sensory neuron is implicit in the *identity* of the neuron, and variations in the *magnitude* of the response carry information about stimulus amplitude (see, for example, Barlow 1972 or Georgeson 1980). This modern version of the Doctrine of Specific Nerve Energies is known as the *principle of labeled lines*. Each neuron is considered to bear a label that is related to its tuning characteristics, such that the message conveyed by its activity is that the stimulus to which that neuron is most sensitive (or most responsive) is present. The stimulus to which a neuron is most sensitive is sometimes termed the *adequate stimulus*. If neurons act as labeled lines, then to determine the character of the *adequate stimulus* is to determine the way in which the visual system analyzes spatial patterns in the world. The adequate stimulus becomes the basic unit of spatial information.

One intuitively appealing notion is that neurons act as feature detectors, signaling the presence of particular natural objects or easily identified features of objects. Such a system would require dedicated circuitry to ensure both that the cells were able to determine the presence of their particular features and that these could be successfully discriminated from all other possible features in the world. If there are only a few objects of visual interest, and if the organism can afford to ignore the presence of all other objects, then feature detectors might be a reasonable solution to the problem of characterizing objects. Indeed, there have been suggestions that some simpler animals (e.g., frogs; see Lettvin, Maturana, McCulloch, and Pitts 1959) use dedicated feature detectors. It could be that naturalistic feature detectors occur at some post-striate level in cats and primates, but they clearly do not exist at or before the striate cortex. Neurons in V1 respond to patterns in ways that are not simply related to obvious spatial features of objects such as edges or angles, and a given neuron will respond to a wide variety of patterns that have no apparent commonality of features. This raises the question of what alternate form of information coding could be used at early levels of the visual system.

SPATIAL FREQUENCY ANALYSIS

One possibility is that a more abstract analytic code is used—for example, the visual system could perform a spatially localized, two-dimensional spatial frequency analysis of the visual scene (Robson 1975). A given neuron could act as a spatial frequency filter, responding to a pattern, any pattern, to the extent that it contains power within a localized two-dimensional spatial frequency band. Such a system would have certain very powerful advantages. It would be universal, in the sense that any visual stimulus could be analyzed by the same set of filters. It would also be efficient, in that only a limited number of such filters would be required, unlike the very large to infinite number that would be necessary to encode the presence of the potentially infinite number of naturalistic features.

If the visual system were to analyze the retinal image in terms of the two-dimensional spatial frequencies present within a localized region, neurons in V1 might be expected to show selectivity along these dimensions. These neurons have been well characterized in terms of their selectivity for spatial frequency and orientation. The vast majority of such cells show band-pass tuning for two-dimensional spatial frequency, that is, for orientation and spatial frequency (Movshon, Thompson, and Tolhurst 1978; De Valois, Albrecht, and Thorell 1982; De Valois and De Valois 1988). Selectivity along both dimensions is significantly greater than that found at earlier neural levels, and the total range of both orientations and spatial frequencies represented by the whole ensemble of responding neurons is much greater than the range of either to which a typical neuron responds. Since most cells in V1 have little if any spontaneous activity, activity of a particular cell represents the presence of one stimulus drawn from a fairly restricted portion of all possible stimuli.

In a sample of some hundreds of V1 neurons in the macaque monkey, the average spatial frequency bandwidth was found to be 1.4 octaves (De Valois, Albrecht, and Thorell 1982) and the average orientation bandwidth 45° (De Valois, Yund, and Hepler 1982). The significance of this can be seen in figure 13.2, which represents the selectivity of a neuron with these "average" tuning

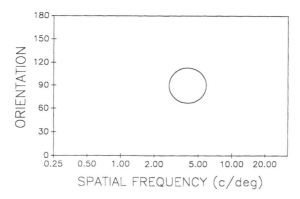

Figure 13.2 The two-dimensional spatial frequency sensitivity range of an average neuron in VI of macaque monkey. The range of spatial frequencies and orientations to which macaques show significant sensitivity is represented as the total area of the figure. The area covered by the tuning function of this one neuron is about 3 percent of the total area.

characteristics in the frequency domain. The figure illustrates the region within which an effective stimulus for this cell could fall, which is shown as the circumscribed area within the total range of spatial frequencies and orientations to which macaque monkeys show significant sensitivity on behavioral tests (De Valois, Morgan, and Snodderly 1974). (Here we consider an effective stimulus to be one that produces a response at least half as great as that produced by the cell's "best" stimulus—i.e., one that lies within the cell's pass-band as described above.)

The area covered by such a cell's sensitivity function is about 3 percent of the total sensitivity range. Thus this one neuron, in combination with a set of 32 other cells with similar but nonoverlapping tuning functions and identical receptive field (RF) centers, could signal the presence of any visible stimulus in one region of the visual field. Further, the identity of the responding neuron could localize the stimulus to one of 33 possible bands within the full two-dimensional region of visual sensitivity. This could form the basis for a true labeled-lines mechanism. (Of course, if this were an accurate representation of the neuron's selectivity function, more than 33 neurons would be required, because no set of circular and nonoverlapping subregions could actually tile the area. In order to tessellate this region with nonoverlapping units, the neural sensitivity functions would have to be of a different shape, hexagonal for example, or rectangular.)

This approach to the question of the encoding of spatial patterns has been a powerful one. To the extent that neurons behave in a linear fashion, it should be possible to predict a cell's response to any arbitrary pattern based upon a knowledge of its tuning function for sine waves, just as the detectability of a pattern can be predicted from a knowledge of the subject's contrast sensitivity function (Campbell and Robson 1968; Campbell, Carpenter, and Levinson, 1969). Although a relatively small number of complex stimuli have been used and certain manifest nonlinearities are present (e.g.,

De Valois and Tootell 1983; Bauman and Bonds 1991), attempts to predict responses to complex patterns have been surprisingly successful (De Valois, De Valois, and Yund 1979; Albrecht, De Valois, and Thorell 1980).

We wish to consider two questions that are raised by this approach to the encoding of visual spatial information. First, if we assume that neurons in V1 act as two-dimensional spatial frequency filters, how is this information read out? Do observers perceive spatial frequency directly based on the activity of these neurons, or is V1 simply a nonaccessible way station on the way to some higher cortical representation? Second, how might the important characteristics of objects—their invariances—be encoded by a spatial frequency analytic system? We shall consider these questions separately.

SPATIAL FREQUENCY: LABELED LINES

To ask whether observers can access information about the spatial frequency of a pattern by reading out the activity of V1 neurons is equivalent to asking whether these cells act explicitly as labeled lines and what their labels are. Although few would argue that visual perception takes place in the striate cortex, it is not unusual to find models of spatial vision that assume that information about spatial frequency is directly available to the observer (e.g., Georgeson 1980, 1985; Davis, Kramer, and Yager 1986). Since the narrowest spatial frequency tuning appears to be available by V1, and since we have considerably more information about cell-tuning characteristics at that level than at later levels, modeling of visual behavior based on spatial frequency-tuning functions most often assumes tuning like that seen in V1. We have examined the question of how observers gain information about spatial frequency using a simple psychophysical matching task. We asked subjects to match the spatial frequencies of sine waves and square waves, because these are two patterns for which we have considerable information about the responses of V1 cells.

Neurophysiology

We recorded from 31 individual neurons in the striate cortices of anesthetized, paralyzed cats and macaque monkeys (Elfar, De Valois, and De Valois 1990 and in preparation), comparing the spatial frequency tuning functions for luminance-varying sine waves and square waves of optimal orientation and various contrasts. In 36 percent of the individual comparisons we made, the peak spatial frequencies for sine and square waves were identical. In 45 percent of the comparisons, the peak frequency for square waves was lower than that for sine waves in the same neuron and at the same pattern contrast. This difference was systematic and occurred reliably within individual neurons. The average ratio of square wave peak frequency to sine wave peak frequency was 0.94 across all cells and all conditions. In the 19 percent of individual comparisons in which the peak frequency for square waves was higher than that for sine waves, no systematic trend was found. When the same set of conditions was repeated more than once, no reliable shift toward a higher peak for square waves was ever seen, and the individual instances appeared to result from short-term response variability.

The reduction in peak spatial frequency for square waves appeared to occur in two ways. In broadly tuned cells, the lower peak frequency for square waves presumably reflects the inclusion of one or more higher harmonic components with the cell's pass-band. This can be seen as a broadening of the frequency-tuning function toward the low frequencies. In the remaining cells, the shift to lower peak frequencies appears to be the result of inhibition from the higher harmonics present in the square wave. This is seen as a narrowing of the frequency-tuning function resulting from a reduced response to higher spatial frequencies. An example of such a response function can be seen in figure 13.3.

Many neurons also respond, though less vigorously, to a square wave of fundamental frequency significantly lower than the peak. Such responses are correlated with the presence and temporal frequency of the higher harmonics in the square wave pattern. An example of the contrast sensitivity of a V1 neuron to square waves of different spatial frequencies is shown in figure 13.4. The contrast sensitivities corresponding to responses to the fundamental third and fifth harmonic components are shown separately.

These observations allow us to make some simple predictions about the perceived spatial frequencies of sine waves and square waves based upon a labeled lines model. This model is very similar to—indeed, largely based upon—other suggestions in the current literature (see, for example, Georgeson 1985; Davis, et al. 1986). We report in brief the results of tests of predictions based upon the following assumptions:

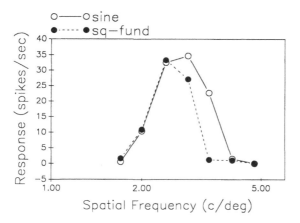

Figure 13.3 Responses of a VI neuron to spatial sine waves and square waves of identical pattern contrast. The spatial frequency of the square wave is that of its fundamental frequency component. Note that the responses to square waves of higher fundamental frequencies are reduced, producing a narrower frequency pass-band and a shift of the peak toward lower frequencies.

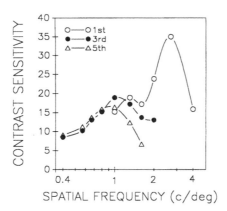

Figure 13.4 Contrast sensitivity of a VI neuron to the various harmonic components of a square wave. Plotted are the amplitudes of the first, third, and fifth harmonic components of the peristimulus time response wavefrom, as a function of the spatial frequency of the fundamental frequency component of the stimulus. Note that the third harmonic component of the response is maximum to a square wave grating of approximately one-third the frequency of that which produces the greatest response at the fundamental. At this frequency, the thrid harmonic component of the stimulus is within the most sensitive region of the cell's spatial frequency pass-band.

1. Each cell carries an invariant label such that activity in the cell signals the presence of the particular stimulus characteristics associated with its label.

2. For any cell, the spatial frequency signaled by it is that of the sine wave to which the cell is most sensitive—that is, the peak of its spatial frequency tuning function for sine waves at the optimal orientation.

3. When an observer is asked to compare the spatial frequencies of two patterns, he or she will do so by comparing the labels of the cells that are most responsive to each pattern. When the labels are identical, the observer will say that the two frequencies are identical. If one pattern produces maximum activity in cells whose frequency label is higher, that pattern will be identified as having a higher spatial frequency.

With these propositions in mind, we can make the following prediction from the physiological results. If a sine wave grating and a square wave grating, both of moderate to high contrast and fundamental spatial frequency, are compared, their spatial frequencies should appear to be identical either when their fundamental frequencies are identical or when the square wave fundamental is slightly lower in frequency than the sine wave. Since the square wave component with the greatest amplitude is the fundamental, neurons that respond to the fundamental component will, for most square wave spatial frequencies, be the most responsive. Here we explicitly exclude spatial frequencies below the peak of the spatial contrast sensitivity function. Thus observers should match spatial periods (and therefore fundamental frequencies) of sine waves and square waves accurately if the cells most responsive to the square wave are identically tuned for sines and squares. Note that this predicts that the presence of the higher harmonics in the square wave pattern should have no effect on the matching procedure. If the most responsive neurons prefer square waves of lower frequency (recall that many cells do), then sine waves should appear to match square waves of slightly lower frequencies. In other words, either the apparent spatial frequency of a square wave should be identical to that of a sine wave of its fundamental frequency or the apparent spatial frequency of a square wave should be higher than that of a sine wave of the same frequency.

Psychophysics: Sine/Square Wave Matching

In psychophysical experiments, we have examined the way in which human subjects match the spatial frequencies of sine waves and square waves (De Valois, Switkes, and Kooi, in preparation). The two patterns to be compared on a given trial were displayed on a 19-inch Mitsubishi color monitor with a 30-Hz interlaced raster rate, under computer control. The addition of specially designed attenuators on the RGB video outputs permitted the rentention of the full 8-bit intensity resolution over a reduced dynamic range so that threshold and near-threshold patterns could be produced. All patterns were identical in space-averaged luminance (27.4 cd/m²) and chromaticity (CIE coordinates x = .3101, y = .3162). The circular aperture subtended 8.7 deg at the 172-cm viewing distance. The two patterns to be compared were matched in Michelson contrast but, because it has been reported that grating contrast can affect the apparent spatial frequency under certain conditions (Georgeson 1980, 1985; Gelb and Wilson 1983; Davis, Kramer, and Yager 1986), the contrast of the reference grating varied randomly over a range of ±5 percent of its nominal contrast. In addition, at various times we also equated the sine and square waves for amplitude of the fundamental components or for multiples of the detection threshold contrasts. None of these manipulations made any significant difference as long as the pattern contrast was well above the threshold range.

We presented the two patterns in a two-alternative, spatial forced-choice paradigm, using a staircase procedure designed to converge on the test frequency that appeared to match the frequency of the reference pattern. The two gratings were presented above and below a 1 deg horizontal strip of the same average luminance and chromaticity, on which a fixation target was displayed. The reference and test gratings changed positions randomly from trial to trial. In order to prevent possible quantization effects due to the use of a digital display, the square wave was always the pattern of fixed frequency. In the forced-choice experiments the subject's task was to say which of the two gratings presented on each trial appeared to be higher in spatial frequency.

On this task most subjects make systematic, reliable, and often large errors. The matches inevitably deviate from veridical in the same direction. If a square wave grating is of a particular fixed spatial frequency, the sine wave grating that appears to match it must be of a *lower* spatial frequency. To put it another

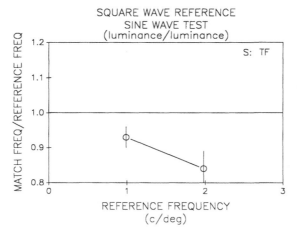

Figure 13.5 The ratio of matching frequency to reference frequency as a function of the reference spatial frequency. The subject was asked to judge the relative spatial frequencies of a sine wave grating and a square wave grating of approximately equal contrast. When the two matched in perceived spatial frequency, the sine wave was actually lower in retinal spatial frequency.

way, if the square wave and the sine wave are actually and appropriately matched in fundamental frequency, the square wave will appear to be lower in frequency. Figure 13.5 shows an example of data from one naive subject. This "error" persists across a range of spatial frequencies up to about 4 c/deg, and it is largely unaffected by contrast as long as the square wave contrast is high enough to make it appear to be a square wave—that is, its higher harmonics are above their independent detection thresholds. The presence of the higher harmonic components in the square wave has a significant effect upon the perception of the grating period (thus, fundamental frequency), even though the neuron(s) giving the greatest response must usually be the same for both sine and square waves.

This failure suggests a revision to the simple labeled-lines model proposed above. Perhaps the perceptual decision depends not simply upon the identity of the cell(s) that are most responsive, but upon some combination of all the neurons responding to a particular pattern. Consider what this would predict for the sine-square comparison. The square wave contains power at all odd harmonic frequencies, and the physiological data shown earlier illustrate neuronal responses to those components. Thus, if the fundamental frequency of the square wave is, say, 1 c/deg and the pattern contrast is high, then neurons sensitive to 3 and 5 c/deg, respectively, might be expected to show some activity, in addition to those neurons that respond to the presence of the fundamental frequency. (Depending on the contrast, of course, even higher harmonics could produce detectable activation.) If the response of any given cell signals the presence of a stimulus that corresponds to the cell's "best" frequency, then there would be messages saying that frequencies of 1, 3, and 5 c/deg were present, as they are. (Here we are ignoring the further complication produced by the neurons tuned to various intermediate spatial frequencies, but also responding to one or more of the square wave components.) The subject, however, is asked to judge the single frequency corresponding to the periodicity of the square wave. How would those diverse signals be combined?

One reasonable suggestion is that each would be weighted according to its magnitude, and the ultimate decision would reflect the weighted average of all the inputs. Another possibility is that each would be weighted by some factor proportional to the reciprocal of its spatial frequency label in order to selectively amplify the signal corresponding to low spatial frequencies in the stimulus. (See Davis et al. 1986 for a discussion of several possible combination rules.) In either case, the perceptual decision should be that the frequency of the square was higher than the frequency of its fundamental. How much higher would depend upon the relative magnitudes of the responses to the various components and the actual combination rule adopted. In any case, though, the apparent frequency of the square wave would be higher than the apparent frequency of a sine wave with the same period and thus the same fundamental frequency.

The data, however, showed just the opposite. Refer back to figure 13.5. The square wave, if it appears to differ from the sine wave, always appears to be *lower* in frequency when the two are actually equated in fundamental frequency, not *higher* as it should if its apparent frequency were determined by some combination of the frequency labels of all the responding units. Thus, even a modification of the labeled-lines model that takes into account the presence of the higher harmonics in the square wave fails to predict performance on this very simple psychophysical task.

Missing Fundamental

One counterargument could be based upon the fact that V1 neurons, as we noted above, do not directly encode the contrast of the whole pattern. Rather, their responses can be more readily predicted from the amplitude of the particular frequency components for which they are selective. In the case of sine waves and square waves that are matched in pattern contrast, the amplitude of the square wave fundamental exceeds that of the sine wave by a factor of $4/\pi$. Thus the "effective contrast" of the fundamental component of the square wave should be higher than that of the sine wave.

Georgeson (1980, 1985) reports that any stimulus manipulation that takes a grating nearer its detection threshold will increase its apparent spatial frequency, and Davis et al. (1986) also affirm the significance of contrast in determining apparent spatial frequency. Although we included a number of control conditions to reduce the possibility that our results could be due to this factor, the possibility is still of concern. Therefore, we asked our subjects to match the spatial frequency of a sine wave to that of a square wave from which the fundamental component had been removed. The missing fundamental pattern has the same spatial period as the full square wave, but it contains no power at the fundamental frequency. Any version of a frequency labeled-lines model, therefore, should predict that the apparent frequency of the missing fundamental pattern should be higher than that of a sine wave of the same period. In fact, the missing fundamental, like the full square wave, appears to be lower, not higher, in frequency than a sine wave matched for spatial period.

Matching Chromatic and Luminance Patterns

A similar and probably related failure occurs if subjects are asked to match the spatial frequencies of two sine waves, one of which varies in luminance, the other in chrominance. Thorell, De Valois, and Albrecht (1984) and Lennie, Krauskopf, and Sclar (1990) have examined the selectivity of V1 neurons in macaque monkey to grating patterns varying in either luminance or chrominance. They report that neurons that respond to both tend to be similarly tuned for spatial variations in both dimensions. However, Thorell et al. note that a significant subclass contains cells that are tuned differently for color and luminance. When they differ, it is virtually always in the same direction. A given neuron will have a *lower* peak frequency for color, it will be frequency band-pass for luminance but low-pass for color, or both. If we assume that a cell carries a single set of labels (i.e., one spatial frequency, one orientation, etc.), then a cell that has a high peak frequency for luminance and a lower peak frequency for color should indicate that a high-frequency luminance grating matches a low-frequency chromatic grating. Similarly, because of the presence of significant numbers of neurons with low-pass characteristics for color, the population of neurons responding to an isoluminant grating of some particular spatial frequency should include many that are tuned to (and thus presumably signal the presence of) higher spatial frequencies. Both factors would lead to the prediction that the apparent frequency of a chromatic grating should be higher than the apparent frequency of a luminance grating that is veridically matched.

We have tested these predictions by the same method described above, with the addition of certain control measures. Subjects viewed the patterns through an air-spaced achromatizing lens designed to correct for longitudinal chromatic aberrations. Contrast sensitivity for each pattern was measured for each observer, and test and reference patterns were equated for multiples of threshold contrast at the reference frequency. Two chromatic axes were used. These corresponded to an axis of equal and opposite L and M cone activation, with constant absorption by the S cones and a tritanopic confusion axis, the so-called cardinal color axes (Krauskopf, Williams, and Heeley 1982).

We found that, if luminance and chromatic gratings are actually identical in spatial frequency, the apparent frequency of the chromatic grating will be lower. Thus, in order for the two to appear identical, the chromatic grating must be increased in frequency, not decreased. The error of the setting may

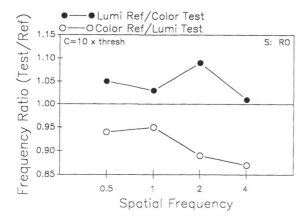

Figure 13.6 Spatial frequency matching of an isoluminant chromatic grating a luminance-varying grating. The ration of matching frequency to reference frequency is shown as a function of the reference spatial frequency. Note that regardless of which pattern is used as the reference, the isoluminant grating must be higher in retinal spatial frequency in order for the apparent frequencies of the two sinusoidal gratings to match.

reach 25 to 30 percent of the reference frequency. An example of spatial frequency matches by one naive observer is shown in figure 13.6. As in the case with sine waves and square waves, a simple labeled-lines model can predict either that the two patterns should be veridically matched (if only the most responsive subset of neurons is used) or the matches should deviate from accuracy, but in a direction opposite to that actually seen. In neither case does any manipulation of the combination rules allow for accurate prediction. Thus we conclude that some mechanism other than a straightforward system based upon labeled lines with the response characteristics of V1 neurons is involved in making these judgments.

The fact that V1 neurons are selective for two-dimensional spatial frequency does not imply that all spatial information about the stimulus is encoded in this way. These neurons have spatially localized RFs, and their responses can signal visual location as well as spatial frequency and orientation. Each neuron could be tagged with a "local sign," an idea derived from the work of Lotze (1886) and Hering (1879). It is easy to see how the period or spatial frequency of a grating could be determined if each active neuron transmitted precise information about the spatial location of the stimulus to which it was responding. Models of spatial vision often incorporate local signs assumptions, and Georgeson (1980) has explicitly discussed the manner in which such information could be used to determine grating frequency. A local signs model has not been successful in predicting the change of apparent spatial frequency produced by changes in contrast (Georgeson 1980), however, and it gives no promise of explaining our observations on the apparent spatial frequency of sine versus square waves or of luminance sine waves versus chromatic sine waves.

SPATIAL REPRESENTATIONS

Neither a labeled-lines mechanism based on the spatial frequency selectivity of V1 neurons nor a local signs mechanism based on the spatial positional selectivity implied by their delimited RFs has provided a basis for understanding the anomalous spatial frequency judgments described above. Both models have been successfully applied to a variety of other psychophysical and perceptual phenomena, however, and the evidence in support of the existence and utility of each is convincing. This leads us to suggest that, with regard to the analysis and encoding of pattern spatial characteristics, the visual system may use a variety of different mechanisms. A clear example of the use of multiple kinds of information by the visual system is in the task of object segregation, where luminance, color, depth, and motion can all be used either individually or in combination to segment a scene. Similarly, spatial frequency labels, local signs, or other (yet unknown) kinds of information may be used to identify the spatial character of a visual stimulus. With this possibility in mind, we wish to describe one additional way in which spatial information about an object might be encoded. Although the mechanism we shall suggest does not explicitly solve the problem we raised earlier, modifications of it could potentially do so.

A third kind of spatial information that is present in the representation in V1 is due to the fact that there is a consistent functional anatomical organization within the individual cortical modules. The large number of neurons with identical (or nearly identical) RF centers are grouped together anatomically to form a cortical module with two subunits, each half-module mainly related to one eye. Consider a simplified representation of the arrangement of neuronal selectivities within a single V1 module as shown in figure 13.2. Here we have illustrated a module in which the peak orientation and spatial frequency of individual neurons vary systematically in a rectangular array. This is probably a reasonable representation of the organization of a module in the cat striate cortex (De Valois and De Valois 1988). In the monkey the organization may be polar rather than rectangular (De Valois and De Valois 1988), but the important assumption is that the two dimensions are orthogonal, irrespective of the precise geometric form. Several interesting kinds of information can be derived by looking at the pattern or profile of activity within such an array.

First consider the case that would occur if the array were rectangular, with orientation one dimension and log spatial frequency the other. A pattern of a single spatial frequency and orientation would produce a single peak of activity. A pattern of slightly greater complexity, a plaid pattern composed of three spatially overlapping gratings of different orientations and spatial frequencies, might produce the activation pattern shown in figure 13.7a. Magnifying the stimulus pattern by a constant factor would shift the response pattern either right or left within the "module" represented in the figure, but it would not change the spacing between the local activity maxima (see figure 13.7b). The essential similarity of the two stimuli—the original and its

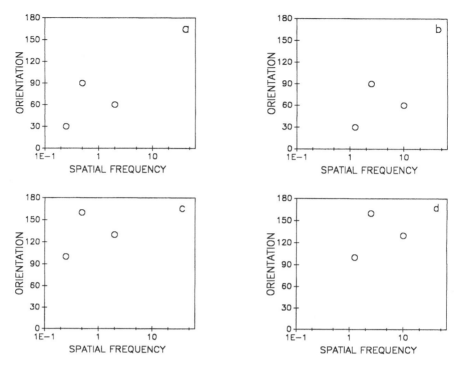

Figure 13.7 Rectangularly arrayed modules in which orientation is represented along one axis and (log) spatial frequency along the other. (a) The local activity peaks that would result from the presence of a three-component plaid, with all components of different spatial frequencies and orientations. (b) The local activity peaks that would result from a minification of the pattern. (c) The activity pattern that would result from a rotation of the original stimulus. (d), the stimulus has been both minified and rotated, producing the pattern of activity shown. Note the essential similarity of all four response patterns.

magnified fellow—can immediately be seen by noting the relationship between the three response maxima, *without any information as to the precise spatial frequencies of either*. Similarly, a plaid composed of three gratings of the same spatial frequency but different orientations could also be recognized despite a pattern rotation, which would result in a vertical translation as shown in part c, and a combination of magnification and rotation would produce a translation in x and y, as in part d.

Within a single rectangularly arrayed module such as that described here, stimulus complexity can be increased to any desired degree in terms of numbers of components without sacrificing the essential similarity of the representation under any combination of magnification and/or rotation in two-dimensional space. The pattern of activation produced by the transformed figure will be congruent with the pattern of activation produced before the transformation. Thus two essential conditions for object constancy, invariance under magnification and planar rotation, are satisfied by virtue of the characteristics of spatial representation within a single rectangularly arrayed cortical module.

If the dimensions of spatial frequency and orientation are represented in a polar space with spatial frequency increasing along the radius and orientation varying with angle, the situation is somewhat different. Under rotation without magnification, the two patterns of activity will still be congruent. Under magnification, the distance separating two corresponding points in the activity array will differ and the resulting patterns will not only not be congruent, they will not be geometrically similar. If spatial frequency is scaled linearly along the radius, however, the total pattern of activation within the module will form a figure that is geometrically similar to the original pattern. That is, corresponding angles in the two activity patterns will be identical, and the distances between corresponding points will be proportional. This is illustrated in figure 13.8, in which the object represented by points Y_1, Y_2, and Y_3 undergoes both a magnification and a rotation. After transformation it is represented by points X_1, X_2, and X_3, which together form a pattern that is geometrically similar to the original.

Whether the functional organization within a single cortical module is rectangular or polar, as long as spatial frequency and orientation are appropriately represented some of the essential conditions for high-level object constancy can be met. A subsequent analytic mechanism need not deal with information

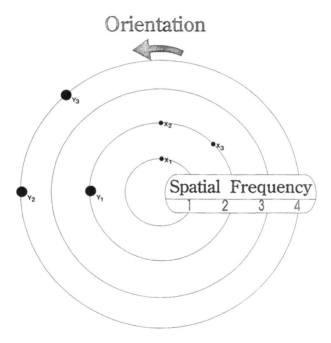

Figure 13.8 Radially arrayed module in which spatial frequency increases linearly along the radius and orientation varies around the circumference. A three-component plaid, with all components of different spatial frequencies and orientations, might produce the local activity peaks shown as points X_1, X_2, X_3. A combined rotation and minification of the stimulus would produce the local activity peaks shown as Y_1, Y_2, and Y_3. Although the resulting pattern is not congruent with the original pattern of activity, the two are geometrically similar.

respecting absolute spatial frequency or absolute orientation. The relative spatial frequencies and orientations that comprise the essence of the object's identity are preserved, while the absolute values of each dimension become irrelevant.

Two cautionary notes are in order here. First, note that we have been discussing the representation of activity within a single cortical module. The region of visual space subtended by the RFs of neurons within a single module varies with the retinal position represented by the module. In any case, however, the area is relatively small, and when it is foveal it is very small indeed. Thus, the analysis of and neural encoding representing objects that subtend large visual angles surely cannot be carried out within a single module. The activation produced by such a large object must involve a great number of modules. Many visual objects of interest are not large, though, and even physically large objects may be seen and recognized at great distances, at which their images subtend only a small visual angle. Further, even large objects have small features that may in themselves aid the observer in object identification. Thus it does not seem inherently unreasonable to suggest that analysis of the pattern or profile of responses within a single module might be useful.

The second cautionary note is both more interesting and perhaps more controversial than the first, particularly in light of the general topic of this volume. By suggesting that the relevant information is carried in the relative positions of the local activity maxima, we imply that effective contrast is of minor importance. Recall our earlier discussion about the effect of a non-flat contrast sensitivity function on the effective contrasts of different components in a complex pattern. When a simple three-component plaid like that described is translated in depth, the relative effective contrasts of its components can change dramatically.

What effect would such a change have on the pattern of activity within a V1 module? For a given stimulus (spatial frequency and orientation), as effective contrast increases the number of responding units also increases. Neurons tuned to more and more distant spatial frequencies and orientations will be recruited. The result will be, in terms of the illustrations in figure 13.7, that the sizes of the circles corresponding to suprathreshold activity will increase with increasing contrast. What will not change, however—or at most will shift only very minimally due to small asymmetries in tuning functions—is the center of each of the local regions of activation. As long as a component retains sufficient contrast to produce any discriminable neural activation, the spatial pattern produced within a module by localization of the various centers of activation will remain essentially constant, and the internal relationships that define the object will be preserved in the geometry of its representation.

REFERENCES

Albrecht, D. G., De Valois, R. L., and Thorell, L. T. (1980). Visual cortical neurons: Are bars or gratings the optimal stimuli? Science 207: 88–90.

Barlow, H. B. (1972). Single units and sensation: A neuron doctrine for perceptual psychology? Perception 1: 371–394.

Bauman, L. A., and Bonds, A. B. (1991). Inhibitory refinement of spatial frequency selectivity in single cells of the cat striate cortex. Vision Res. 31: 933–944.

Campbell, F. W., Carpenter, R. H. S., and Levinson, J. Z. (1969). Visibility of aperiodic patterns compared with that of sinusoidal gratings. J. Physiol. (Lond.) 204: 283–298.

Campbell, F. W., and Robson, J. G. (1968). Application of Fourier analysis to the visibility of gratings. J. Physiol. (Lond.) 197: 551–566.

Cannon, M. W. (1979). Contrast sensation: A linear function of stimulus contrast. Vision Res. 19: 1045–1052.

Davis, E. T., Kramer, P., and Yager, D. (1986). Shifts in perceived spatial frequency of low-contrast stimuli: data and theory. J. Opt. Soc. Amer. A 3: 1189–1202.

De Valois, K. K., De Valois, R. L., and Yund, E. W. (1979). Responses of striate cortex cells to grating and checkerboard patterns. J. Physiol. (Lond.) 291: 483–505.

De Valois, K. K., and Tootell, R. B. H. (1983). Spatial-frequency-specific inhibition in cat striate cortex. J. Physiol. (Lond.) 336: 359–376.

De Valois, R. L., Albrecht, D. G., and Thorell, L. T. (1982). Spatial frequency selectivity of cells in macaque visual cortex. Vision Res. 22: 545–559.

De Valois, R. L., and De Valois, K. K. (1988). Splatial Vision. New York: Oxford University Press.

De Valois, R. L., Morgan, H., and Snodderly, D. M. (1974). Psychophysical studies of monkey vision III. Spatial luminance contrast sensitivity tests of macaque and human observers. Vision Res. 14: 75–81.

De Valois, R. L., Yund, E. W., and Hepler, N. K. (1982). The orientation and direction selectivity of cells in macaque visual cortex. Vision Res. 22: 531–544.

Elfar, S., De Valois, K. K., and De Valois, R. L. (1990). Sine waves, square waves. Invest. Ophthalmol. Vis. Sci. Ann. Supp. 31: 397.

Gelb, D. J., and Wilson, H. R. (1983). Shifts in perceived size as a function of contrast and temporal modulation. Vision Res. 23: 71–82.

Georgeson, M. A. (1980). Spatial frequency analysis in early visual processing. Philos. Trans. R. Soc. London Ser. B 290: 11–22.

Georgeson, M. A. (1985). Apparent spatial frequency and contrast of gratings: separate effects of contrast and duration. Vision Res. 25: 1721–1727.

Georgeson, M. A., and Sullivan, G. D. (1975). Contrast constancy: Deblurring in human vision by spatial frequency channels. J. Physiol. (Lond.) 252: 627–656.

Graham, N., and Nachmias, J. (1971). Detection of gratings patterns containing two spatial frequencies: A comparison of single channel and multichannel models. Vision Res. 11: 251–259.

Hering, E. (1879). Der Raumsinn und die Bewegungen des Auges. In: Hermann, L.: Handbuch der Physiologie 3 (Part 1). English translation, Radde, C. A. (Ed.), Spatial Sense and Movement of the Eye. Am. J. Optom., 1942.

Krauskopf, J., Williams, D. R., and Helley, D. W. (1982). Cardinal directions of color space. Vision Res. 22: 1123–1131.

Lennie, P., Krauskopf, J., and Sclar, G. (1990). Chromatic mechanisms in striate cortex of macaque. J. Neurosci. 10: 649–669.

Lettvin, J. Y., Maturana, H. R., McCulloch, W. S., and Pitts, W. H. (1959). What the frog's eye tells the frog's brain. Proceedings of the Institute of Radio Engineers 47: 1940–1951.

Lotze, H. (1886). Outline of Psychology. Translated and edited by Ladd, G. T. Boston: Ginn.

Movshon, J. A., Thompson, I. D., and Tolhurst, D. J. (1978). Spatial and temporal contrast sensitivity of neurones in areas 17 and 18 of the cat's visual cortex. J. Physiol. (Lond.) 283: 101–120.

Mueller, J. (1826). Zur Vergleichenden Physiologie des Gesichtssinnes des Menschen und der Thiere, nebst einen Versuch ueber die Bewegungen der Augen und ueber den menschlichen Blick. Leipzig: Knobloch.

Robson, J. G. (1975). Receptive fields: neural representation of the spatial and intensive attributes of the visual image. In E. D. Carterette and M. P. Friedman (Eds.), Handbook of Perception: Vol. 5 (pp. 81–112). New York: Academic Press.

Rushton, W. A. H. (1972). Visual pigments in man. In Dartnall, H. J. A. (Ed.), Handbook of Sensory Physiology, VII/I, pp. 364–394. Photochemistry of Vision. Heidelberg: Springer-Verlag.

Thorell L. T., De Valois, R. L., and Albrecht, D. G. (1984). Spatial mapping of monkey V1 cells with pure color and luminance stimuli. Vision Res. 24: 751–769.

IV Human Contrast Sensitivity and Its Clinical Applications

Finally we consider human vision and its dependence on contrast. The authors in section IV also intentionally covered the clinical utility of studying contrast sensitivity from their or own experience. This is where the interface between basic and applied research becomes apparent.

J. G. Robson first offers us a history of the measurement of contrast sensitivity, particularly in the clinic. This is a story told with relish by the author. Next we read a fascinating chapter about reading and the role of contrast by Gordon Legge. This reveals the fundamental sensory limits on reading, while providing sober reminders of how valuable normal vision is for communication. Robert Hess then provides the reader with many major insights about the pattern ERG and the difficulty in pinning down mechanisms in a system in which there are many thousands of active interacting neurons. He also shows how the ERG may be useful in diagnosing retinal disease. Finally D. Regan offers many examples of how concepts about contrast sensitivity have been useful in studying and analyzing diseases that produce visual deficits. Using psychophysical and electrophysiological tools, Dr. Regan has done a remarkable job of characterizing the visual deficits due to disease.

14 Contrast Sensitivity: One Hundred Years of Clinical Measurement

J. G. Robson

While our extraordinary ability to detect small differences in the luminance of adjacent regions in the visual field has long been a matter for remark, the first numerical estimate of the luminance difference threshold was provided by the French hydrographer Pierre Bouguer in his *Traité d'Optique sur la gradation de la lumière*, which was published in 1760. Using only the simplest apparatus (figure 14.1), Bouguer was able to show that the luminance difference threshold for a dark stripe on a uniform brighter background lay between 1 part in 49 and 1 part in 64 (i.e., around 2 percent). This he did by demonstrating that the shadow of a rod cast by a distant candle on a white screen remained visible until this distant candle was more than seven but less than eight times as far removed from the screen as a nearer candle just one foot away from it. This rather low value for what would become known first as the "light-difference threshold" and then much later as the "contrast threshold" resulted, of course, from the rather low level of illumination produced by a single candle at a distance of one foot (1 footcandle, giving a luminance of about 3 cd/m^2).

MASSON'S DISCS

Nearly a hundred years later another Frenchman, the physicist Masson (1845), used rapidly rotating discs of white paper marked with short black sectors of various lengths to examine how the contrast threshold for an annular dark stripe depended upon the light level. When a disc like this is rotated sufficiently fast (more than 50 or so times a second) the black sector is visible only as a gray stripe, the effective contrast of the stripe depending exactly on the proportion of a complete circle occupied by the black sector. As a result of viewing a set of such discs under different conditions of illumination, Masson concluded that his own contrast threshold, as well as that of several other observers, was essentially independent of absolute luminance, being slightly less than 1 percent in any good light.

Masson's interest in the differential sensitivity of the visual system was primarily related to his attempt to devise a precise method of photometry for the brief flashes produced by spark discharges, and his measurements of visual sensitivity were limited to those appropriate for this task. However, it is

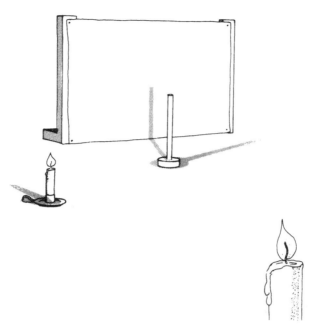

Figure 14.1 Bouguer's apparatus for determining the light-difference threshold. The white paper screen is mainly illuminated by the candle on the left (1 foot away from it), while the shadow of a rod is cast on it by a second candle (on the right). The second candle is moved away until the shadow becomes invisible. This happens when the second candle is somewhere between 7 and 8 feet from the screen, indicating that a luminance difference of between about 1 part in 49 and 1 part in 64 is required to produce a perceptible difference in brightness. This luminance difference corresponds to a contrast of about 0.02 (or 2 percent).

intriguing to note Masson's suggestion that contrast sensitivity measurements of this kind might be applied by doctors to the study of visual disorders or used to advance physiology. "Nous n'avons examiné, dans ce travail, que les effets physiologiques qu'il nous importait de connaître pour la suite de nos recherches, laissant aux médecins le soin d'appliquer notre instrument dans l'étude des affections de la vue ou pour les progrès de la physiologie."

The clinical application of contrast sensitivity testing using Masson's disc was indeed not long delayed. Although Aubert (1876), in his chapter on physiological optics in Graefe and Saemisch's great *Handbook of Ophthalmology*, had pointed out that the luminance difference threshold was not quite as exactly independent of background luminance as Masson had suggested, Snellen and Landolt (1874), in their chapter on the functional examination of the eye in the same handbook, appear to have had no hesitation in recommending that the light-difference threshold should be measured using a version of Masson's disc that had been described by Donders. By this time the measurement of visual acuity using Snellen's test types (Snellen 1862) had already become established as a routine part of every ophthalmological examination, largely as a result of Donders' (1864) advocacy. However, since Snellen, Landolt, and Donders, the three great pioneers in the clinical measurement of visual acuity, all seem to have been involved in encouraging the measurement of the light-difference threshold as well, we may assume that they all believed that such a measurement could be a useful adjunct to a measurement of visual acuity.

Unfortunately a measurement of the light-difference threshold using Masson's disc was not as rapid, as convenient, or as precise as a measurement of visual acuity using Snellen's chart. This prompted various attempts to devise a more satisfactory practical method of measuring the light-difference threshold for use in the clinical setting. One such attempt was that of a Norwegian ophthalmologist, Ole Bull (1881).

Bull's main objections to the use of Masson's disc related not only to the inconvenience of having an apparatus to rotate the disc, but, more important, to the difficulty of explaining the nature of the required observation to the patient and to the lack of any control of the patient's report. In these latter respects the measurement differed greatly from that of visual acuity using a chart of test types. With the letter acuity chart the task was both readily explained and easily understood, and the correct naming of a letter provided a more or less unambiguous indication that the patient had in fact seen the test letter. (That these were all highly desirable features of a practical test was clearly understood by Snellen and Donders.) Therefore Bull proposed to make a letter chart to measure the light-difference threshold using letters of various shades of gray on a uniform white or black background. Bull's chart was to be constructed by cutting letters from papers that had previously been painted to match the appearance of the rings made by appropriate sectors on a rotating disc and that would then be mounted on a suitable background. The grays to be used were intended to correspond to sectors subtending 2°, 3°, 5°, 7°, 10°, etc at the center of the disc. In reality Bull made only a chart with dark gray letters on a black background and not one with light gray letters on a white background, pleading rather lamely that "a white background is to be regarded as less expedient, since the amount of light reflected by it can dazzle the eye." In fact, we may suppose that painting the necessary very light grays turned out to be too difficult for him.

BJERRUM'S LETTER CHARTS

A rather different approach was taken by Bjerrum (1884) in Copenhagen. Bjerrum also appreciated the special advantages of letter charts, and he quite simply proposed that acuity should be measured using several charts of Snellen's design with letters printed in various tones of gray as well as using a normal chart with black letters (figure 14.2). Bjerrum's charts were made of letters with contrasts of 9, 20, 30, and 40 percent, and he reported many measurements made with each of these charts, every one at several light levels, on patients with various ocular disorders.

In Britain, George Berry (of Edinburgh) seems to have been the first ophthalmologist to report the use of light-difference measurements. Berry, who initially used Masson's disks to examine the light-difference threshold in a

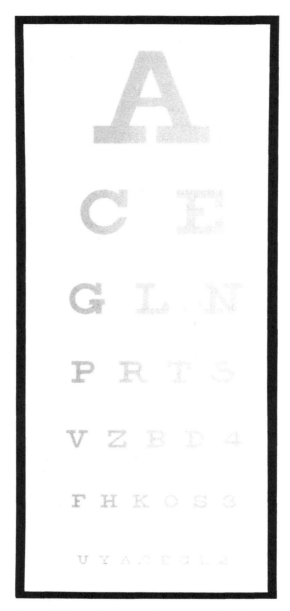

Figure 14.2 A low-contrast test chart of the kind suggested by Bjerrum (1884). The letter chart reproduced here is from Snellen's book published in 1862 and has a contrast of about 10 percent.

Human Contrast Sensitivity and Its Clinical Applications

study of tobacco amblyopia (Berry 1880), later adopted Bjerrum's charts to study the visual defect in retrobulbar neuritis (Berry 1889). In connection with this latter study, Berry noted that he found the chart with letters of 9 percent contrast to be the "most practical," a comment much in keeping with modern experience with Regan's low-contrast letter charts (Regan 1988). Berry also emphasized the point that in certain pathological cases it was possible to have a very greatly reduced low-contrast acuity (in exceptional cases reduced even to a level at which letters of 9 percent contrast could not be read at all) without any obvious reduction of normal (high-contrast) acuity.

Bjerrum's charts, the first low-contrast letter acuity tests, clearly achieved some degree of general acceptance, as they were one of the two methods of examining the light-difference threshold recommended in the fifth (1895) edition of Henry Swanzy's *Handbook of the Diseases of the Eye*, which was the standard manual of practical ophthalmology in Britain at that time.

GEORGE YOUNG'S INK SPOTS

Despite the interest in clinical measurement of the light-difference threshold that was apparent in the last decades of the nineteenth century, interest subsequently seems to have waned until temporarily revived in England in 1918 by George Young. In that year Young, an ophthalmologist in practice in Colchester, described to the Opthalmological Society a new method that he had devised of measuring the light-difference threshold. Young (1918a,b) made no great claims for his method, admitting that it could be "easily contested on scientific grounds." Nevertheless, he felt justified in bringing it to the attention of his colleagues on the grounds that it was rapid, handy, inexpensive, and of sufficient accuracy. "Its main object is practical," wrote Young, and he hoped it would serve those who did not have the time "to go through what may be called laboratory tests."

Young's method was based on a small album on each page of which he had mounted a square of blotting paper with an ink spot at its centre. The ink spots were made with various dilutions of black ink; the palest spot, the one made with the most dilute ink, appeared at the front of the book, while on each succeeding page the spot was made with ink that had been diluted only half as much as for the preceding page. As the pages were turned, the patient was first presented with spots of too low a contrast to be seen, but then at some stage the spot became visible and the dilution of the ink used to make the spot was recorded as the patient's threshold. In addition to spots made with black ink for measuring the light-difference threshold, Young's test book also had spots made with colored inks, thus providing a novel test of chromatic contrast threshold as well.

George Young's threshold test was indeed a particularly convenient one, and a version of it was subsequently commercially produced by John Weiss and Son and later, after Young's death in 1934, a second improved version was published by Raphael's in London. In the improved version the spots were directly printed on the leaves of the book and randomly positioned on each page so that, if the patient was able to indicate the position of a spot correctly, it could reasonably be assumed that the contrast of the spot was really above threshold. This incorporation into Young's test of a simple multiple forced-choice procedure for determining the threshold must have been a great improvement over simply asking for a subjective report of whether or not the spot was visible, as this would inevitably have left the patients too much freedom to vary their threshold criteria and to indulge their imaginations.

Although George Young's threshold test seems to have gained some acceptance with both ophthalmologists and also optometrists, it clearly never caused contrast-sensitivity testing to become the routine procedure Young had thought it should.

There were two difficulties with Young's ink spot test; one was the absence of any absolute calibration of the contrast of the spots (and also possibly a lack of calibration stability), and the other was the coarseness of the contrast steps (each step a factor of two). Young was well aware of these deficiencies, but in the absence of photoelectric photometers, he was able to suggest only that, if more precise measurements were required, they should be made with a version of Masson's disc that could provide infinitely variable low contrasts of defined absolute value.

At roughly the same time that George Young was encouraging his fellow members of the U.K. Ophthalmological Society to measure contrast threshold using his new ink spot method, Archibald Percival, an ophthalmologist from Newcastle-upon-Tyne, was encouraging them to make more use of Masson's disc in their normal practice. Percival (1920, 1922) described how useful he had found a very simple form of this device, a small disc of white card with a hole in the middle, with three black sectors on each side designed to produce contrasts of 8, 4, and 2 percent on one side and 2, 1, and 0.5 percent on the other. These values spanned the normal threshold (between 0.5 and 1 percent) as well as the increased levels to be expected in optic neuritis and toxic amblyopias. To use his disc, Percival would spin it on an ordinary dissecting needle and ask his patients how many dark rings they could see. Percival's contribution was not in itself of great consequence, but is of interest because it seems to have been Percival who first proposed that measurements of the light-difference sense could most conveniently be recorded not directly in terms of the threshold contrast required for perception, but as the reciprocal of this number, the quantity we now know as contrast sensitivity. (For the author it is also intriguing that Percival's version of Masson's disc could be supplied to anyone who wished to have one by Robson and Co. of Newcastle.)

Also about this same time, Carsten Edmund, a young ophthalmologist working in Tscherning's department in Copenhagen, was encouraged to examine the effect of lowering the light level on contrast sensitivity (Tscherning's "power of distinction").[1] Although this could be done quite satisfactorily in normal subjects using Masson's disc (Edmund, 1924a), measurements in patients were more difficult, and so, in collaboration with his colleague Ulrik

Möller, Edmund (1924b) devised for this purpose a simple test chart of large letters having nine different contrasts spanning the range from 100 percent to 1 percent in equal logarithmic steps. While it appears from a subsequent joint publication (Edmund and Möller, 1925) that a version of this chart may have been commerically available, neither Edmund or Möller published anything further about its use nor am I aware of any report of its use by others.

No new method of measuring contrast threshold or contrast sensitivity appears to have been suggested until 1946, when Hecht, Hendley, Frank, and Shlaer described the apparatus they had devised during the Second World War to demonstrate the reduction in vision produced by hypoxia. This apparatus used low-contrast Landolt rings of different contrasts that were produced photographically by varying the exposure time and then calibrated using a photoelectric cell and a galvanometer system. In the most satisfactory version of their apparatus, Hecht et al. arranged 18 pairs of Landolt rings of different contrasts side by side around the periphery of a large disc. The contrasts of these targets were approximately uniformly spaced through the 1 to 4 percent range of contrasts that were relevant at the low light levels involved in the demonstration. The small step size and duplication of the targets were necessary in order to provide the resolution required to demonstrate the definite, but quite small, effect of hypoxia (roughly a doubling of contrast threshold).

While an apparatus of the kind described by Hecht et al. could obviously have been used to make clinical measurements, it does not appear that it was ever used in this way. In fact, following the revival of interest in the early 1920s, it was to be about fifty years before the measurement of contrast sensitivity was again seriously considered in a clinical context. During this time, however, there were to be major changes in the way contrast sensitivity would come to be regarded as a result of revolutionary developments in both image science and image engineering, as well as in basic vision science.

E. W. H. SELWYN AND SINE WAVE GRATINGS

The beginning of this revolution is to be found in the work of E. W. H. Selwyn, who was a scientist at Kodak's Research Laboratories in England. Selwyn's contribution, like that of Hecht et al. (1948) that I have already referred to, was also prompted by the operational requirements of the air forces in the Second World War. As part of his involvement in efforts to improve aerial reconnaissance photographs intended for visual interpretation, Selwyn (1948) devised a novel test object that could be used to examine in a theoretically simple and unifying way the sensitivity of the human observer as well as the imaging performance of lenses and photographic film.

This new test object was the sine wave grating, a target whose luminance varies in one direction as a sinusoidal function about its mean level but is invariant in the direction at right angles to this. Selwyn made his sine wave test gratings by photographing the appropriate black and white profile through a cylindrical lens. As Selwyn explained in his report, a test object of this kind has the peculiar property that, whenever it is imaged by a lens and whatever the image-forming properties of the lens may be, the image is of exactly the same kind as the test object; i.e., the image of a sine wave grating is always another sine wave grating, albeit one whose contrast is always less than that of the original test object.

Having made a set of sine wave test gratings, Selwyn was able, using an optical system that allowed both the apparent size and the contrast of a test grating to be varied, to find out what contrast was required for an observer to see the stripes of a grating when the bars subtended different angles at the eye. In this way Selwyn provided the first measurements of the way in which the threshold contrast for sine wave gratings varies as a function of spatial frequency. Selwyn was not at all surprised to find that the threshold rose when the width of the bars was small (when the spatial frequency was high), attributing this to "the structure of the retina, or some similar cause," but he was puzzled to find that the threshold also rose when the period of the pattern became greater than about 12 minutes of arc. Selwyn's suggested explanation for this rise in threshold at spatial frequencies below about 5 cycles per degree was that it resulted from "the disturbing effects of scratches and specks of dust" that became particularly obvious under these conditions. While we now know that an increase in contrast threshold at low spatial frequencies can be observed even with stimulus gratings that do not have the defects of those available to Selwyn, it is interesting to note that even he, working in Kodak's no doubt well-equipped photographic laboratory, was unable to obtain entirely satisfactory grating stimuli using photographic methods.

Selwyn's work does not seem to have attracted the attention of vision scientists, and it cannot really be said to have been responsible for the later explosion of interest in the human contrast threshold function.

OTTO SCHADE AND GRATINGS ON CATHODE RAY TUBES

A more significant contributor was Otto Schade (1956). Schade was deeply involved in optimizing the design of television systems for RCA, and in this context he felt that it would be highly desirable to find a way of describing human visual characteristics that would make it possible to assess the overall performance of a complete television system comprising a camera, signal transmission, display, and human observer. Realizing the enormous power of describing the performance of the physical components of such a system in terms of their spatial and temporal frequency response functions, Schade decided to describe human visual performance in the same way. Finding that the information then available about human vision was inadequate for his purpose, Schade set about making his own measurements of the contrast thresholds for sine wave gratings of different spatial frequencies at different luminance levels.

Being familiar with the necessary electronic techniques, Schade was able to generate the sine wave gratings to be employed as stimuli by electronically modulating a raster displayed on the screen of a cathode ray tube, thereby gaining an almost ideal experimental system in which it was very easy to change both the contrast and the spatial frequency of the stimulus patterns by simple electronic means. Moreover it was also relatively easy, again using purely electronic means, to cause the grating pattern to drift continuously across the screen.

While Schade's new analytic approach to imaging systems was of the utmost importance and was recognized as such by those scientists and engineers who were involved with instrumental imaging systems, the impact of his work on vision science was much less direct. Schade's seminal paper (1956), which encompassed an almost extraordinarily wide range of topics relating to spatial vision, was unfortunately written in a manner that was certainly obscure (to vision scientists anyway), if not actually opaque. Gerald Westheimer, however, was one of the few vision scientists who quickly realized the significance of Schade's work, and it was largely as a result of his prompting that Fergus Campbell and I decided in the early 1960s to make our own measurements of the human contrast threshold for sine wave gratings. Just as we were starting to do this, we read a report from the Kodak Research Laboratories in the United States (DePalma and Lowry 1962) claiming that sine wave gratings were more visible than square wave gratings of the same spatial frequency and contrast and that the threshold contrast for gratings depended not only on the spatial frequency subtended at the observer's eye, but also on the actual viewing distance. On both physical and physiological grounds this all seemed rather unlikely, and Fergus Campbell and I decided to take another look at these particular aspects of grating visibility.

CAMPBELL AND ROBSON: CONTRAST SENSITIVITY FUNCTIONS

Using a cathode ray tube display in much the same way that Schade had, Campbell and I were able to show that, as was to be expected on simple optical grounds, the threshold contrast for square wave gratings at high spatial frequencies was in reality just slightly less than that for sine wave gratings (Robson and Campbell 1963; Campbell and Robson 1964, 1968). However, we had not expected to find that the relative visibility of sine and square wave gratings would remain very much the same until the spatial frequency was made very low indeed. This, as well as observations on the visibility of various other periodic patterns, led us to suggest that the measured contrast sensitivity function was in fact the envelope of the contrast sensitivity functions of a number of independent parallel detecting mechanisms, all coexisting within the visual system.

This work, as well as other studies that helped to define the relative importance of optical and neural factors in determining the visibility of sine wave gratings (particularly the work of Campbell and Green 1965; Enroth-Cugell and Robson 1966; Blakemore and Campbell 1969), seemed to catch the attention and imagination of many people, including some with clinical interests, and it soon led to studies of alterations in contrast sensitivity in various disease states, starting with Bodis-Wollner's (1972) examination of patients with cerebral lesions. Bodis-Wollner's study, and the great majority of the large number of clinical studies of altered contrast sensitivity that followed, used some kind of cathode ray tube display system to provide the required stimuli, and all involved measurements of the threshold contrast for sine wave gratings at several different spatial frequencies (eg., see review by Storch and Bodis-Wollner, 1990).

While these studies served to show that there was almost certainly some real utility in clinical measurement of contrast sensitivity, they also made it clear that the standard laboratory method of measuring contrast sensitivity was not really suitable for routine clinical use. As the early innovators in the clinical measurement of the light-difference threshold had been at pains to point out, routine testing is really practicable only with a method which is easy, quick, accurate, and cheap, and ideally, portable as well. Thus began a series of attempts to devise some method that met these desiderata.

Prior to the definitive publication in 1968 of the work that Fergus Campbell and I had done on sine and square wave gratings, we had presented our findings at various meetings and very quickly discovered that, if we wanted the audience to understand what we were talking about, it was necessary to provide some visual demonstration that could help to explain what was meant by a "contrast sensitivity function." We therefore, and with some difficulty, made a demonstration picture showing a sine wave grating whose spatial frequency increased from left to right and whose contrast increased from top to bottom. Simple inspection of such a pattern shows how contrast sensitivity has a maximum at some intermediate spatial frequency but falls off at both higher and lower frequencies. Fergus and I were very pleased with ourselves for making this picture, and for a very short time we thought that we had not only made a good demonstration, but that we could also use such a picture to measure a subject's contrast sensitivity function by getting the subject to mark the boundary between the region in which a grating was visible and the region that appeared uniform. It even occurred to us that this might be the basis of a method that would be suitable for clinical measurement of contrast sensitivity. It did not take long, however, for us to see that for several reasons this was not at all a satisfactory procedure, and we did not pursue it.

CONTRAST SENSITIVITY CHARTS

However, a modified version of this method was later introduced by Geoffrey Arden (1978), and its effectiveness was examined in several subsequent studies. Arden's method involved the use of a set of six printed cards ("Arden plates"), each bearing a vertical grating of a different spatial frequency whose contrast was graded from a low value at the bottom of the card to a high value at the top. The threshold measurement was made by showing the patient one of the cards that was initially completely covered with a second uniformly gray card and then steadily moving the gray card upward so as successively to uncover regions of the concealed grating of higher and higher levels of contrast. As soon as the patient reported being able to see the stripes of the grating, the position of the edge of the obscuring card was noted and this position used to provide a measure of the threshold contrast at the spatial frequency of that particular card. This process was then repeated for each of the six cards. While this method was indeed relatively easy, cheap, quick, and certainly portable enough to allow measurements to be made at the bedside, it employed a very unsatisfactory psychophysical procedure for determining the threshold and was unable to provide sufficiently reliable measurements.

More recently another printed chart for measuring contrast sensitivity at six different spatial frequencies was introduced by Arthur Ginsburg (1984), who had previously been a student of Campbell's in Cambridge. Ginsburg's chart (subsequently published as the "Vistech" chart) is also related to the variable spatial frequency, variable contrast arrangement referred to earlier. However, in Ginsburg's chart a grating pattern with continuously variable contrast and spatial frequency has been replaced with a matrix of discrete round patches of grating, each individual patch having a particular spatial frequency and contrast. This makes it possible to introduce that important refinement, the use of a multiple-alternative forced-choice procedure for finding the threshold. In each of the patches on the chart, the orientation of the grating is randomly chosen to have one of three distinctly different values, either vertical or rotated 15° clockwise or counterclockwise. For any patch to be judged as being above the subject's threshold, the subject must correctly report its orientation. While this is a good feature, in normal use only one identification at each contrast is used in determining a subject's threshold for each of six spatial frequencies, and this unavoidably introduces a fair degree of variability into the measurements. Even so, the whole procedure is reported as typically taking about 6 minutes. While this may not seem too long a time, it must be remembered that in a clinical situation it will nearly always be necessary to make measurements on each eye separately, and the total time required for this then appears to be severely inhibiting, if not completely prohibitive, for a routine procedure.

While no doubt modifications could be made to Ginsburg's method to improve its accuracy and speed the testing, it seems unlikely that there is any way in which measurements at as many as six spatial frequencies can be made with adequate reliability in any time short enough to be acceptable for routine use. Nor is there any obvious way in which more elaborate instrumentation could be used to change this. Psychophysical determinations of threshold inevitably require a minute or so each if useful accuracy is to be achieved, and it has therefore seemed to various workers in this field that, if routine contrast sensitivity measurements are to be made clinically, the number of thresholds to be determined must be reduced.

With this in mind, various proposals have been made in the past few years that, rather than assessing visual function on the basis of measurements of contrast sensitivity for sine wave gratings at several different spatial frequencies, routine assessments should instead be based on two measurements only, a standard measurement of visual acuity using high contrast optotypes and just one other measurement to augment it. In particular, Regan and Neima

(1983) have proposed that this second measurement should also be one of acuity but made should be using a letter chart of low contrast, while others have suggested that the second measurement should be a contrast sensitivity determination made with a single kind of test object of a large size.

Each of these latter proposals has involved the use of books or charts with targets of various contrasts. Thus Wilkins and Robson (see Della Sala, Bertoni, Somazzi, Stubbe, and Wilkins 1985) have suggested measuring contrast sensitivity for a square wave grating of 3 cycles per degree, Verbaken and Johnston (1986) have suggested measuring the contrast required to see the edge between the two halves of a circular bipartite disc, while Pelli and Robson (1989) have suggested measuring the contrast necessary to recognise letters subtending 3 degrees at the eye. Interestingly, none of these most recent proposals involves the use of sine wave gratings, the authors making the proposals all taking the view that, however theoretically appealing the idea of measuring contrast sensitivity using sine wave gratings may be, there is little or no evidence to show that measurements made with this particular test pattern are of any especially great clinical relevance and that practical considerations are of overriding significance.

At this stage one may perhaps be forgiven for feeling a strong sense of déjà vu, as these various proposals for the single extra measurement to be made in addition to a normal acuity determination all, in effect, simply recapitulate the actual or proposed methods for measuring the light-difference threshold that were current at the end of the last century. Regan's low contrast letter charts really differ from Bjerrum's only in being more like modern acuity charts than Snellen's original one. The Cambridge Low-Contrast Gratings and the Melbourne Edge Test are really nothing more than the low-contrast stripes of a Masson's disc presented as printed charts. While a chart with letters of varying contrasts was never actually produced in the nineteenth century, Ole Bull's proposed chart would no doubt have looked not too unlike the Pelli-Robson version if Bull had only had access to the necessary techniques to make one (it is not clear how Möller and Edmund's variable contrast letter chart was produced).

So how does the present situation differ from that a hundred years ago? In many ways. Unlike those who proposed the clinical measurement of contrast thresholds in the nineteenth and early twentieth centuries, we now have much better methods of generating test stimuli, be they static patterns on a printed chart or dynamic patterns on a cathode ray tube display, as well as electronic instruments of high precision to calibrate them photometrically. Moreover, we now know far more about the many factors that can affect measurements of contrast sensitivity and that must be controlled if reliable results are to be obtained.

But, more important, we now have a very different idea about the nature of the visual threshold itself. Whereas in earlier times there is no doubt that a visual threshold was viewed much as the threshold of a nerve for electrical stimulation, as a rather precisely defined level below which no effect is produced and above which a definite response will be obtained, it is now tacitly

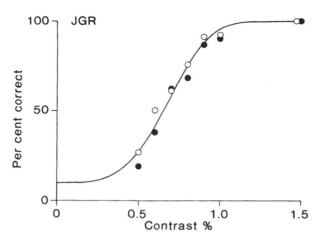

Figure 14.3 A typical psychometric function relating the probability of correctly naming low-contrast letters to the contrast at which they are viewed. To obtain these results each of the ten different Sloan letters used on the PelliRobson chart was quasi-randomly presented (with slow turn-on) 100 times at each of seven different contrast levels; the open and filled symbols are results obtained on two different days. Because the 10 different letters are presented with equal frequency, the probability of correctly naming a letter that is unseen is 0.1; hence the asymptotic level of the curve at the lefthand side must also be 0.1. When the contrast is high, the probability of correctly naming each letter becomes 1. At intermediate contrasts the probability goes from its zero-contrast asymptote to its maximum level over a contrast range of about 1:2 (0.5 to 1 percent in this case). A Weibull function (see Pelli, Robson, and Wilkins 1988) with an exponent of 3.8 has been drawn through the points, though other formulations can probably be used to describe the experimental results just as well.

accepted that visual detection and visual discrimination are stochastic processes. The strength of a visual stimulus required for its detection or discrimination from another stimulus can be defined only in a statistical way (e.g., figure 14.3) This means that accurate measurement of a contrast threshold, for example, is not simply a matter of testing using enough different stimuli with sufficiently closely spaced levels of contrast. It is more a matter of making a large enough number of judgments to allow for statistical reliability; in practice it is a matter of spending enough time making the measurements.

This greater appreciation of the problem and the more sophisticated tools that we have available for its solution mean that we can be more certain when we devise a method of measuring some aspect of visual function that we have adopted a good strategy. However, it does not mean that we can necessarily always find a clinically acceptable method of measuring any given visual function, nor even that there is necessarily any measurement of visual function, however accurate, that will be diagnostically useful. Moreover, the unfortunate fact is that, although we now know a great deal more about the workings of the visual mechanisms than was known a hundred years ago, we still don't know enough about normal physiology, or about the exact nature of the defects associated with disease, to proceed in an entirely logical way to develop diagnostic testing procedures. Until we do, we can only combine what knowledge we have with our best guesses to suggest procedures to try. As George Young wrote in 1918, "As a clinician I mean to continue exploring the thresholds for clinical purposes. The question to decide, as far as our work is concerned, is: Does studying the threshold of light lead to diagnostic signs and what are they? This can [only] be settled empirically. Quantities of tests, quantities of earnest collaborators, will reveal the scope and limitations of the method." Some things change, but the need for careful empirical observation does not.

NOTE

1. I am grateful to John Mollon and Gabriele Jordan for drawing my attention to Edmund's work.

REFERENCES

Aubert H. (1876) Physiologische Optik. in Handbuch der gesammten Augenheilkunde. Vol 2, 393–690. Eds. Alfred Graefe and Theod. Saemisch. Wilhelm Engelmann, Leipzig.

Berry G. A. (1880) On central amblyopia. Ophthalmic Hospital Reports. 10:44–55.

Berry G. A. (1889) Remarks on retro-bulbar neuritis with special reference to the condition of the light sense in that affection. Ophthalmic Hospital Reports. 12:244–254.

Bjerrum J. (1884) Untersuchungen über den Lichtsinn und den Raumsinn bei verschiedenen Augenkrankheiten. Albrecht von Graefe's Archiv für Ophthalmologie. (See Ophthalmic Review (1886) 5:170–172 for a précis in English.)

Bodis-Wollner I. (1972) Visual acuity and contrast sensitivity in patients with cortical lesions. Science, 178:769–771.

Bouguer P. (1760) Traité d'Optique sur la gradation de la lumière. publ. M l'Abbé de la Caille, Paris.

Bull O. B. (1881) Studien über Lichtsinn und Farbensinn. Albrecht von Graefe's Archiv fur Ophthalmologie. 27:54–154.

Campbell F. W. and Green D. G. (1965) Optical and retinal factors affecting visual resolution. Journal of Physiology, 181:576–593.

Campbell F. W. and Robson J. G. (1968) Application of Fourier analysis to the visibility of gratings. Journal of Physiology. 197:551–566.

Della Sala S., Bertoni G., Somazzi L., Stubbe F., and Wilkins A. J. (1985) Impaired contrast sensitivity in patients with and without retinopathy: a new technique for rapid assessment. British Journal of Ophthalmology. 69:136–142.

DePalma J. J. and Lowry (1962) Sine-wave response of the visual system II. Sine-wave and square-wave contrast sensitivity. Journal of the Optical Society of America. 52:328–335.

Donders F. C. (1864) On the anomalies of accommodation and refraction of the eye. New Sydenham Society, London.

Edmund C. (1924a) The dependence of the light sense on the adaptation of the eye. Acta Ophthalmologica. 2:125–136.

Edmund C. (1924b) Uber hemeralopia idiopatica mit besonderem hinblick auf untersuchung und behandlung. Acta Ophthalmologica. 2:225–238.

Edmund C. and Möller (1925) Vision in light of reduced intensity. Archives of Ophthalmology. 54:531−544.

Enroth-Cugell Ch. and Robson J. G. (1966) The contrast sensitivity of retinal ganglion cells of the cat. Journal of Physiology. 187:517−552.

Ginsburg A. P. (1984) A new contrast sensitivity vision test chart. American Journal of Optometry and Physiological Optics. 61:403−407.

Hecht S., Hendley C. D., Frank S., and Shlaer S. (1949) Contrast discrimination charts for demonstrating the effects of anoxia on vision. Journal of the Optical Society of America. 39:922−923

Masson M. A. (1845) Études de photometrie électrique. Annales de Chimie et de Physique. 14:129−195.

Pelli D. G., Robson J. G., and Wilkins A. J. (1988) The design of a new letter chart for measuring contrast sensitivity. Clinical Vision Sciences. 2:187−199.

Percival A. S. (1920) Light-sense. Transactions of the Ophthalmological Society of the United Kingdom. 40:311−329.

Percival A. S. (1922) Notes on light-sense. Transactions of the Ophthalmological Society of the United Kingdom. 42:285−288.

Regan D. (1988) Low-contrast letter charts and sine-wave grating tests in ophthalmological and neurological disorders. Clinical Vision Sciences. 2:235−250.

Regan D. and Neima D. (1983) Low-contrast letter charts as a test of visual function. Ophthalmology. 90:1192−1200.

Schade O. H. (1956) Optical and photo-electric analog of the eye. Journal of the Optical Society of America. 46:721−739.

Selwyn E. W. H. (1948) The photographic and visual resolving power of lenses. Photographic Journal, Section B. 88B:6−12 and 46−57.

Snellen H. (1862) Test types for the determination of the acuteness of vision. Printed by P. W. van de Weijer, Utrecht.

Snellen H. and Landolt E. (1874) Ophthalmometrologie. Die Functionsprüfungen des Auges. in Handbuch der gesammten Augenheilkunde. Vol 3, 1−248. Eds. Alfred Graefe and Theod. Saemisch. Wilhelm Engelmann, Leipzig.

Storch R. L. and Bodis-Wollner I. (1990) Overview of contrast sensitivity and neuro-ophthalmic disease. in Glare and Contrast Sensitivity for Clinicians. Eds. M. P. Nadler, D. Miller and D. J. Nadler. Springer-Verlag, Heidelburg.

Swanzy H. R. (1895) A handbook of the diseases of the eye and their treatment. 5th edition H. K. Lewis, London.

Verbaken J. H. and Johnston A. W. (1986) Population norms for edge contrast sensitivity. American Journal of Optometry and Physiological Optics. 63:724−732.

Young G. (1918a) Suggested clinical tests of the threshold of light and colour. Transactions of the Ophthalmological Society of the United Kingdom. 38:279−281.

Young G. (1918b) Threshold tests. British Journal of Ophthalmology 2:384−392, 430−433.

15 The Role of Contrast in Reading: Normal and Low Vision

Gordon E. Legge

Text usually consists of high-contrast black letters on a white page. The corresponding retinal images produce strong neural signals. People with normal vision read quickly and effortlessly, unaware of the role of vision unless the letters are tiny, the lighting poor, or the typescript bad. For almost all of the three million Americans with low vision (Tielsch et al. 1990), however, reading is always difficult. In fact, one definition of *low vision* is the inability to read the newspaper (with best lens correction) at a normal reading distance (40 cm).

What role does vision play in reading? How do eye disorders affect reading? How should text be tailored to maximize its legibility for people with impaired vision? Beginning with the seminal studies by Enroth-Cugell and Robson (1966), Campbell and Robson (1968), and Hubel and Wiesel (1968), our basic knowledge of pattern vision has matured to the point at which we can begin to understand how visual signals participate in complex perceptual tasks like reading. (Prior to the 1960s, perceptual studies of reading had no sensory foundation upon which to build. This was true of the pioneering work of Tinker (1963).)

For several years my colleagues and I have used psychophysical methods to study visual factors in reading. Our two major goals have been to understand the roles played by sensory mechanisms in reading and to understand how visual impairment affects reading. In this paper I will review our work on contrast and reading. I will focus on four main questions: How does text contrast affect reading speed? What is the relationship between contrast sensitivity and reading performance? Can the effects of contrast in reading be linked to principles of contrast coding in vision? Can losses in retinal image contrast (or contrast sensitivity) account for the reading difficulties experienced by people with low vision?

MEASURING READING PERFORMANCE

Our primary measure is reading speed in words/minute. We have developed two measurement techniques.

In the *drifting text* method (Legge et al. 1985a) a line of text (80 characters) drifts smoothly across the face of a TV monitor, much like the drifting text in

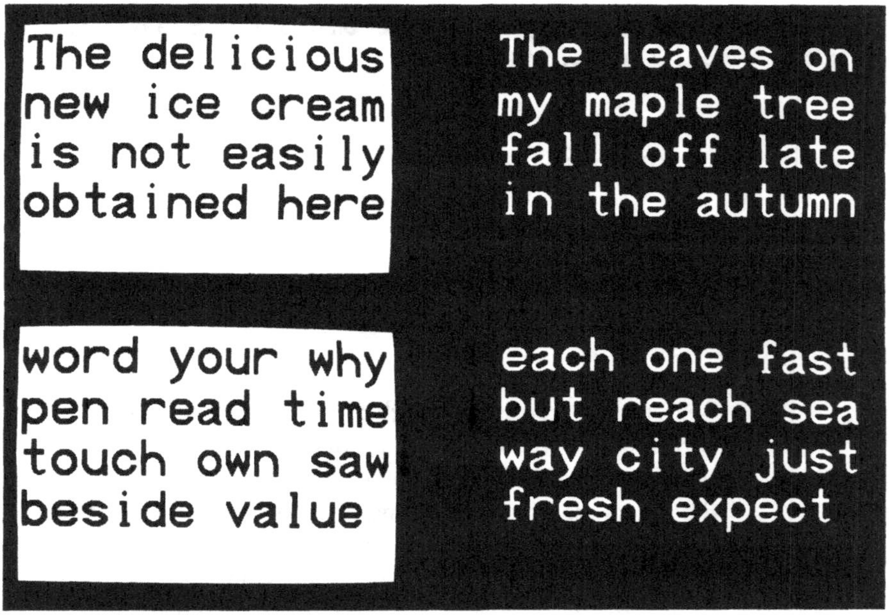

Figure 15.1 Illustration of the four types of text displays that are used in the stationary text procedure. (From Legge et al. 1989.)

Times Square, New York. The subject reads the line aloud as it drifts by. If no errors are made, the experimenter increases the drift rate on the next trial. When the drift rate is high enough so that the subject consistently makes a small number of errors, we compute reading speed in words per minute from the drift rate and the number of errors made.

A second method for measuring reading speed uses *stationary text* (Legge et al. 1989). The test stimuli are sentences or random words that are displayed as black-on-white or white-on-black (figure 15.1). The text is presented on a computer screen for a specified period. If the subject reads the complete text aloud without missing any words, the exposure period is decreased. When the period is too short for the subject to finish, reading speed is computed as the number of words read correctly divided by the exposure time. The test is quick (5 minutes) and easy to administer. The results are highly reproducible (R = 0.9).

In our studies of contrast, we have used both methods for measuring reading speed. Although there are small differences in performance levels,[1] the functional dependence on contrast is the same for the two presentation modes.

We have used two methods to vary text contrast. In one, contrast was controlled by analog attenuation of video signals (Legge et al. 1987a). In the other, contrast was controlled by look-up table assignment of gray levels in binary text images (Legge et al. 1990). In both, the luminance of the dark letters was increased while holding background luminance constant in order

Human Contrast Sensitivity and Its Clinical Applications

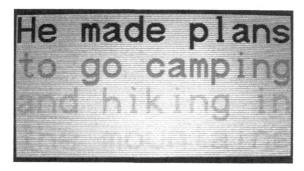

Figure 15.2 Illustration of four contrast levels for text. The display was photographed with contrasts of 0.9 ("he made plans"), 0.3 ("to go camping"), 0.10 ("and hiking in"), and 0.03 ("the mountains"). In a given experimental trial, the entire sentence would be displayed at a single contrast level.

to reduce contrast (figure 15.2). We use the Michelson definition for text contrast:

$$C = (L_b - L_c)/(L_b + L_c),$$

where L_b and L_c are the luminances of the background and the characters, respectively. Text contrast ranges from 0 to 1.0.

The effects of contrast polarity (white-on-black vs. black-on white text) will not be considered in this chapter. Polarity effects have been discussed elsewhere (Legge et al. 1985a,b, 1987b).

CONTRAST LEVEL AND READING SPEED

How rapidly could you read text displayed with the contrast levels illustrated in figure 15.2? The four lines have contrasts of 0.9, 0.3, 0.1, and 0.03. The data in figure 15.3 show how reading speed depends on text contrast for four subjects. For high contrasts, above 0.1 (10 percent) the curves are quite flat. Normal reading has a contrast reserve of about a factor of 10. Below a contrast of about 0.1, reading speed drops quite steeply.

Curves for different character sizes have approximately the same shape. In figure 15.4, text contrast has been normalized by the threshold contrast for letter recognition. This means that reading speed is plotted against multiples of threshold contrast. Data are shown for one subject at three character sizes (0.25, 1, and 6 deg). By normalizing, we factor out differences due to contrast sensitivity (see the discussion of contrast sensitivity in a later section). The three sets of data are qualitatively similar and superimpose up to a normalized contrast of 10. At higher levels there is some divergence.

What accounts for the shape of the speed-vs.-contrast curves? Psychophysical models of contrast coding typically include a nonlinear transformation from stimulus contrast to visual response (see Legge and Foley 1980; Wilson and Gelb 1984). The solid curve in figure 15.4 is the compressive function used in the Legge and Foley model, which is derived from contrast masking

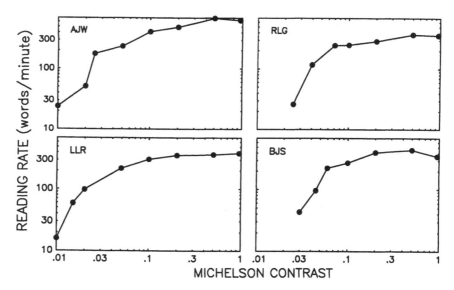

Figure 15.3 Data are shown for four subjects with normal vision. Reading rate is plotted as a function of luminance contrast for characters that subtend 1 deg of visual angle. Data were collected using the stationary text method. (Adapted from Legge et al. 1990)

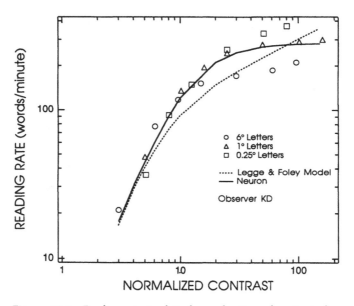

Figure 15.4 Reading rate is plotted as a function of contrast after normalization by the contrast threshold for recognizing letters of the appropriate size. Data for three character sizes are shown for observer KD. The dotted curve, eq. (15.1a), has the form of the compressive nonlinearity proposed by Legge and Foley (1980) to describe suprathreshold contrast coding. The solid curve, eq. (15.1b), has the form of a contrast-response function for a cortical neuron. (Adapted from Legge et al., 1987a)

Human Contrast Sensitivity and Its Clinical Applications

and discrimination data. It is nonsaturating because human subjects retain the ability to discriminate between contrasts, even at the highest levels. This function has the form

$$R = aC^{2.4}/(C^2 + b^2),$$ (15.1a)

where R is the magnitude of internal response, C is stimulus contrast, and a and b are constants. Contrast-response functions of simple and complex cells in cat and monkey visual cortices have similar compressive form except that they saturate (Sclar et al. 1990; Albrecht and Geisler 1991). The dashed curve in figure 15.4 has the shape of a contrast-response function for a cortical neuron[2]:

$$R = R_{max}C^2/(C^2 + C_{50}^2),$$ (15.1b)

where R is neuron response, C is stimulus contrast and R_{max} and C_{50} are constants.

Both curves in figure 15.4 have the same qualitative features as the data. Quantitatively, the saturating neuron curve better represents the flattening of the reading data at high contrast. It is premature to conclude that the contrast independence of reading speed at high levels is due to cell saturation. Smith, and Thomas (1989) described a psychophysical model containing compressive but nonsaturating contrast-response functions to account for contrast-independent pattern discrimination. Heeger (1991) presented another model in which contrast dependence is factored out by the cortical cells through a normalization process.

COLOR CONTRAST AND READING

Letters can be rendered with color contrast—such as green letters on a red background—as well as luminance contrast. There is evidence for differences in the sensory coding of color and luminance. Can color contrast support the high-speed pattern-recognition process in reading?

Figure 15.5 illustrates how separate red and green templates can be added either (1) in register to produce yellow text (luminance contrast), or (2) out of register to produce equiluminant red and green text (color contrast). We produced equiluminant text (i.e., the letters and background were matched in luminance) by video addition of separate red and green templates (Legge et al. 1990). Equiluminance was based on heterochromatic flicker photometry for each subject.

To compare the effects on reading of color contrast and luminance contrast, we expressed both as multiples of a threshold value. We adopted a threshold criterion for reading of 35 words/minute. We took the luminance contrast of the red and green templates at this threshold to be unity (in register for luminance-contrast text, out of register for color-contrast text) and expressed other contrasts as multiples of this value. The open and closed circles in figure 15.6 show reading speed vs. normalized contrast for text rendered by luminance contrast and color contrast. The luminance-contrast data have been

Legge: The Role of Contrast in Reading

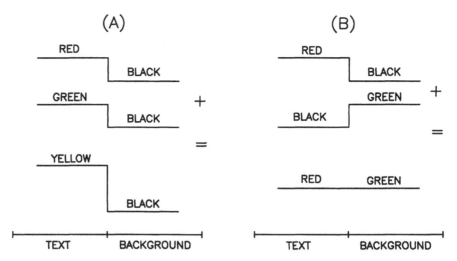

Figure 15.5 Luminance profiles of red and green images are summed to produce stimuli with either luminance contrast or color contrast. In (A) the bright portion of both the red and green images fall on the text and the dark portions fall on the background. When summed, the background remains dark and the text becomes yellow; there is no chromatic difference between the text and background. In (B) the bright portion of the red image falls on the text, whereas the bright portion of the green image falls on the background. When summed, there is a chromatic difference between the text and the background, but no luminance difference. (From Legge et al., 1990)

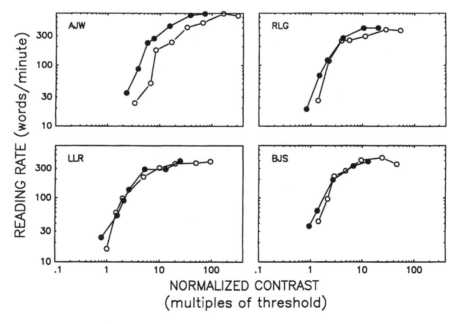

Figure 15.6 The contrast of the red and green templates making up the text has been normalized by a threshold value, the contrast required to read 35 words/min. In these units, plots of reading rate vs. luminance contrast and color contrast nearly superimpose. (From Legge et al., 1990)

Human Contrast Sensitivity and Its Clinical Applications

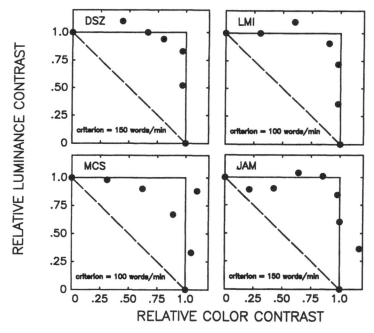

Figure 15.7 Data are shown for four subjects for whom text and background varied in both color contrast and luminance contrast. The circles show the relative color and luminance contrasts that combined to yield a criterion reading rate of 100 or 150 words/min. A relative contrast of 1.0 refers to the color contrast (or luminance contrast) needed to read at the criterion rate. The solid lines in each panel show the prediction of an independent channel model, and the dashed lines show the prediction of a linear summation model. (From Legge et al. 1990)

replotted from figure 15.3. The curves for color and luminance superimpose, apart from some deviation in the data of subject A.J.W. Switkes, Bradley, and De Valois (1988) also found superposition when masking curves for color contrast and luminance contrast were expressed in multiples of threshold.

The data in figure 15.6 clearly demonstrate that color contrast can support rapid reading. Knoblauch et al. (1991) found the same result. It is likely that the strongest sensory signals carrying information about equiluminant text are transmitted by the parvocellular pathway. Because this pathway is said to be temporally sluggish (Livingstone and Hubel 1988), it may be surprising that reading rates in excess of 340 words/minute are possible for equiluminant text. However, a dominant temporal frequency in reading is about 4 Hz (corresponding to about 4 saccades/sec), and this is well within the temporal resolution limit of the parvocellular pathway (Derrington and Lennie 1984).

The superposition of curves in figure 15.6 indicates that color contrast and luminance contrast are processed in the same way in reading. Could they be processed in a single pathway after all, not independent pathways? If so, we would expect an additive interaction. Imagine text in which letters and background differ in both luminance and color. Would two threshold multiples of luminance contrast and two threshold multiples of color contrast yield a reading rate corresponding to four threshold multiples of either one? Figure 15.7 shows the results of an additivity experiment in which we set a criterion reading speed of 100 or 150 words/minute and found the combinations of color and luminance contrast yielding the criterion speed (Legge et al. 1990). Data for four normal subjects are shown with relative color contrast plotted against relative luminance contrast. A scale value of 1.0 represents the amount of pure color contrast (or pure luminance contrast) required to read at the criterion rate. The solid lines show the predictions of an *independence* model in which reading rate is determined by the pathway that yields highest performance and is unaffected by the other. The diagonal dashed line shows the predictions of a *linear summation* model.

It is clear from the data that color contrast and luminance contrast act independently in their effects on reading. For all four subjects, the data lie close to the independence prediction, and far from the linear summation model. Of necessity, this test of independence was conducted at quite low contrasts (typically <0.10) to avoid ceiling effects. Therefore, our finding of independence applies only to low contrasts.

CHARACTER SIZE EFFECTS AND CONTRAST SENSITIVITY

Figure 15.8 shows reading rate as a function of angular character size for one normal subject (Legge et al. 1987a). The four curves are for the four text contrasts illustrated in figure 15.2. Character size ranges from 0.1 deg (near the

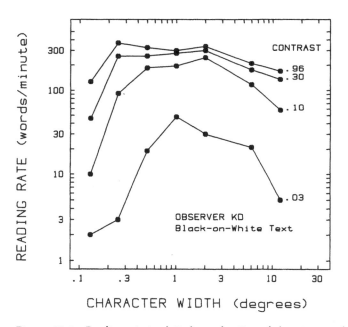

Figure 15.8 Reading rate is plotted as a function of character size for four contrasts. The contrasts correspond to those shown in figure 15.2. (From Legge et al. 1987a)

Human Contrast Sensitivity and Its Clinical Applications

acuity limit) to 12 deg. Reading speeds are highest (about 300 words/minute) on a plateau from about 0.3 to 3 deg. Reading has a tolerance of about a factor of 10 in character size as well as contrast. There is a sharp decline in reading rate for small characters near the acuity limit and a more gradual decline for large ones. Of relevance to low vision, it is noteworthy that normal vision can achieve moderately rapid reading for enormous characters (around 100 words/minute at 12 deg).

What determines the shapes of these curves? High performance for middle-size characters and lower performance for small and large characters is reminiscent of the contrast-sensitivity function (CSF) for gratings. For comparison, we created CSFs for reading (Legge et al. 1987a). In figure 15.9 the lower horizontal scale gives the "fundamental spatial frequency." It is the reciprocal of the angular character size shown on the upper scale. We defined the *threshold for reading* as the contrast required to read 35 words/minute. Contrast sensitivity is the reciprocal of this threshold contrast. (A lower criterion would be inconvenient because the measurements are more variable and difficult to obtain. The shape of the reading CSF is not much affected by modest changes of the criterion.) Data are shown for two subjects. The highest sensitivity of about 50 (corresponding to a lowest threshold of about .02) occurs for char-

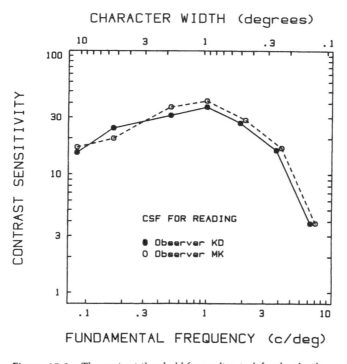

Figure 15.9 The contrast threshold for reading is defined to be the contrast required to read 35 words/min. Contrast sensitivity is the reciprocal of threshold contrast. Values of threshold contrast in this figure have been interpolated from curves like those shown in figure 15.3. The fundamental spatial frequency is equal to the reciprocal of the character width (i.e., one cycle/character). CSFs are shown for observers KD and MK. (From Legge et al. 1987a)

acters subtending 1 deg. Sensitivities decline slowly for low frequencies (large characters) and more rapidly for high frequencies (small characters).

These reading CSFs are qualitatively similar in shape to sine wave grating CSFs, but what about a quantitative comparison? We measured sine wave CSFs with stimulus conditions similar to those of the reading experiments. (This included 4 Hz flicker as a rough match to the temporal spectrum of reading, which is dominated by about 4 saccades/sec.) In figure 15.10, the data points are grating CSFs. The solid curve is an average CSF for reading. Since the threshold criteria are different, the vertical positioning is arbitrary. The reading curve has been shifted vertically so its peak sensitivity matches the grating curve. There is also a horizontal shift by a factor of 2. (Studies with spatially filtered letters and text have shown that a bandwidth of at least 2 cycles/character is required for reading [Legge et al. 1985a; Parish and Sperling 1991]. For this reason, reading contrast sensitivities have been compared with grating sensitivities at spatial frequencies equal to 2 cycles/ character.) In the left panel the match of the reading and grating CSFs is very good, and in the right panel it is fair. These results indicate that the mechanisms responsible for grating contrast sensitivity play a role in limiting reading speed and help to explain character-size effects.

These contrast sensitivity results, along with the shape invariance of the speed-vs.-contrast curves discussed in the previous sections, reveal an impor-

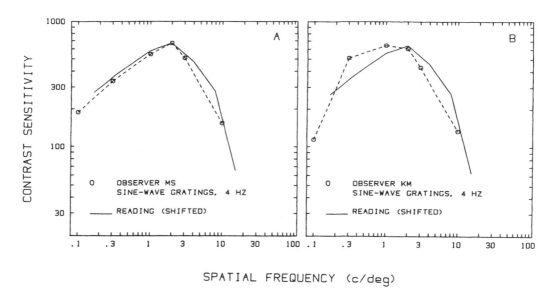

SPATIAL FREQUENCY (c/deg)

Figure 15.10 The data points show contrast sensitivity functions for the detection of sine wave gratings with 4 Hz sinusoidal flicker. Spatial frequency was varied by changing viewing distance so that all the stimuli had six cycles. The solid curve in each panel is the mean reading CSF from figure 15.9 based on the data of observers KD and MK. The reading CSF has been shifted vertically so that its peak value is equal to that of the grating CSF and shifted rightward by a factor of two for reasons described in the text. (From Legge et al. 1987a)

Human Contrast Sensitivity and Its Clinical Applications

tant principle. Differences in *contrast sensitivity* are equivalent to differences in *text contrast* in their effects on reading speed.

LOW-VISION READING AND CONTRAST

High contrast is often critical for successful low-vision reading. The data points in figure 15.11 show reading speed vs. contrast for a low-vision subject with congenital cataracts. The filled and open symbols are for black-on-white and white-on-black text, respectively. Like many patients with cloudy ocular media, this subject reads faster with reversed-contrast print (Legge et al. 1985b; Legge et al. 1987b). The upper curve shows average data for three normal subjects. The subject with the cataract does not have the normal contrast reserve. Reading speed drops sharply for any reduction in text contrast. This subject's high contrast data resemble the steep low-contrast portion of the normal curve. This makes sense because an eye with cataract scatters light, thereby reducing retinal image contrast.

This explanation follows from a *contrast-attenuation* model of low-vision reading deficits (Rubin and Legge 1989). According to the model, reading is slow because of reduced retinal image contrast or, equivalently, because of reduced contrast sensitivity. More specifically, the model predicts that (1) curves of low-vision reading differ from the normal curve only by a contrast attenuation factor (i.e., a horizontal shift on a log contrast axis), and (2) the

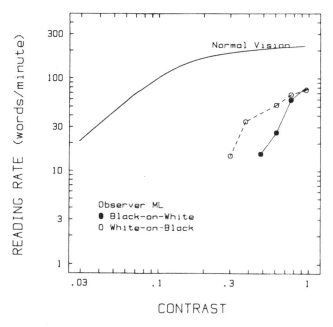

Figure 15.11 Reading rate is plotted as a function of contrast for 6-deg characters. The upper curve is average data from three normal subjects. The data points are for a low-vision subject with cloudy media due to congenital cataracts.

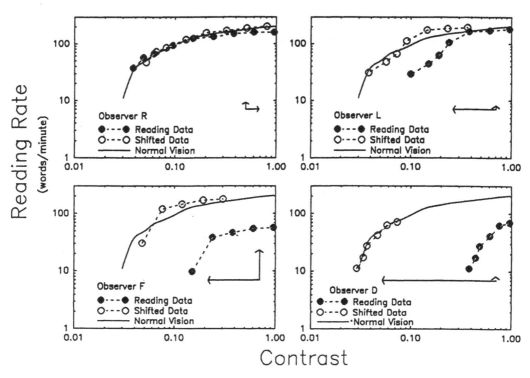

Figure 15.12 Reading rate is plotted as a function of contrast for four low-vision subjects. The filled symbols show the data, and the open symbols show the same data shifted horizontally and vertically to overlap the normal curve. In each panel arrows represent the horizontal (contrast) and vertical (reading rate) shifts. The character size was 6 deg. Subjects: D, optic neuropathy; F, age-related maculopathy; L, optic nerve hypoplasia; R, congenital cataract and surgical aphakia. (From Rubin and Legge 1989)

contrast attenuation factor is predictable from a measurement of contrast sensitivity.

To evaluate this model, we measured reading speed as a function of contrast for 19 low-vision subjects with a wide range of pathologies (Rubin and Legge 1989). The filled symbols in the four panels of figure 15.12 show data for four low-vision subjects. The solid curve in each panel shows normal performance. In each case we found the horizontal and vertical shifts of the low-vision data that produced the best match to the normal data. The open circles show the shifted low-vision data. The two arrows in each panel show the size of the horizontal (contrast) and vertical (reading speed) shifts. For most of our subjects, the shifted data closely match the normal curve.

One prediction of the model is that contrast attenuation alone is sufficient to account for differences in reading between normal and low-vision subjects. This is equivalent to claiming that only horizontal shifts, and no vertical shifts, are required to bring low-vision curves into coincidence with the normal curve. This was true of a subset of our subjects, those with cloudy ocular media. Their contrast attenuation factors ranged[3] from 0.8 to 20.8, with a

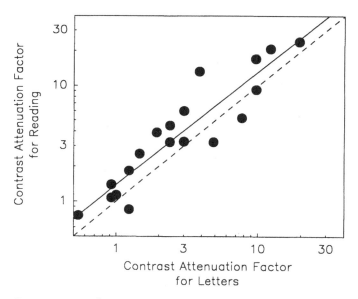

Figure 15.13 The contrast attenuation factor for reading is the size of the contrast shift required for the low-vision data to overlap the normal data in figure 15.12. This factor is plotted against the contrast attenuation factor for letters, which is the ratio of low-vision contrast threshold to normal threshold. The dashed line shows where the data would fall if the two factors were in perfect agreement. The solid curve is the actual regression line fit to the data. Each point is for a different low-vision subject. (From Rubin and Legge 1989)

mean of 6.9. For them, no statistically significant vertical shift was required. Subjects with clear media but central field loss (due to optic nerve damage, age-related maculopathy, and other retinal diseases) required vertical shifts as well as horizontal shifts. For them the contrast attenuation factors ranged from 0.8 to 23.9, with a mean of 7.3, and the "reading rate attenuation factors" (i.e., vertical shifts) ranged from 0.7 to 8.3, with a mean of 2.64, significantly greater than one.

A leftward shift in figure 15.12 is equivalent to a contrast reduction. A second prediction of the contrast attenuation model is that the horizontal shift is equal to a loss in contrast sensitivity. For each of the low-vision subjects we measured contrast sensitivities for recognizing letters of the size used in the reading experiments (6 deg). We took a low-vision subject's contrast sensitivity relative to mean normal contrast sensitivity as a *contrast attenuation* factor for letter recognition. Figure 15.13 is a scatter plot of the contrast attenuation factor for reading (horizontal shift in figure 15.12) vs. the contrast attenuation factor for letter recognition. The dashed line shows where data would fall if the two measures were identical, and the solid line is a regression fit to the data. The two factors are highly correlated, R = 0.92. The high correlation indicates that the dependence of reading on contrast can be predicted from a simple measure of contrast sensitivity for letters. The Pelli-Robson chart could serve such a purpose (Pelli, Robson, and Wilkins 1988).

The results indicate that changes in effective contrast due to media opacities or neural losses in contrast sensitivity play an important role in limiting low-vision reading speed. The contrast attenuation model, which equates losses in contrast sensitivity with a reduction in stimulus contrast, explains the deficits of people with cloudy media. The model accounts for some, but not all, of the deficits in reading experienced by people with field loss.

Normal vision has a contrast reserve of about a factor of ten for reading. If a patient's contrast sensitivity indicates that the reserve has been depleted (i.e., sensitivity reduced by a factor of 10 or more), we can be quite sure that the patient will read slowly because of inadequate contrast. Every effort must be made to provide such patients with high-contrast text of suitable angular size.

The contrast attenuation model has recently been applied successfully to another clinical problem. Modern cataract surgery usually involves replacement of a patient's crystalline lens with an artificial intraocular lens (IOL). The IOL is monofocal (i.e., has a fixed focus) and is selected for clear focus of distant objects. The patient wears reading glasses for near tasks. Recently several designs of multifocal IOLs have been introduced that are intended to increase depth of field and reduce the cataract patient's postoperative need for glasses (Holladay et al. 1990). The multifocal IOLs split the light entering the eye into two or more images on the retina that are conjugate with two or more depth planes. An object in one depth plane—such as a page of text—will produce a focused image on the retina that is superimposed on a highly defocused image of the same object. The defocused image is thought to act like a veiling source of light that reduces the contrast of the focused image.

Akutsu et al. (1992) measured sine wave grating CSFs for multifocal patients and compared them with CSFs for age-matched normal subjects and monofocal IOL patients. From their results they estimated contrast attenuation factors at different spatial frequencies (MTFs) of the multifocal IOL. The results closely matched the optical MTF measured by Holladay et al. (1990) and revealed contrast attenuation factors averaging about two. Akutsu et al. then asked how this contrast attenuation would affect reading performance. Considerations of the contrast reserve and character size dependence of normal vision suggest that a two-fold reduction in image contrast should affect reading only for low text contrasts or tiny letters. This is exactly what Akutsu et al. found. Multifocal patients had deficits in reading speed only for text that was low in contrast (< 30 percent) and had small characters (0.2 and 1 deg).

Can color contrast play a helpful role for low-vision readers who are contrast limited? According to Mullen (1985), color-contrast sensitivity is higher than luminance-contrast sensitivity at low spatial frequencies. People with low vision usually read large letters for which the important spectral content has low spatial frequencies. It is possible that low-vision readers are more sensitive to color contrast at low frequencies and would read faster using text rendered by color contrast. We evaluated this possibility by measuring reading speeds for 10 low-vision subjects (Legge et al. 1990). (Many low-vision patients have acquired color defects. We restricted our study to patients with normal or nearly normal color vision.) Unfortunately, none read faster with color contrast than with luminance contrast. Most read more slowly, even with the maximum color contrast we could produce.

Color contrast by itself may not be advantageous for low-vision reading, but could color contrast be added to luminance contrast to help? This question was part of the motivatlon for the "additivity" study described in connection with figure 15.7. Our finding that color contrast and luminance contrast act independently on normal reading speed makes it highly unlikely that any combination of color contrast and luminance contrast would be beneficial in low-vision reading.

Our findings show that color contrast does not enhance reading for people with low vision. In an earlier study we showed that the color of text per se (i.e., colored letters on dark backgrounds or dark letters on colored backgrounds) rarely has much effect on reading speed in subjects with normal or low vision (Legge and Rubin 1986).

Although color coding does not seem to be helpful in low-vision reading, recent work in my laboratory shows that color improves low-vision object recognition (Wurm et al. 1992). Reaction times were faster (and error rates lower) for recognizing full-color images of food objects compared with corresponding gray-scale images that were matched pixel by pixel in luminance.

Why should reduced contrast result in slower reading? Research in progress provides one possible answer (Ahn et al. 1991). In this research we are using a different procedure for measuring reading speed, the *rapid serial visual presentation* (RSVP) method. Words are presented one after the other at the same place on the screen. In one study we measured RSVP reading speeds as a function of word length from three to twelve letters. A trial consisted of the presentation of four random words of a fixed length. In a series of trials, each with a new set of words, exposure time was decreased until subjects could no longer read the words accurately. Words of different lengths were equated for frequency in English.

Figure 15.14 shows reading time/word as a function of word length. Reading time is the reciprocal of rate (shown on the right scale), so a high value means slow reading. The filled symbols are average data for six normal subjects measured at three levels of text contrast (100 percent, 10 percent, and 5 percent). The open symbols are data for one low-vision subject with cloudy media due to corneal vascularization.

For normal subjects the curve for 100 percent contrast text is nearly flat—that is, there is only a weak dependence of reading time on word length. The curves are steeper for lower-contrast text. The low-vision data were collected with 100 percent contrast text, but they rise on a line close to the 5 percent contrast normal data. This is consistent with this subject's 17-fold reduction in contrast sensitivity for letters of the corresponding size (6 deg).

The slopes of straight lines fit to the data give time/letter. If we assume a constant time/fixation of about 250 msec,[4] we can convert the slopes to letters/fixation. The slope of the nearly flat 100 percent contrast line for normal subjects converts to 4.9 letters/fixation. This suggests that normal subjects require more than one fixation to read the longer words in the RSVP

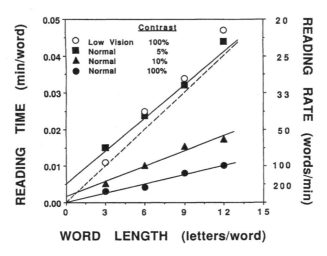

Figure 15.14 Reading time per word (left scale) is plotted as a function of word length using the RSVP method. Reading time per word is the reciprocal of reading rate (right scale). The solid symbols and regression lines show average data for six normal subjects and three contrast levels (100, 10 , and 5 percent). The open symbols and dashed regression line show data for a low-vision subject with cloudy ocular media due to corneal vascularization. Although he was reading high-contrast text, his data closely resemble those of normal subjects reading text with 5 percent contrast.

task. The slopes of the steeper 10 percent and 5 percent contrast lines convert to 3.0 and 1.3 letters/fixation, respectively. The line through the low-vision data has a slope that converts to 1.1 letters/fixation.

These preliminary findings fit the following interpretation. When text contrast drops (for normal vision) or when contrast sensitivity declines (in low vision), the visual span for reading grows narrower; the reader recognizes fewer letters per fixation. As a consequence, the reader saccades through the text in smaller and smaller steps with a corresponding reduction in reading speed. In effect, the capacity of normal vision to process several letters in parallel deteriorates with loss of either text contrast or contrast sensitivity.

CONCLUSIONS

Psychophysical techniques can be used to study the role of vision in reading. The dependence of reading speed on text variables, especially contrast and character size, can be related to the spatiotemporal filtering properties and contrast coding properties of vision. The findings are consistent with the view that text stimuli are first passed through an early stage of linear filtering that determines contrast sensitivity. Subsequent signal processing is invariant in form across character size and for color contrast and luminance contrast. The large contrast reserve enjoyed by normal readers may be a consequence of compressive or even saturating contrast response functions in the visual pathway.

An understanding of the role of contrast in reading is helpful in understanding the reading deficits of people with low vision. Deficits of contrast sensitivity in low vision can be modeled as a reduction in text contrast (contrast attenuation model). For one group of low-vision subjects, those with media opacities, the contrast attenuation model accounts for reading deficits. For people with central field loss, contrast attenuation must be coupled with other factors to explain fully their reading deficits.

ACKNOWLEDGMENTS

I would like to thank the co-organizers, Dominic Man-Kit Lam and Robert Shapley, for the opportunity to present this work at the symposium honoring Dr. Christina Enroth-Cugell. I would also like to thank Paul Beckmann, Andrew Luebker, and Sonia Ahn for help in preparing the figures; Carrie Rentschler for help with manuscript preparation; and many colleagues, cited in the text, who participated in the research described here. This work was supported by NIH grant EY02934.

NOTES

1. For normal subjects, reading speeds obtained with the stationary text method are usually a little faster than with the drifting text method. The reverse is true for many subjects with low vision (Legge et al. 1989).

2. I have used an exponent of 2.0 for simplicity. There is considerable variation in this parameter from cell to cell. Sclar et al. (1990) found a median value of 2.4 for a sample of V1 cells in the macaque monkey.

3. These are multiplicative factors, so a value of 1.0 means no shift. A value of less than one means a rightward shift (contrast attenuation factor) or a downward shift (reading rate attenuation).

4. Not much is known about the effect of reduced contrast on fixation time and saccade length in reading. More generally, as text difficulty increases, fixation times do not change much, but saccades tend to get shorter.

REFERENCES

Ahn, S., Legge, G. E., and Luebker, A. (1991). Reading speed and serial/parallel processing in vision. Suppl. Invest. Ophthalmol. Vis. Sci., 32, 1041.

Akutsu, H., Legge, G. E., Showalter, M., Lindstrom, R. L., Zabel, R. W., and Kirby, V. M. (1992) Contrast sensitivity and reading through multifocal intraocular lenses. Arch. Ophthalmol., 110, 1076–1080.

Albrecht, D., and Geisler, W. S. (1991). Motion selectivity and the contrast response function of simple cells in the visual cortex. Vis. Neurosci., 7, 531–546.

Campbell, F. W., and Robson, J. G. (1968). Application of fourier analysis to the visibility of gratings. J. Physiol. (London), 197, 551–566.

Derrington, A., and Lennie, P. (1984). Spatial and temporal contrast sensitivities of neurones in lateral-geniculate nucleus of macaque. J. Physiol. (London), 137, 219–240.

Enroth-Cugell, C., and Robson, J. G. (1966). The contrast sensitivity of retinal ganglion cells of the cat. J. Physiol. (London), 187, 517–552.

Heeger, D. J. (1991). Non-linear model of neural responses in cat visual cortex. In Landy, M., and Movshon, J. A., ed. *Computational Models of Visual Processing*, Cambridge, Mass.: MIT Press.

Holladay, J. T., van Dijk, H., Lang, A., et al. (1990). Optical performance of multifocal intraocular lenses. J. Cataract Refract. Surg., 16, 413–422.

Hubel, D. H., and Wiesel, T.N. (1968). Receptive fields and functional architechture of monkey striate cortex. J. Physiol. (London), 195, 215–243.

Knoblauch, K., Arditi, A., and Szlyk, J. (1990). Effects of chromatic and luminance contrast on reading. J. Opt. Soc. Am., A, 8, 428–439.

Legge, G. E., and Foley, J. M. (1980). Contrast masking in human vision. J. Opt. Soc. Am., 70, 1458–1471.

Legge, G. E., Parish, D. H., Luebker, A., and Wurm, L. (1990). Psychophysics of reading. XI. Comparing color contrast and luminance contrast. J. Opt. Soc. Am., A, 7, 2002–2010.

Legge, G. E., Pelli, D. G., Rubin, G. S., and Schleske, M. M. (1985a). Psychophysics of reading. I. Normal vision. Vision Res., 25, 239–252.

Legge, G. E., Ross, J. A., Luebker, A., and LaMay, J. M. (1989). Psychophysics of reading. VIII. The Minnesota low-vision reading test. Opt. Vis. Sci., 66, 843–853.

Legge, G. E., and Rubin, G. S. (1986). Psychopyhsics of reading. IV. Wavelength effects in normal and low vision. J. Opt. Soc. Am., A, 3, 40–51.

Legge, G. E., Rubin, G. S., and Luebker, A. (1987a). Psychophysics of reading. V. The role of contrast in normal vision. Vision Res., 27, 1165–1171.

Legge, G. E., Rubin, G. S., Pelli, D. G., and Schleske, M. M. (1985b). Psychophysics of reading. II. Low vision. Vision Res., 25, 253–266.

Legge, G. E., Rubin, G. S., and Schleske, M. M. (1987b). Contrast-polarity effects in low-vision reading. Low Vision: Principles and Applications. (Ed.) G.C. Woo. Springer-Verlag (New York), 288–307.

Livingstone, M., and Hubel, D. (1988). Segregation of form, color, movement, and depth: anatomy, physiology, and perception. Science, 240, 740–749.

Mullen, K. T. (1985). The contrast sensitivity of human colour vision to red-green and blue-yellow chromatic gratings. J. Physiol. (London), 359, 381–400.

Parish, D., and Sperling, G. (1991). Object spatial frequencies, retinal spatial frequencies, noise and the efficiency of letter discrimination. Vision Res., 31, 1399–1415.

Pelli, D. G., Robson, J. G., and Wilkins, A. J. (1988). The design of a new letter chart for measuring contrast sensitivity. Clin. Vis. Sci., 2, 187–199.

Rubin, G. S., and Legge, G. E. (1989). Psychophysics of reading. VI. The role of contrast in low vision. Vision Res., 29, 79–91.

Sclar, G., Maunsell, J., and Lennie, P. (1990). Coding of image contrast in central visual pathways of the macaque monkey. Vision Res., 30, 1–10.

Smith, B., and Thomas, J. (1989). Why are some spatial discriminations independent of contrast? J. Opt. Soc. Am., A, 6, 713–724.

Switkes, E., Bradley, A., and De Valois, K. K. (1988). Contrast dependence and mechanisms of masking interactions among chromatic and luminance gratings. J. Opt. Soc. Am., A, 5, 1149–1162.

Tielsch, J. M., Sommer, A., Witt, K., Katz, J., and Royall, R. M. (1990). Blindness and visual impairment in an American urban population: The Baltimore eye survey. Arch. of Ophthalmol. 108, 286–290.

Tinker, M. A. (1963). *Legibility of Print*. Ames: Iowa State University Press.

Wilson, H. R., and Gelb, D. J. (1984). Modified line-element theory for spatial-frequency and width discrimination. J. Opt. Soc. Am., A, 1, 124–131.

Wurm, L., Legge, G. E., Isenberg, L., and Luebker, A. (1993). Color improves object recognition in normal and low vision. J. Exp. Psychol.: Human Perception and Performance, in press.

16 Assessing Human Retinal Function Beyond the Receptors

Robert F. Hess

There have been many attempts to devise psychophysical measures of retinal function. These have been successful in the investigation of the receptoral limits on performance—for example, directional sensitivity (Stiles and Crawford 1933), cone action spectra (Stiles 1949), bleaching adaptation (Lamb 1990), and cone sampling (Williams 1988). As far as postreceptoral function is concerned, there are no adequate psychophysical means for separating retinal from postretinal contributions. To do this one must rely on the potentially hazardous task of interpreting visually evoked retinal potentials.

Retinal evoked potentials have had a long and checkered history, dating back to Holmgren (1865). However, it is only recently, through our emerging understanding of retinal function as the result of single-cell neurophysiology, that there has been renewed interest in using the retinal evoked potentials to assess postreceptoral retinal function in humans. Two major obstacles remain: first, the selection of the most appropriate stimulus, and second, proving that the recorded potential represents postreceptoral processes. We have come a long way in terms of the first of these, and I believe that the initial steps that have been made toward the second are encouraging.

METHODS AND RESULTS

The Stimulus

Technical innovation has played an important role in the history of vision research, particularly in terms of stimulus design. For example, it was not until the 1950s that stimuli were sinusoidally modulated in time about a mean light level (de Lange 1958). This provided the advantage of being able to test temporal modulation sensitivity while keeping light adaptation constant. Before this time, incremental sensitivity and light adaptation were confounded. Furthermore, the sinusoidal nature of the stimulus provided the basis for the application of linear systems analysis to visual function.

It was not until the 1960s that the spatial properties of the stimulus were also adequately controlled (Robson 1966). The combination of these refinements to the stimulus and the then-developing technique of single-cell recording resulted in a totally new way of thinking about retinal function. The view that retinal function could be analyzed using a linear systems approach was quite novel and controversial yet, as a result of this approach, we now know the extent of the linearity of some retinal cells. This approach has led to the now-accepted notion that stimuli of reduced incremental contrasts are particularly useful for demonstrating linear operations (Rodieck and Ford 1969).

There are a variety of stimuli that may be used for evoked potential measurements. The spatial and temporal properties of these stimuli are under tight control, and light adaptation is held constant (figure 16.1). Although a com-

A Uniform field

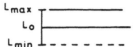

$$L(s,t) = L_0 \left[1 + C \cos 2\pi f_0 t \right]$$

B Contrast reversal

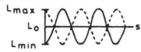

$$L(s,t) = L_0 \left[1 + C \cos 2\pi f_0 t \sin 2\pi g_0 s \right]$$

C Flickering pattern

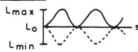

$$L(s,t) = L_0 \left[1 + C \cos 2\pi f_0 t \left(\frac{1 + \sin 2\pi g_0 s}{2} \right) \right]$$

D Pattern on-off

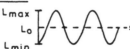

$$L(s,t) = L_0 \left[1 + C \left(\frac{1 + \cos 2\pi f_0 t}{2} \right) \sin 2\pi g_0 s \right]$$

E White pattern on-off

$$L(s,t) = L_0 \left[1 + C \left(\frac{1 + \cos 2\pi f_0 t}{2} \right) \left(\frac{1 + \sin 2\pi g_0 s}{2} \right) \right]$$

F Black pattern on-off

$$L(s,t) = L_0 \left[1 + C \left(\frac{-1 + \cos 2\pi f_0 t}{2} \right) \left(\frac{1 + \sin 2\pi g_0 s}{2} \right) \right]$$

Figure 16.1 The set of spatiotemporal stimuli that could be used to evoke retinal potentials. In each graph, luminance (L) is plotted against distance (S) along a horizontal spatial profile. Solid and dashed profiles represent the spatial profile at extremes of a temporal cycle.(From Baker and Hess 1984)

Human Contrast Sensitivity and Its Clinical Applications

plete understanding necessitates appreciating the interrelationships between the retinal responses evoked by all of these stimuli (Baker and Hess 1984), I will concentrate on the sinusoidally contrast-reversing stimulus (figure 16.1B) and to a lesser extent on the sinusoidally modulated uniform field (figure 16.1A).

It will be obvious that for the former stimulus, in which there is spatio-temporal symmetry for each half temporal cycle, the response of any purely linear mechanism would cancel if the responses were averaged over each complete temporal cycle. Thus one would not expect to see a direct contribution from the linear photoreceptor response in the electroretinogram evoked by such a stimulus. However, any nonlinearity, such as separate neurons carrying "light-on" and "light-off" information (Kuffler 1952), would be expected to be specifically revealed, as would any photoreceptor nonlinearity of this form, in the evoked response as a frequency doubling. This is exactly what is found, although the response picked up at externally placed electrodes (for example, an active lid electrode and a reference temple electrode) is quite small, only a few microvolts at best.

Key Properties of the Retinal Evoked Response

The main properties of the retinal potential evoked by the previously de-scribed stimulus are shown in figure 16.2. The stimulus is modulated sinu-soidally in space and time, and fixation is symmetrically located with respect to the spatial structure of the stimulus. Otherwise the spatiotemporal sym-metry would be disrupted and significant response energy would result at the fundamental stimulus frequency. The response is sinusoidal, but at twice the stimulus frequency. The average amplitude of the second harmonic is measured; it is approximately equal to half the peak-to-peak amplitude of the unfiltered waveform.

In the upper left-hand part of the figure (A) we see the relationship between the evoked potential and the stimulus temporal frequency. Two peaks are seen in the response, one at 1.5 Hz and another larger one at around 10 Hz. The significance of these two peaks is obscure, and they are likely to represent a composite response since the temporal phases associated with these amplitude responses vary dramatically as a function of temporal frequency. We chose to work at a stimulus frequency of 8 to 10 Hz since this maximizes the response and was well outside the bandwidth of pupillary dynamics. The relationship with the stimulus spatial frequency is shown in the upper right-hand part of the figure (B). Note that there is a small but definite (6 dB/decade) decrease in the evoked response amplitude as stimulus spatial frequency is lowered. A similar but steeper decline is seen at spatial frequencies above 5 c/deg (data not shown), mainly due to a contrast dependence that we will see shortly.

The decline in the response at low spatial frequencies is best understood in terms of postreceptoral retinal processes that have spatial antagonism. Further support for the view that this response is postreceptoral in origin comes from

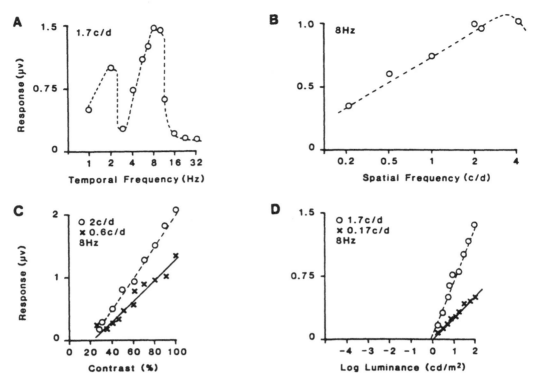

Figure 16.2 The four key properties of the human retinal evoked potential to a sinusoidally contrast-reversing pattern are illustrated. (A) Temporal response; (B) spatial response; (C) contrast response; (D) luminance response. (From Hess et al. 1986)

the fact that the peak location, but not the shape of this spatial response function, is shifted to progressively lower spatial frequencies for stimuli imaged on progressively more eccentric regions of the retina (Hess and Baker 1984b).

The results in part B were obtained at high contrasts. However, the shape of the spatial response function is not dependent on this choice, as is seen in the results in the lower left-hand part of the figure (C). Here we see that the amplitude of the evoked response is proportional to stimulus contrast up to 98 percent contrast, which was the limit of our equipment. Responses are displayed for two spatial frequencies, one representing the peak of the spatial response (1.7 c/deg) and another representing a point on the low-frequency decline (0.17 c/deg). The response is attenuated at the low spatial frequency regardless of the stimulus contrast at which it is measured. This type of proportional contrast response is found for all spatiotemporal combinations of steady-state stimuli.

Finally, in the lower right-hand part of figure 2(D), results are shown for the relationship between the mean retinal illumination, previously held constant at

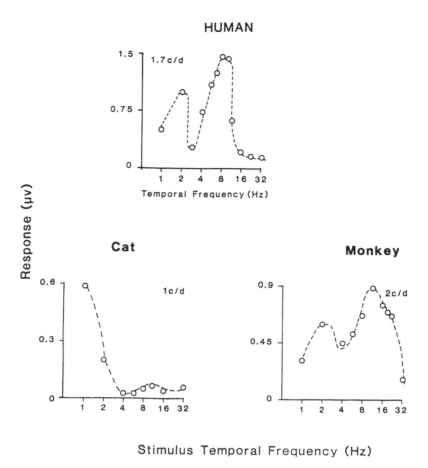

Figure 16.3 A comparison of the relationship between evoked potential amplitude and stimulus temporal frequency in human, cat, and monkey for a contrast-reversing pattern (figure 16.1B). Both human and monkey display a dominant response peak at 8–16 Hz, but the cat does not.

100 cd/m², and the response amplitude for two stimulus spatial frequencies (1.7 c/deg and 0.17 c/deg). Surprisingly, there is a rather steep decline in the response amplitude within the photopic region with no evidence of a scotopic component at either spatial frequency. This is remarkable because psychophysical sensitivity remains unaltered for both stimuli within this same luminance range. Note that these results also confirm that the low spatial frequency decline in response is not critically dependent on the photopic light level under which it is measured so long as there is a response present.

The picture that emerges from these properties of the overall potential as measured from external electrodes is one that, by its very nature, is likely to reflect the rectifying properties of either the photoreceptors or, more likely, the ON and OFF postreceptoral pathways that are known to exist in the mammalian retina (Kuffler 1952). The spatial tuning of the response and the way in which this changes with retinal eccentricity tips the balance in favor of the latter, i.e., a postreceptoral nonlinearity. Its strong dependence on mean luminance and retinal locus (Hess and Baker 1984b) suggests generators with exclusive input from cones. Although I have put forth the argument in favor of a foveal cone-only postreceptoral generator for this evoked response, the argument as it stands is not conclusive. The location of the generators must be verified directly in the living retina. This first requires a suitable animal model for the human evoked potential. Equipped with the "fingerprint" of its key properties, we are in an excellent position to assess the suitability of different animal models.

Establishing a Suitable Animal Model

In order to assess the suitability of cat and monkey (*Macaca fascicularis* and *Macaca mulutta*) models we recorded gross retinal potentials in these animals in a way as similar as possible to that in which we had obtained this data in

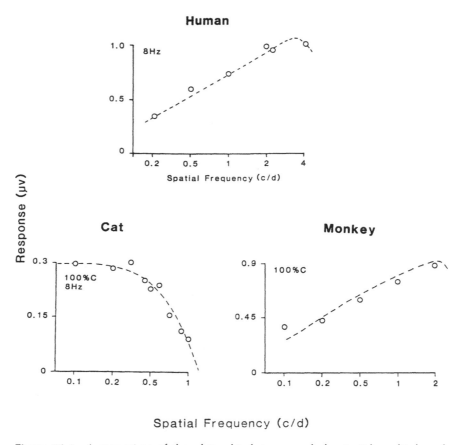

Figure 16.4 A comparison of the relationship between evoked potential amplitude and stimulus spatial frequency in human, cat, and monkey for a contrast-reversing pattern (figure 16.1B). Both human and monkey display similar spatial tuning, but the cat does not.

humans, with the exception that the animals were paralyzed and anesthetized (Hess et al., 1986). The properties of the evoked potential in the monkey were quite similar to those previously found by Baker and me in humans. For example, two clear peaks (at 1.5 Hz and 10 Hz) were seen in the monkey's temporal response (figure 16.3), a similar low spatial frequency decline in response was evident (figure 16.4), and a proportional contrast response was present (figure 16.5). Last, in both humans and monkeys there was a strong dependence of the response on mean luminance without evidence of a scotopic component, regardless of the spatial frequency (figure 16.6).

Somewhat to our initial surprise, these relationships were very different in the cat. First, the temporal response is dominated by a strong response at low temporal frequencies (figure 16.3). Second, the spatial response in the cat is essentially low-pass (figure 16.4), even when one takes into account the fact that the cat's contrast sensitivity function covers a lower spatial frequency

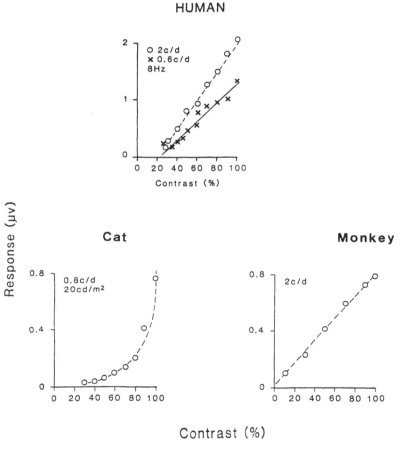

Figure 16.5 A comparison of the relationship between evoked potential amplitude and stimulus contrast in human, cat, and monkey for a contrast-reversing pattern (figure 16.1B). Both human and monkey display a proportional contrast dependence, but the cat does not.

Hess: Retinal Function Beyond the Receptors

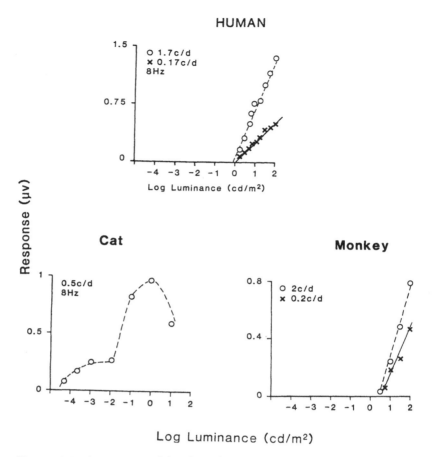

Figure 16.6 A comparison of the relationship between evoked potential amplitude and mean luminance in human, cat, and monkey for a contrast-reversing pattern (figure 16.1B). Both human and monkey display a strong dependence within the photopic region with no evidence of a scotopic component, but the cat does not.

range than that of the primate. Third, the cat's response-contrast relationship is logarithmic rather than linear as in the primate (figure 16.5). Last, the feline response as a function of mean luminance, in contrast to that of the primate, displays a peak at a midphotopic luminances, and there is clear evidence of a scotopic component (figure 16.6)

This comparison clearly indicates that the monkey rather than the cat is a more suitable model for the purposes of localizing the site of the human evoked potential. The reasons for these differences in the cat are unclear. One possibility is that the responses from the cat may reflect mixed rod-cone input to the generators and, possibly a different regional distribution rather than a fundamentally different site of generation of the response. Such optimism is supported by the recent findings of Sieving and Steinberg (1987) in the cat.

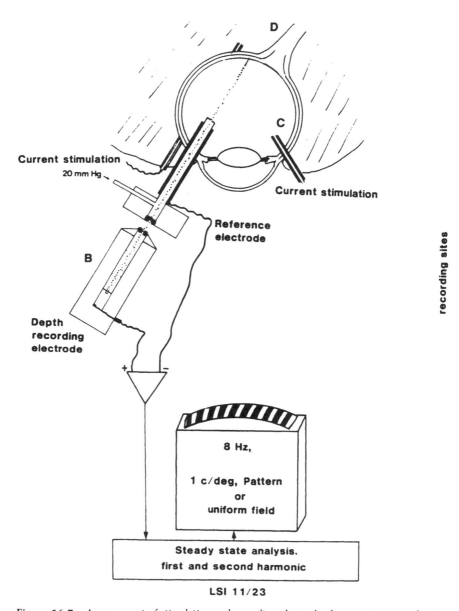

Figure 16.7 Arrangement of stimulating and recording electrodes for current source density measurements. For recording local evoked potential measurements electrode B is used. A constant current is passed between stimulating electrodes C and D, and the resultant voltage drop is recorded at B. The two stimuli used are illustrated below.

Locating the Site of Generation

In order to obtain the source of the membrane currents responsible from the evoked potentials, it is necessary to locate within the retina the site at which the current density is changing most rapidly (termed the current source density). To do this one needs a recording arrangement similar to that illustrated in figure 16.7, namely one pair of electrodes for measuring the local visual evoked potential as a function of retinal depth and another pair that can supply a constant current across the retina for the resistance measurement. Since our evoked potential measurements were in sinusoidal steady state, which affords the best signal-to-noise ratio, we adapted the standard current source density analysis (Nicholson and Freeman 1975) to handle steady-state signals. This provides a result that can be specified entirely by one-dimensional operations on the Fourier coefficients of the response without considering the temporal variation (Baker et al. 1988).

We compared two stimuli, first a spatial sinusoid that was sinusoidally contrast reversing, and second a sinusoidally modulated uniform field. The

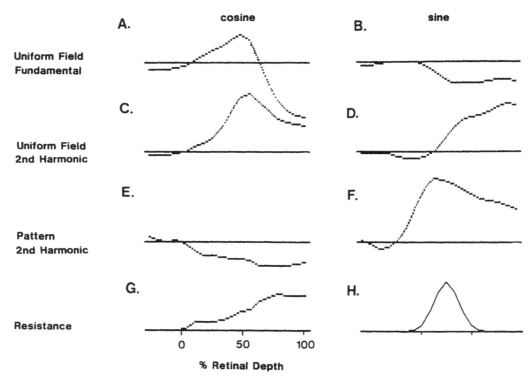

Figure 16.8   An example of the complete set of signal-averaged data obtained from one penetration of the retina. (A–F) Profiles of the Fourier coefficients (rectangular coordinates) of the voltages of each of the response components for the two stimuli used as a function of depth, with distal retina to the right. All profiles have been 1-2-1 smoothed twice. H represents the smoothing kernel. (From Baker et al. 1988)

first stimulus evokes a response at the second harmonic of the stimulus frequency, and its properties have been discussed above. The second, unlike the first, produces a significant response at the stimulus frequency (the fundamental linear response), as well as a response at twice the stimulus frequency (the second harmonic, non-linear response). The linear component of the uniform field response is suggestive of a photoreceptor contribution to the evoked potential.

At each of a number of retinal depths we collected the following data using signal averaging; the amplitude and phase of each response component for the fundamental and second harmonic components of the uniform field, for the second harmonic component of the contrast reversing grating, and for the integrated resistance (figure 16.8). The results were analyzed in rectangular coordinates in terms of the sine- and cosine- phase amplitudes in the following way. Resistivity was calculated as the reciprocal of the integrated resistance

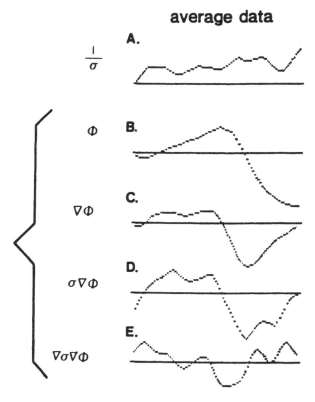

Figure 16.9 An example of the analysis undertaken to go from recorded voltages to underlying current source density (which was undertaken for the sine and cosine parts of the three components resulting from the two types of stimulation illustrated in figure 16.7), here illustrated only for the cosine component of the fundamental response to a sinusoidally modulated uniform field. (A) Resistivity; (B) voltage depth profile for the cosine component of the fundamental response to a uniform field; (C) current density uncorrected for resistivity variations; (D) current density corrected for resistivity; (E) current source density. (From Baker et al.1988)

Hess: Retinal Function Beyond the Receptors

(figure 16.9A), and current density was computed as the first derivative (figure 16.9C) with respect to the depth of the voltage amplitude (figure 16.9B). This current density profile was then corrected for resistivity variations by multiplying it by the resistivity at each depth (figure 16.9d) and the current source density obtained by a second differentiation with respect to depth (figure 16.9E). This analysis was undertaken for the sine and cosine components of each of the three components arising from the two stimuli described above. The resulting data were smoothed by a 1-2-1 operator that was applied four times. Its associated spatial kernel is illustrated in figure 16.8H.

One curious finding was that there were often variations in the temporal phase of the current source density profile. This is illustrated in its most extreme form in figure 16.10 for the two components of the uniform field response and for the one component of the contrast reversing grating. These are represented in the rectangular coordinates (A, B, D, E, G, and H) as sine- and cosine-phase components and in the polar coordinates (C, F, and I)

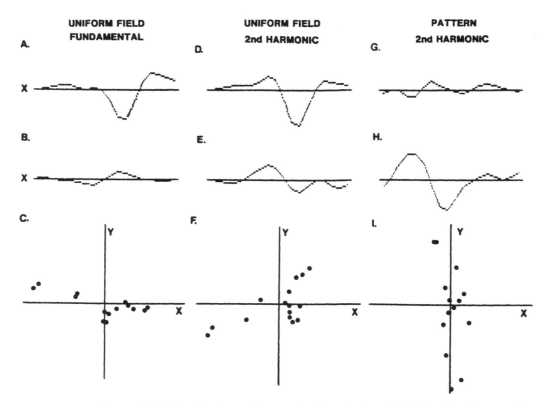

Figure 16.10 Results of current source density analysis applied to the six voltage profiles resulting from the uniform field stimulus (fundamental and second harmonic responses) and the contrast-reversing grating (second harmonic response). In (A, D, and G) cosine-phase CSDs are displayed. In (B, E, and H) sine-phase CSDs are displayed. In (C, F, and I) the same responses are displayed in polar coordinates. Note the different absolute temporal phases for these CSDs and hence the need for their normalization (see text). (From Baker et al. 1988)

as amplitude and phase. The fact that there is a constant phase offset does not undermine the analysis, but it does mean that before one can average the CSDs obtained across electrode tracks and across animals and before the CSDs for the three different components can be compared, one needs to normalize all the CSDs to the same absolute phase. This displaces the energy into one or other of the two quadrature components.

The results of this normalization and subsequent averaging of CSD profiles within and across animals are shown in figure 16.11. The success of the normalization procedure can be assessed by the extent to which all of the significant response energy could be successfully displaced to one or the other of the two quadrature components, in this case the cosine component. The reproducibility of CSD profiles from different tracks and different animals can be assessed by the standard error bars associated with each sample on the profile. Since each of the individual CSD profiles was obtained from slightly different areas of retina, we have also normalized them for depth prior to averaging, so that the x-axis in figure 16.11 is in terms of percentage depth.

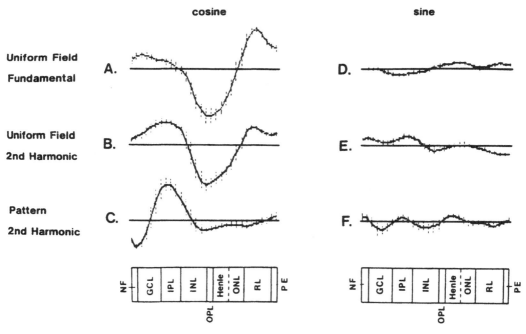

Figure 16.11 Averaged CSD profiles for the three components of the two stimuli used (figure 16.7). Each profile represents the average of 10 individual profiles, each normalized for temporal phase to facilitate averaging and subsequent comparison. The vertical bars are standard errors at each of 30 depth locations. The success of the phase normalization is shown by the extent to which most of the significant response energy is in one of the two quadrature components, in this case the cosine component. The x-axis is the percentage depth. Note the different dipole positions for the fundamental component of the uniform field (distal retina) and the second harmonic of the contrast-reversing stimulus (proximal retina). All stimuli were temporally modulated at 8 Hz. (From Baker et al. 1988)

It is clear that the dipole associated with the uniform field fundamental has a different distribution from that of the second harmonic of the contrast-reversing grating; the former is located in the distal two-thirds of the retina corresponding to the location of the photoreceptors, whereas the latter is located in the proximal one-third of the retina where ganglion cells, bipolar cells, and amacrine cells are located. The second harmonic's CSD profile for the uniform field is quite similar to that of the fundamental, although it may get a contribution from the generators of the second harmonic response from the contrast-reversing grating. Unlike the fundamental response of the uniform field whose CSD profile makes the photoreceptors a likely candidate for its generation, the contrast-reversing grating has a very different CSD profile, one that is located in the more proximal retinal layers. This supports the view, suggested above on the basis of indirect evidence, that the generators of this potential are postreceptoral (see also Sieving and Steinberg 1987 as well as Maffei et al. 1985).

TWO CLINICAL APPLICATIONS

Amblyopia

The question as to whether the retina is normal in humans with amblyopia has been an important issue in recent years. The findings of Ikeda and colleagues (Ikeda and Wright 1976; Ikeda and Tremain 1979) have shown that, in some animal models of amblyopia (surgically induced strabismis and atropine-induced anisometropia), a disorder of retinal ganglion cell function can be observed. This was followed by the claim by Arden and colleagues (Arden et al. 1980; Arden and Wooding 1985) that the retinal evoked potential to a contrast-reversing pattern was reduced in amplitude in the amblyopic eyes of human amblyopes.

This question about the retinal function of human amblyopes can be resolved only using methods based on the retinal evoked potential, since this is the only means available to assess retinal function in the living eye. The situation for animal models of amblyopia is interesting but model-dependent. The properties and postreceptoral site of the retinal evoked potential to a contrast-reversing grating make it an ideal means of addressing this issue. However, before rushing in let us recall what we know of the properties of this potential in normal eyes.

First, the amplitude of the potential varies proportionally with contrast, and second, the potential is foveally dominated. Previous studies (Arden et al. 1980; Arden and Wooding 1985; Persson and Wanger, 1982) have not considered these factors. The first relationship is important because it means that even small refractive errors will attenuate the response (Hess and Baker 1984a,b). This will be most influential in severe amblyopia because the cortical loss makes it difficult to do sufficiently accurate refractions to ensure that the retinal contrast is optimized. This problem can be rectified by doing the refraction at the retinal level using the evoked potential itself (Hess and Baker 1984a; Hess et al. 1985).

The second relationship, that of the regional retinal distribution of the potential, is important because a large proportion of human amblyopes, particularly strabismics in which ERG abnormalities had been previously reported, have nonfoveal fixation. If not taken into account, this will result in reduced responses. Again the best way to ensure that the foveas of normal and fellow amblyopic eyes are comparably positioned with respect to the stimulus is to use the evoked potential itself as the means of assessment. A significant misalignment will not only reduce the amplitude of the second harmonic response, but will also introduce a spurious response at the fundamental of the stimulus frequency.

These two factors turn out to be critical in the assessment of amblyopic function, because in the majority of the amblyopic eyes that we (Hess and Baker 1984a; Hess et al. 1985) have studied, responses have been significantly reduced for one reason or another, neither of which is relevant to whether retinal function per se is anomalous in amblyopia.

In figure 16.12 we see a comparison of the evoked potentials between the normal and amblyopic eyes of two human observers with severe amblyopia,

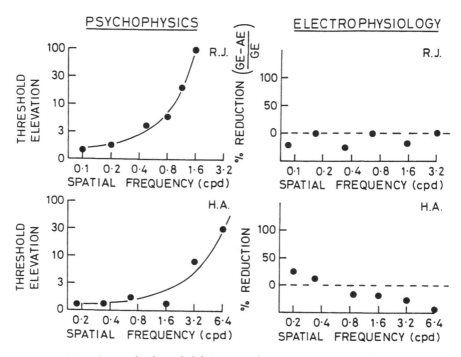

Figure 16.12 The psychophysical deficit (ratio of contrast sensitivities of good and amblyopic eyes) is compared with the electroretinographic deficit (percent reduction of ERG for good and amblyopic eyes) to the same 8-Hz contrast-reversing sine wave grating over a range of spatial frequencies. Note that normal ERG responses can be obtained for stimuli that are psychophysically invisible to the amblyopic visual system as a whole. (From Hess and Baker 1984a)

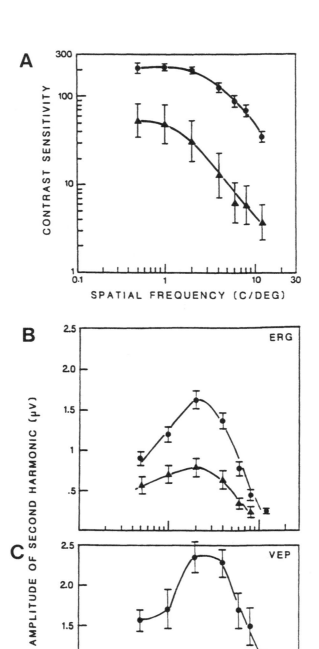

Human Contrast Sensitivity and Its Clinical Applications

indeed so severely affected that some of the stimuli were invisible. This again illustrates why focus and fixation must be optimized at the level at which the potential is generated. For comparison we show the contrast sensitivity abnormality to the same stimuli (figure 6.12). Using this technique, there is no indication of any retinal abnormality that might underlie the form of the amblyopic loss measured psychophysically using same stimuli.

Optic Neuritis

This is a condition that is characterized by demyelination of the optic nerve and, in its later stages, axonal degeneration. Recent evidence (Rucker 1972; McDonald 1983) suggests that the retina may be affected in the early stages and indeed that the primary pathology may be vascular. Since the retinal evoked potential to a contrast-reversing stimulus has its origin in the proximal retina layers, it is an ideal means of assessing any possible retinal involvement resulting from an anomaly of the retinal vasculature. In order to address this question we simultaneously recorded retinal and cortical evoked potentials to a contrast-reversing grating and compared this result with the psychophysical data (figure 16.13). We did this for a population of 24 patients with optic neuritis and 40 with normal eyes. The results show that, even though the cortical potential reflects a larger abnormality, the retinal potential is also abnormal. This is sufficient to challenge the previously held view that optic neuritis solely involves retrobulbar pathology in the early stages.

In the light of this finding a second question of interest concerns whether the long "conduction" delays that are observed in the cortical evoked potential in this condition are solely due to postretinal factors (nerve conduction and cortical temporal integration) or whether, in the light of our results indicating retinal involvement, significant intraretinal delays are also involved. A comparison of the simultaneously recorded retinal and cortical evoked potentials in this patient group, which had characteristically large cortical delays, is shown in figure 16.14. We show the phase of the second harmonic of the pattern ERG after first verifying that the phase delay was a function of temporal frequency, that is, a single time delay (Plant and Hess 1986), and this is plotted as a function of the spatial frequency of the stimulus. The dashed lines represent the ± 99 percent confidence limits for a group of normal observers. There is no evidence of any additional delay within the retina, and we conclude that the delay that is characteristic of the cortical evoked potential in this condition must arise proximal to the generators of the retinal response.

Figure 16.13 A comparison of the contrast sensitivity deficit (A), the electroretinographic deficit (B) and the electrocorticographic deficit (C) for a control group (n = 40) and 24 eyes with a history of optic neuritis. The error bars represent ± 2 SE. The stimulus is a contrast-reversing sine wave grating, temporally modulated at 8 Hz. Note that the deficit is retinal as well as postretinal. (From Plant, et al. 1986)

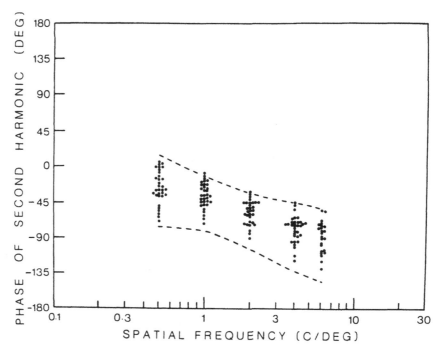

Figure 16.14 The relationship between the temporal phase of the ERG and spatial frequency is plotted for 24 eyes with a history of optic neuritis. The dashed lines represent the 99 percent confidence limits for a normal population (n = 40). Many of the patients exhibited long delays in their cortical evoked potentials that are not seen in the retinal responses to the same stimuli; hence they do not have a retinal origin. (From Plant et al. 1986)

CONCLUSIONS

Evoked potentials provide the only means presently available of assessing the postreceptoral function of the human retina. Their usefulness depends on the type of stimulus that is used and the extent of our knowledge of where the underlying generators are located in the retina. Our understanding of both of these factors is in its infancy, although we have made significant progress since the days when the accepted stimulus was an abruptly presented blinding flash of light in an otherwise totally dark room. The stimuli that are currently in use are physiologically based and have the ability to reveal the distal and proximal processes of the retina. The clinical application of this approach is potentially very fruitful, but as yet largely unexplored.

ACKNOWLEDGMENTS

I am grateful to have collaborated with the following people in this area of research: Curtis Baker, Eberhart Zrenner, Gordon Plant, Ulker Tulunay-Keesey, Jim Verhoeve, Borgor Olsen, and Thomas France. This work was supported by the Medical Research Councils of Great Britain and Canada, the Natural Science and Engineering Research Council of Canada, and the Wellcome Trust of Great Britain. I am grateful to John Robson, whose skepticism about the properties and origin of the ERG evoked by a contrast-reversing stimulus compelled Curtis Baker and me to deviate from our current areas of research to measure our first retinal potentials in 1983.

REFERENCES

Arden, G. B. Vaegan, Hogg, C. R., Powell D., and Carter, R. M. (1980) Pattern ERGs are abnormal in many amblyopes. Trans. Ophthal. Soc. UK 308: 82−83.

Arden, G. B., and Wooding S. L. (1985) Pattern ERG in amblyopia. Invest. Ophthal. Vis. Sci. 26: 88−92.

Baker, C. L., and Hess, R. F. (1984) Linear and nonlinear components of human electroretinogram. J. Neurophysiol. 51: 952−967.

Baker, C. L., Hess, R. F., Olsen, B. T., and Zrenner, E.(1988) Current source density analysis of linear and nonlinear components of the primate electroretinogram. J Physiol. 407: 155−176.

Hess, R. F., and Baker, C. L., (1984a) Assessment of retinal function in severely amblyopic individuals. Vision Res. 24: 1367−1376.

Hess, R. F., and Baker, C. L. (1984b) Human pattern-evoked electroretinogram. J. Neurophysiol. 51: 939−951.

Hess, R. F., Baker, C. L., Verhoeve, J., Tulunay-Keesey, U., and France, T. (1985) The pattern evoked electroretinogram: Its variability in normals and its relationship to amblyopia. Invest. Ophthal. Vis. Sci 26: 1610−1628.

Hess, R. F., Baker, C. L., Zrenner, E., and Schwarzer, J. (1986) Differences between electroretinograms of cat and primate. J Neurophysiol. 56: 747−768.

Holmgren, F. (1865) Metod att objektivisera effekten av ljusintryck pa retina. Upsala Lakareforen. Forh. 1: 177−191.

Ikeda, H., and Tremain, K. E. (1979) Amblyopia occurs in retinal ganglion cells of cats reared with convergent squint without alternating fixation. Exp. Brain Res. 35: 559−582.

Ikeda, H., and Wright, M. J. (1976) Properties of LGN cells reared with convergent squint: A neurophysiological demonstration of amblyopia. Exp. Brain Res. 25: 63−77.

Kuffler, S. W. (1952) Neurons in the retina; organization, inhibition and excitation problems. Cold Spring Harbor Symp. Quant. Biol. 17: 281−292.

Lamb, T. D. (1990) Dark adaptation; A re-evaluation. In Night Vision eds R. F. Hess, L. T. Sharpe, and K. Nordby. Cambridge University Press.

de Lange, H (1958) Research into the dynamic nature of the human foveal cortex systems with intermittent and modulated light 1: Attenuation characteristics with intermittent coloured light. J. Opt. Soc, A m. 48: 777−784.

Maffei, L., Fiorentini, A., Bisti, S., and Hollande, H. (1985) Pattern ERG in monkey after section of optic nerve. Exp. Brain Res. 59: 423−425.

McDonald, W. I. (1983) The significance of optic neuritis. Trans. Ophthal. Soc. UK 103: 230−246.

Nicholson, C., and Freeman, J. A. (1975) Theory of current source density analysis and determination of conductivity tensors for anuran cerebellum. J. Neurophysiol. 38: 356−368.

Persson, H. E., and Wanges, P., (1982) Pattern reversal electroretinograms in squint amblyopia, artificial anisometropia and simulated eccentric fixation. Arch. Ophthamol. 60: 123–132.

Plant, G. T, and Hess, R. F. (1986) The pattern evoked electroretinogram in optic neuritis. Brain 109: 469–490.

Robson, J. G. (1966) Spatial and temporal contrast sensitivity functions of the visual system J Opt. Soc. Am. 56: 1141–1142.

Rodieck, R. W., and Ford, R. W. (1969) The cat local electroretinogram to incremental stimuli. Vision Res. 9: 1–24.

Rucker, C. W. (1972) Sheathing of the retinal veins in multiple sclerosis: a review of pertinent literature. Mayo Clinic Proc. 47: 335–340.

Sieving, P. A., and Steinberg, R. H. (1987) Proximal retinal contribution to the intra-retinal 8 Hz pattern ERG of cat. J Neurophysiol. 57: 104–120.

Stiles, W. S. (1949) Increment thresholds and the mechanisms of colour vision. Ophthalmology 3: 138–163.

Stiles, W. S., and Crawford, B. H. (1933) The luminous efficiency of rays entering the eye pupil at different points. Proc. Roy. Soc. 112B: 428–450.

Williams, D. R. (1988) Topography of the foveal cone mosaic in the living eye. Vision Res. 28: 433–454.

17 Detection and Discrimination of Spatial Form in Patients with Eye or Visual Pathway Disorders

D. Regan

INTRODUCTION

A serious reduction of one's ability to see and recognize objects can compromise self-sufficiency and remove many of the more agreeable aspects of life. This crucial visual capability has traditionally been assessed in terms of visual acuity alone, and in clinical practice the Snellen chart has been the most favored of the acuity tests. It is instructive to spell out the rationale of the Snellen test. The rationale is that the smaller the high-contrast letters that can be read correctly, the better is macular form vision. This is an adequate rationale for correcting refractive errors. But it is flawed when visual loss has a retinal or visual pathway component or when there are corneal irregularities, lens opacities, or turbidity of the ocular media. In such cases the Snellen test for the ability to see and recognize high-contrast luminance-defined shapes can usefully be supplemented by an additional test for the ability to see and recognize low-contrast luminance-defined shapes.

Five Kinds of Contrast that Allow Us to See and Recognize an Object

An object is said to be perfectly camouflaged when it is visually identical to its surroundings. Such an object can be neither seen nor recognized, and for this reason many species of predators and prey have evolved so as to merge more or less perfectly into their surroundings. Humans are able to see and also recognize objects when they differ from their surroundings along any one of the following five visual dimensions: luminance, color, motion, texture, or disparity (reviewed in Regan 1991 and Bergen 1991). As noted above, clinical tests of form vision are usually restricted to the ability to process luminance contrast, and this chapter will focus on failures in this specific ability. However, a broader approach to spatial form vision should consider all five kinds of contrast, because it has become clear that intersubject differences in the processing of the different kinds of contrast are only loosely correlated. For example, it is well known that the ability to process color contrast can fail, while the processing of luminance contrast and disparity contrast remain normal. It has also long been known that the ability to process disparity contrast can fail, while Snellen acuity and color vision remain normal. More recently we have found that the ability to detect and/or recognize motion-defined form can be degraded by white matter lesions that spare the ability to detect and recognize luminance-defined form (Regan et al. 1991, 1992; Giaschi et al. 1991, 1992). Currently we are investigating whether a selective loss of ability to detect and/or recognize texture-defined form can be degraded without affecting the ability to recognize or detect form defined by luminance contrast, color contrast, motion contrast, or disparity contrast (Regan and Hong 1992).

Detecting versus Recognizing an Object

It is well known in neurology that brain damage can cause a general failure of the ability to recognize objects. This general failure is usually described as a cognitive abnormality. Less well known is the evidence that a defect of sensory rather than cognitive processing can degrade the ability to spatially discriminate and recognize objects while leaving detection sensitivity unimpaired. For example, a unilateral hemispheric lesion can impair recognition of motion-defined letters while leaving detection sensitivity unaffected (Regan et al. 1992). For luminance-defined form also. spatial discrimination can be dissociated from detection sensitivity. The evidence is as follows. Figure 17.1A

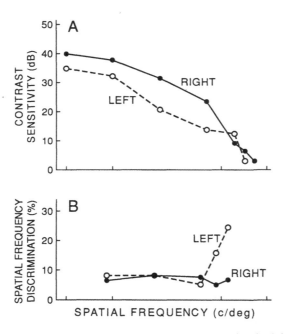

Figure 17.1 (A) Contrast sensitivity curves for the left and right eyes of a patient with multiple sclerosis. The reciprocal of the contrast detection threshold for a sine wave grating was plotted as the ordinate on a logarithmic scale. (B) Spatial frequency discrimination for the same patient. The percentage difference in spatial frequency between two gratings that were just distinguishable is plotted as the ordinate. (Modified from Regan et al. 1982. Reprinted with permission)

shows grating contrast detection sensitivity curves for the left and right eyes of a patient with multiple sclerosis (MS), and figure 17.1B shows spatial frequency discrimination curves for the same patient. This patient had a lower contrast sensitivity in her left eye than in her right eye for sine wave gratings whose spatial frequencies were less than about, 10 c/deg, while the two eyes had similar sensitivities above, 10 c/deg. Testing spatial frequency discrimination revealed the converse pattern of loss. Below about, 10 c/deg, discrimination was similar for the two eyes, but above, 10 c/deg discrimination was worse for the left eye; the frequency difference between two gratings had to

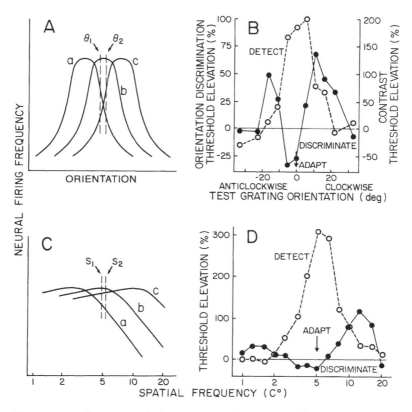

Figure 17.2 Detection and discrimination. The continuous lines in (A) and (C) represent tuning curves of three neurons that are driven from the same retinal location. (A) When the orientation of a stimulus grating changes slightly from θ_1 to θ_2 (arrows), the response of the most active of the orientation-tuned neurons (b) changes negligibly, but there is a substantial change in the relative activations of neurons a and c. (B) Postadaptation changes in orientation discrimination (continuous line) and contrast detection (dashed line) caused by inspecting a vertical grating (0 on abscissa). (C) Test grating spatial frequency changes from S_1 to S_2 c/deg. A small change in the spatial frequency of the test grating produces little change in the firing of the most excited neuron (b), but a considerable change in the balance of activity between the neurons a and c, the greater contribution to this change in balance coming from neuron a. (D) Postadaptation changes in spatial frequency discrimination (continuous line) and contrast detection (dashed line) caused by inspecting a sine wave grating of frequency 5 c/deg. (Modified from Regan and Beverley 1985. Reprinted with permission)

be as large as 25 percent before the patient could tell them apart (Regan et al. 1982).

A similar dissociation between detection and spatial discrimination can be temporarily produced in normally sighted individuals. The broken lines in figure, 17.2B and D illustrate the well-known finding that adapting to a grating of high contrast and high luminance elevates contrast detection threshold for a subsequently viewed test grating when the test grating has approximately the same spatial frequency and orientation as the adapting grating (Blakemore and Campbell 1969; Blakemore and Nachmias 1971). The effects of adaptation on orientation discrimination and spatial frequency discrimination are, however, quite different. Beverley and I found that orientation discrimination threshold is elevated not at the adapting orientation, but at orientations offset by about 15 to 20 deg from the adapting orientation (figure 17.2B), and that spatial frequency discrimination is elevated not at the adapting spatial frequency, but at spatial frequencies offset from the adapting spatial frequency (figure 17.2D) (Regan and Beverley 1983, 1985). A possible explanation for these dissociations between postadaptation detection and discrimination is that different neurons determine *detection* threshold and *spatial discrimination* threshold for gratings. In particular, the most important neuron for detection is the most excited neuron (b in figure 17.2A and C), while discrimination is chiefly determined by the relative activity of the comparatively weakly excited neurons (a) and (c), whose sensitivity curves differ most in slope (Regan 1982; Regan et al. 1982).

The proposal that opponent-orientation and opponent-size neurons exist in the visual pathway is based on this "relative activity" notion, but the same postadaptation discrimination data can also be explained by a line-element hypothesis (Wilson and Gelb 1984; Wilson and Regan 1984). It will be evident that these opponent-process and line-element hypotheses of spatial discrimination are analogous to the opponent-process and line-element theories of color discrimination (Wyszecki and Stiles 1967). Below we assume that contrast detection threshold and spatial discrimination threshold are determined by different neurons for letters, just as they are for simple gratings.

Different Kinds of Contrast Sensitivity Function Abnormality

This section describes different kinds of abnormal contrast detection threshold curves. There is wide agreement that several retinal and visual pathway disorders can produce a loss of contrast sensitivity to sine-wave grating stimuli and that—as first shown by Bodis-Wollner (1972)—in some cases this loss is relatively more severe at low than at high spatial frequencies. The familiar pattern of contrast sensitivity loss produced by a refractive error in the human eye was described by Campbell and Green (1965) as a loss of contrast sensitivity to sine wave grating stimuli that is relatively more severe at high than at low spatial frequencies. More recently it has been shown that this is not the only possible pattern of loss. The patterns of loss reported in a number of disorders can be regarded as combinations of the five patterns illustrated in

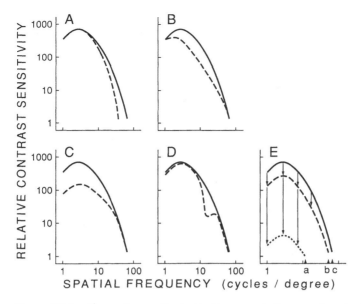

Figure 17.3 The continuous line in (A–E) represents the normal contrast sensitivity curve. The dashed and dotted lines show different kinds of abnormal curves. (Modified from Regan and Neima 1983. Reprinted with permission)

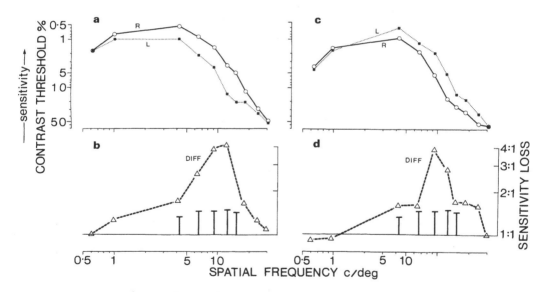

Figure 17.4 Illustrates how multiple sclerosis can selectively degrade contrast sensitivity over a broad range of intermediate spatial frequencies. (A) Visual detection threshold for a grating (ordinate) vs. the grating's spatial frequency (abscissa in c/deg). Continuous line for right eye; dotted for left. Note that the two eyes have similar sensitivities at low and high spatial frequencies.(B) The dashed line plots the ratio between contrast sensitivities for the right and left eyes. The T-shaped bars were calculated from data obtained from 29 control subjects. The ratio was calculated for each individual subject, and the bars show 1 SD. (C and D) Data for a second patient. (From Regan et al. 1977. Reprinted with permission)

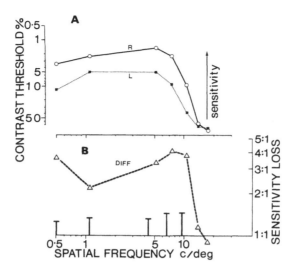

Figure 17.5 Illustrates how multiple sclerosis can degrade visual sensitivity selectively for low spatial frequencies. Details as for figure 17.4. (From Regan et al. 1977. Reprinted with permission)

figure 17.3.[1] The heavy continuous line in figure 17.3A–E represents the normal grating detection contrast sensitivity curve. Figure 17.3A shows the pattern of loss caused by moderate refractive blur. This pattern of loss is also observed in many patients with retinal and visual pathway disorders, even when the retinal image is sharp. Figure 17.3B illustrates the broad, so-called "intermediate-frequency loss" observed in some patients with MS (Regan, Silver, and Murray 1977) and optic neuritis (Hess and Plant 1986; Frisen and Sjöstrand 1978; Zimmern, Campbell, and Wilkinson 1979), and figure 17.4 gives an empirical example. The dashed curves marked "DIFF" in figure 17.4B, D plot the ratio between contrast sensitivities for the left and right eyes. Curves like this have been taken to suggest that the patient had sustained a specific loss of a spatial frequency channel (Regan, Silver, and Murray 1977). Figure 17.3C shows a pattern of loss that is the mirror image of the pattern of loss caused by blur. This so-called low-frequency loss was first observed in patients with MS (Regan, Silver, and Murray 1977), and it seems to be less common than the "intermediate-frequency" pattern of loss. Figure 17.5 gives an empirical example. Selective loss of sensitivity to low-contrast gratings in patients with MS and optic neuritis has since been reported by Zimmern et al. (1979), Bodis-Wollner et al. (1979), Hess and Plant (1986), and by several other groups.

Visual Sensitivity Loss for Low-Contrast Stimuli versus Visual Sensitivity Loss for Low and/or Intermediate Spatial Frequencies

It is important to bear in mind that the grating contrast sensitivity function (CSF) is a plot of the contrast threshold for detecting a grating stimulus. It tells

Human Contrast Sensitivity and Its Clinical Applications

us about the neural mechanism that determines detection threshold for a grating, but it does not necessarily tell us about the visual processing of a grating at contrasts well above detection threshold. In some patients, for example, elevations of contrast threshold are not evident at suprathreshold levels of contrast (Medjbeur and Tulunay-Keesey 1985, 1986), while in other patients contrast sensitivity loss is evident at both threshold and suprathreshold levels (Regan et al. 1981). If the visual system contains mechanisms tuned to low and to intermediate spatial frequencies that are not strongly excited until contrast is high, then these mechanisms may contribute little, if anything, to the grating detection CSF, even though they are important in suprathreshold vision.

Further to this point, the usual way of presenting the detection CSF focuses attention on the spatial frequency at which the visual loss is most evident rather than the contrast at which the visual loss is most evident. Thus, for example, figure 17.5 gives an immediate impression that visual loss is selective for gratings of low and intermediate spatial frequencies rather than being selective for low-contrast gratings. Turning to the case of letter stimuli, I will argue below that in some cases it may be more revealing to regard low-contrast acuity charts as testing vision at different contrast levels rather than testing vision at different spatial frequencies (Paragon 1985).

Caution is necessary with the sharp, so-called "notch" pattern of loss illustrated in figure 17.3D because this can be produced by small-angle monocular diplopia of either optical or neural etiology—a not uncommon condition that can be chronic or temporary. As its name suggests, monocular diplopia manifests itself as a double image when a single target (e.g., a single line or letter) is viewed. However, when a spatially repetitive target (e.g., a grating) is viewed, the dysfunction shows as one or more orientation-tuned dips or notches in the contrast sensitivity curve. It has been suggested that these dips are caused by destructive interference between the two images (Regan and Maxner 1986; Apkarian et al. 1987). Figure 17.6 illustrates this explanation of the effect. For example, if the angular deviation between the two images is about 2 min arc, the contrast sensitivity curve would be expected to show a notch at a spatial frequency of about 15 c/deg.

Monocular diplopia of optical origin is not uncommon. Chronic "notches" of optical origin , are shown in Apkarian et al. (1987). Transient optical diplopia with its associated transient notch can also be produced by mechanically deforming the eye, for example by a tightly fitting eyepatch (Regan and Maxner 1986). In some normally sighted individuals it is also possible to produce transient diplopia of neural origin by occluding one eye while visually stimulating the fellow eye by, for example, a counterphase-modulated pattern of sharp-edged checks (Regan and Maxner 1986). Individuals with a history of oblique astigmatism or surgically corrected strabismus seem especially susceptible. It is possible that some of the notch losses in the literature were associated with monocular diplopia. On the other hand, Travis et al. (1987) described a patient with monocular diplopia who did not have the expected notch in her contrast sensitivity curve. Nevertheless, all patients and

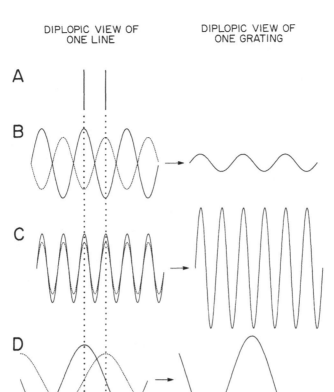

Figure 17.6 Monocular diplopia can cause a sharp "notch" or a ripple in the CSF. (A) In monocular diplopia, a single bright line is seen as double. (B) For a sine wave grating the two images cancel when the grating period is exactly twice the diplopic line separation. Cancellation grows rapidly less as the grating spatial frequency is increased (C) or decreased (D). (From Regan 1991. Reprinted with permission)

control subjects should be tested for monocular diplopia with a sharp-line or single-dot target.

Clearly, however, monocular diplopia cannot explain contrast sensitivity losses that are patchy over the visual field—as they commonly are. Nor can it account for the intermediate-frequency loss that extends over a wide range of spatial frequencies (compare figure 17.3B and D).

Low-Contrast Letter Chart Tests of Spatial Discrimination

After our 1977 article on contrast sensitivity loss caused by MS was published, a number of clinicians asked me to develop some way of testing low-contrast vision that was simple, inexpensive, and suitable for everyday use in the clinic. The most obvious idea was a low-contrast letter-reading chart (Regan 1981; Paragon 1985) because letter charts have many advantages, including familiarity, and the fact that they test spatial discrimination rather than merely testing detection threshold.[2](In everyday life it is often necessary to recognize an object, and detection is not enough.)

Vision theory is not yet sufficiently advanced to accurately predict subject's ability to recognize two-dimensional shapes on the basis of contrast detection thresholds for those very shapes, let alone on the basis of contrast detection thresholds for sine wave gratings. (In any case, responses to complex shapes could not in general be predicted from the CSF alone: in the spatial frequency domain some quite different spatial configurations have similar power spectra, differing only in their phase spectra.) Therefore, if one wishes to assess a patient's ability to discriminate between different two-dimensional shapes, it is simplest to do so directly by using a shape recognition test. The reason for choosing letters as test shapes was that, if it is to be used routinely, a clinical test must be brief and must be well accepted by patients whose intelligence spans the entire range of the general population. The enormous success of Snellen's test indicates that a letter-reading test fits these criteria. The reason for choosing to measure visual performance at several suprathreshold levels of contrast rather than measuring contrast threshold for reading letters was that, in the everyday visual environment, visible objects may have any suprathreshold contrast up to 100 percent. And the reason for using sharp-edged rather than spatially filtered letters was that many important objects in the everyday visual environment (e.g., road signs and automobiles) have sharp-edged retinal images independently of contrast. Furthermore, an empirical study using spatially filtered letters showed no practical advantage over unfiltered letters (Regan et al. 1981).

It was by no means self-evident that a low-contrast letter-reading test would pick up the same patients who were picked by by a sine wave grating detection test. In particular, it was clearly not valid to assume that the ability to discriminate or even detect two-dimensional shapes could be predicted from contrast detection thresholds for one-dimensional sine wave gratings. Therefore we progressed in small steps. First we established that MS patients with elevated contrast detection thresholds for gratings were picked up by measuring reading scores for isolated, spatially filtered letters (Regan et al. 1981). Next we went on to show (Regan et al 1981; Regan and Neima 1983) that low-contrast, spatially unfiltered letters also picked up this detection threshold elevation whether presented in isolation or in a line format. The low-contrast letter charts were made as slides for back or front projection and were provided on request to researchers during 1982–1983.

Because of the difficulty of controlling the contrast of very low-contrast photographs, the next version consisted of charts printed onto cardboard. About 150 sets were made and provided gratis to interested researchers during 1983–1984. The latest design is printed on plastic at contrasts of 96, 50, 25, 11, and 4 percent (available from Paragon Services, P.O. Box 113, Lower Sackville, Nova Scotia, Canada B4C 2S8). Low-contrast acuity charts have been reported to detect visual loss hidden to the Snellen test in patients with neuropathies (Drucker et al. 1988), central serous chorioretinopathy (Lerner et al. 1986), macular degeneration (Kleiner et al. 1988), glaucoma

(Regan and Neima 1984; Moskowitz et al. 1985), diabetes (Regan and Neima 1984; Harnois, Deziel, and Marcotte 1987), multiple sclerosis (Regan and Maxner 1986; Regan and Neima 1983), and Parkinson's disease (Regan and Maxner 1987; Regan and Neima 1984). In Parkinson's disease (PD), however, printed charts have the disadvantage that they are static, and the visual loss resulting from PD is best revealed by temporally modulated stimuli of low contrast (Bodis-Wollner et al. 1987; Regan and Maxner 1987).

The rationale of low-contrast acuity charts is as follows. The everyday visual environment contains objects of many different contrasts and many different sizes. For the purpose of illustration let us separately consider (A) high (near l00 percent)-contrast objects of all sizes, (B) fairly high (50 percent)-contrast objects of all sizes, (C) medium (25 percent)-contrast objects of all sizes, (D) low (11 percent)-contrast objects of all sizes, and (E) very low (4 percent)-contrast objects of all sizes. Visual acuities for letters of 96, 50, 25, 11, and 4 percent contrast tell us the smallest size of object that can be recognized for each of the five classes of real-world object (A through E) just listed (for a specified level of light adaptation and specified glare conditions). In order to predict visual performance in the everyday environment, one mentally divides real-world objects into classes (A through E) above and asks "What is the contrast of the object you wish to see?" Then one states the visual acuity for that class of object. For example, suppose that at a given level of light adaptation and in minimal-glare conditions two eyes have the same acuity for the 96 percent contrast chart, but one of these eyes has a decimal visual acuity of 0.8 for the 11 percent chart while the second eye has an acuity of only 0.4. This suggests that, in minimal glare conditions and at a similar level of light adaptation, the two eyes would recognize a high-contrast object at the same distance, but an 11 percent contrast object (e.g., a light-colored automobile against a light-colored road) that was seen and recognized at a distance of x meters by the first eye would not be seen and recognized by the second eye until it was $x/2$ meters away.

DISEASE-CAUSED ABNORMALITIES OF DETECTION AND DISCRIMINATION OF LUMINANCE-DEFINED FORM

Contrast sensitivity loss can be caused by a large number of diseases and, with the possible exception of PD, no pattern of loss seems to be specific to any particular disease. The following pages will focus on four disease entities—cataract. glaucoma, multiple sclerosis, and Parkinson's disease

Glare Susceptibility and Cataract

Even in young eyes 10 to 20 percent of the light entering the eye is scattered (Miller and Benedek 1973) and reduces the contrast of the foveal retinal image so that a baseball player may experience difficulty in catching a fly ball that is almost in line with the sun, even when the player is careful to fixate the ball and avoid looking directly at the sun. Light scattering within the eye is more severe in the older eye and can severely degrade visual function in patients with certain eye disorders, including cataract (Nadler, Miller, and Nadler 1990). For example, glare-sensitive individuals may be so disabled by oncoming headlights that they are forced to avoid night driving.

Because the high-frequency end of the CSF is steep, it follows that the reduction of high-contrast Snellen acuity produced by glare would be a poor predictor of functional vision in everyday visual environments, and indeed this has been demonstrated experimentally (Nadler, Miller, and Nadle 1990). For that reason it has been suggested that the reduction of sine wave grating contrast sensitivity produced by glare be used as a measure of an eye's glare sensitivity. However, for the following reasons it is not self-evident that this particular measure of glare sensitivity is likely to be a good predictor of the disability caused by glare in everyday visual environments: (1) The retinal image of objects such as an automobile or a tree contains many different spatial frequency components of different orientations, and suprathreshold visual processing is nonlinear; and (2) different neurons determine contrast detection threshold and spatial discrimination thresholds (Regan et al. 1982; Regan and Beverley 1983, 1985). In any case, it is not intuitively obvious how a contrast sensitivity loss at, say, 2 cycles/degree translates into a reduction of ability to see and recognize objects in the everyday visual environment.

The low-contrast acuity procedure for measuring glare sensitivity (Regan 1991) described below is designed to give an intuitive impression of the disabling effect of glare in the everyday visual environment by measuring visual acuity for objects of 96, 50, 25, 11, and 4 percent contrast in the presence of a specified glare source. (A technique with a similar rationale has been developed simultaneously and independently by I. Bailey and M. A. Bullimore 1991.) The rationale can be understood as follows. The effect of scattered light glare is to reduce letter-reading acuity, and there is evidence that the reduction of ability increases progressively as letter contrast is progressively reduced (see figure 17.8). In the everyday visual environment this translates as follows. A low level of scattered-light glare produces a selective invisibility of small, low-contrast objects in the environment. With increased glare, low-contrast objects of all sizes disappear and small objects of medium contrast disappear also. A further increase of glare renders invisible small objects of fairly high contrast as well as rendering invisible low- and medium-contrast objects of all sizes. A still higher level renders invisible or unrecognizable all objects except large objects of fairly high contrast and all objects of high contrast.

In an experimental study, acuity was estimated from the psychometric function (a plot of percent correct reading score against letter size), thus giving credit for each letter read. The BAT™ glare source (Holladay et al. 1987) was used to collect with-glare data. This device is a hemisphere that resembles half a table tennis ball or an ice cream scoop. The hemisphere is held over the eye and diffusely illuminated by a hidden light source so that the entire peripheral visual field is illuminated. The outside world can be viewed through a small hole in the illuminated hemisphere. Figure 17.7A,C shows

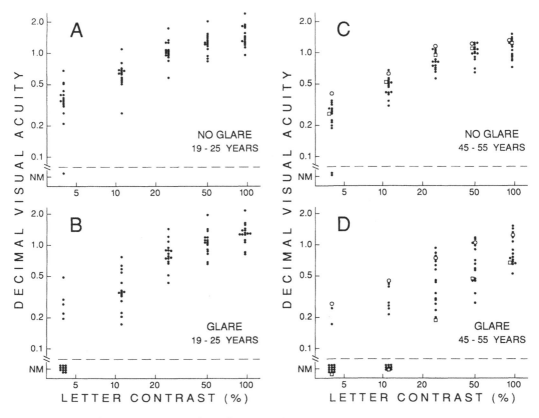

Figure 17.7 Decimal visual acuity (ordinate) vs. letter contrast (abscissa) without glare and with glare for 15 subjects aged 19 to 25 years and for 15 subjects aged 45 to 55 years. Both axes are logarithmic. Viewing was monocular, and one eye per subject was tested. Each symbol represents one eye. In the 45 to 55 years age group, a circle represents the eye shown in figure 17.8 to be least affected by glare, and a square represents the eye most affected by glare. NM on the ordinate signifies "not measurable." (From Regan 1991. Reprinted with permission)

acuity with no glare source, and figure 17.7B,D shows acuity under glare conditions with the BAT™ set at maximum luminance (3,700 cd/m²) Chart luminance remained at 40 cd/m² throughout. Figure 17.7A,B shows 15 subjects aged 19–25 years, and figure 17.7C,D shows corresponding data for 15 subjects aged 45–55. None of the 30 subjects had any history of ocular disorder.

The data for high-contrast (96 percent) Snellen acuity confirm previous findings that glare has little effect on high-contrast Snellen acuity (Nadler, Miller, and Nadler 1990). Figure 17.8, however, brings out the point that glare had a comparatively large effect on visual acuity for low-contrast letters. For some subjects glare produced a much greater loss of functional vision than in other subjects, and these intersubject differences were confirmed on retest. At a viewing distance of 6 m, several subjects were unable to read the largest (0.1 decimal VA) letters on the 4 percent chart under glare conditions, and some were even unable to read the largest (0.1 decimal VA) letters on the 11

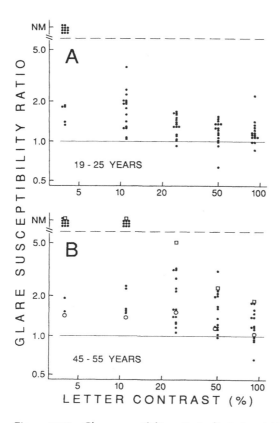

Figure 17.8 Glare susceptibility ratio (ordinates) vs. letter contrast (abscissae) obtained from the date in figure 17.7. Both axes are logarithmic. Glare susceptibility ratio was defined as decimal visual acuity for the no-glare condition divided by decimal visual acuity measured in the glare condition. (A) 15 subjects in the 19 to 25 year age group. (B) 15, subjects in the 45 to 55 year age group. Viewing was monocular. Each symbol represents one eye. NM on the ordinate signifies that acuity under glare conditions was so low that the ratio was not measurable. A circle represents the eye that was least affected by glare, and a square represents the eye that was most affected by glare. (From Regan 1991. Reprinted with permission)

percent chart. The failures are marked NM (not measurable) on the ordinate. Figures 17.7 and 17.8 show that this low-contrast acuity procedure for quantifying susceptibility to glare was sufficiently sensitive to bring out an effect of age. In the presence of glare, four individuals in the older age group were more than 2.5 standard deviations from the mean of the younger age group for the 25 percent letters, whereas no subjects in the older age group fulfilled this criterion for the high (96 percent)-contrast letters (figure 17.7D).

Our preliminary finding is that glare test results correlate with subjective estimates of glare disability caused by approaching headlights in night-time driving (scale of 1 through 3). Note that high susceptibility to glare does not necessarily correlate with poor acuity: in minimal-glare conditions visual acuities were closely similar for the 96, 50, 25, and 11 percent charts for the subjects represented by open squares and open circles in Figure 17.7C, but glare had very different effects on these two subjects (figures 17.7D and 17.8B).

Perhaps functional susceptibility to glare for an object of given contrast might usefully be quantified in terms of ratio $(DVA)_{NG}/(DVA)_G$, where $(DVA)_{NG}$ is decimal visual acuity in minimal glare conditions (no glare source) and $(DVA)_G$ is decimal visual acuity in a specified glare condition. This "glare susceptibility ratio" is plotted as the ordinate in figure 17.8 This index of disability glare might be of use in quantifying intersubject differences in glare disability in relation to night-time driving or driving in low-sun conditions. The index might also be of use in screening aircraft pilots who are required to fly in high-glare environments, and a prospective study of this question is in progress.

Glaucoma and Ocular Hypertension

Contrast Sensitivity Fields for Pattern and Motion in Glaucoma and Ocular Hypertension During the last few years a number of clinical psychophysicists have attempted to find a test that predicts which patients with ocular hypertension will go on to develop glaucoma. Within that restricted context, results have so far been disappointing in that the percentage of OHT patients with psychophysical abnormalities is considerably greater than the percentage of OHT patients who, in longitudinal studies, go on to develop glaucoma. On the other hand, these research efforts should not be regarded as entirely unsuccessful, because they have shown that OHT can produce occult—but, nevertheless, real—abnormalities of visual processing. Such studies can advance our understanding of the mechanisms of glaucoma. For example, when a bright homogeneous spot of light is used as a test target, some patients with OHT and glaucoma have been found to be insensitive to flicker in areas of the peripheral field that seem normal when perimetrically tested with a bright nonflickering spot of light (Tyler 1981; Tytla, Trope, and Buncic 1990); some patients show a reduction of foveal flicker sensitivity at low spatial frequencies (Atkin et al. 1980); and color vision changes have been observed that are not completely predicted by perimetric and visual acuity abnormalities (Drance et al. 1981).

In two studies of the peripheral visual field in patients with OHT and glaucoma, we found that gratings of low spatial frequency can reveal field defects that are not evident when fields are mapped using classical clinical techniques. It was previously known that, in control subjects, contrast sensitivity for a grating of fixed diameter falls off with eccentricity. In particular, log threshold is approximately proportional to eccentricity up to an eccentricity of 24 deg, and the slope of the line increases with spatial frequency (Robson and Graham 1982; Regan and Beverley, 1983). In patients we measured the following four kinds of visual field: (1) contrast sensitivity fields for a 2 c/deg sine wave grating that was counterphase-modulated at 8 Hz; (2) as (1) for a 5 c/deg grating; (3) grating acuity for a sine wave grating of fixed high contrast; (4) clinical fields using an automated (Octopus™) perimeter;

and (5) in selected cases, the modified Drance-Armaly method (Rock, Drance, and Morgan 1971) on the Goldman perimeter.

In glaucoma patients acuity fields merely confirmed the field defects revealed by Octopus™ or Goldman perimetry. But in four patients with glaucoma contrast sensitivity fields revealed field defects that were not evident in the clinical fields. Of 15 patients with OHT, eight had visual field defects at low spatial frequencies. All 15 patients had normal Octopus™ and Goldman fields and, in addition, had normal acuity fields for a grating of high contrast.

In the study just described, the patients' task was merely to detect that the test stimulus (a circular area of 3.5 deg diameter) was not a blank, steadily illuminated patch of light. Historically, this has been a common procedure in clinical studies of contrast sensitivity. However, although the procedure has the advantage of simplicity, the experimenter does not know what the patient saw that distinguished the stimulus from a blank steadily illuminated patch of light. Furthermore, the experimenter does not know whether the patient saw different things when the stimulus had different locations in the visual field and/or had different spatial frequencies.

In an attempt to grapple with this problem we used an approach that was already well known in basic research (Tulunay-Keesey 1972; Kulikowski and Tolhurst 1973; Tolhurst 1973), though less so in clinical studies (MacCana, Kulikowski, and Bhargava, 1983). Patients set two contrast thresholds for each stimulus location in the visual field. In this kind of experiment, ensuring that the experimenter has control over the subject's two sensory criteria presents a problem in psychophysical methodology. We tried to deal with this problem by capitalizing on our finding that, in some situations, as the contrast of a counterphase-modulated grating is slowly raised from zero, the impression of a steady blank field changes to an impression of steady bars extending across the screen, and not until the contrast is somewhat higher than this pattern threshold is there any impression that the bars are flickering or moving. For many subjects this is the situation at 15 to 20 deg eccentricity, especially for a target of moderately high spatial frequency (Regan and Neima 1984).

A different situation usually obtains for a target of low spatial frequency and high temporal frequency, especially in foveal vision. In that case, the initial impression is one of diffuse blobs that move and flicker, and not until contrast is raised somewhat above this "flicker or motion threshold" is there an impression of bars extending across the screen (Tulunay-Keesey 1972). Figure 17.9 illustrates this point. To establish the two threshold criteria we familiarized patients with the appearance of the grating at contrast threshold when viewed foveally and when viewed at an eccentricity of 20 deg, rather than using words to describe the two criteria. We chose a 2 c/deg sine wave grating that was counterphase-modulated at 8 Hz on the grounds that this stimulus provides roughly equal excitation to the sustained and transient channels of human psychophysics (Kulikowski and Tolhurst 1973; Tolhurst 1973). The aim was to find whether visual disorders could have a different effect on visual sensitivity to motion/flicker and to pattern. Visual fields were

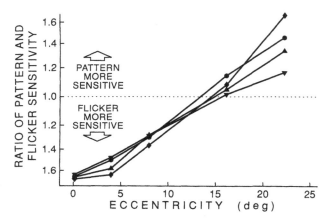

Figure 17.9 Ratios between pattern threshold and flicker threshold plotted vs. eccentricity in the visual field for the four oblique half meridia as follows: circles, upper left; diamonds, upper right; inverted triangles, lower left; triangles, lower right. The horizontal dotted line indicates equality of flicker and pattern thresholds. Above the dotted line, pattern sensitivity was higher than flicker sensitivity. Mean ratios are shown for 10 control subjects. (From Regan and Neima 1984. Reprinted with permission)

mapped for 10 patients with ocular hypertension, 6 patients with glaucoma, 10 patients with MS, and 10 control subjects. Clinical visual fields were obtained using both Octopus™ Goldman perimeters.

For many patients the balance between motion/flicker and pattern thresholds was abnormal in part or all of the visual fields. For example, of 10 patients with OHT and normal clinical visual fields eight had a significantly abnormal ratio between motion/flicker and pattern thresholds at some location in the visual field. In some patients motion/flicker sensitivity was depressed relative to pattern. In other patients the converse was true. The technique revealed diffuse visual field abnormality in both OHT and glaucoma patients.

Two Possible Physiological Bases for Contrast Sensitivity Field Defects in Glaucoma and Ocular Hypertension   The above findings could be understood if the visual field defects revealed in OHT patients by means of the temporally modulated 2 c/deg grating were specific for neurons that respond strongly to low contrasts. In terms of the distinction between magnocellular and parvocellular streams in the monkey's visual pathway, our psychophysical findings imply selective damage to magnocellular-stream neurons, because cells in the magnocellular layers of the LGN have contrast sensitivities for temporally modulated gratings of low spatial frequency (Merigan and Eskin 1986) that are in general considerably higher than those of cells in the parvocellular layers.

At the time we carried out these studies, most authors favored the hypothesis that clinical visual field defects in glaucoma are caused by axonal damage and consequent ganglion cell loss associated with ischemia at the optic disc (Schwartz, Rieser, and Fishbein 1977) or with mechanical stress near the disc

(Quigley, Addicks, and Green 1982; Henkind 1978), though other authors had suggested a second mechanism in glaucoma on the basis both of color vision changes (Drance et al. 1981) and of fundus examination (Henkind 1978). On the basis of our findings we proposed a second mechanism with a retinal site. In particular we reasoned that, if retinal function were moderately compromised by elevated pressure (e.g., by locally reduced blood supply), some neural signals initiated from synapses on dendrites would fail to reach the cell body, and the most vulnerable signals would be those that had farthest to travel. Then, for any given dendritic tree, synapses on the most peripheral dendritic processes would be the first to lose their ability to affect neural firing. We suggested that the biggest dendritic trees would be the most vulnerable, and these presumably belong to the ganglion cells with large receptive fields that govern visual sensitivity to our low spatial frequency test grating (Regan and Neima 1984). Because the biggest dendritic trees are located in peripheral retina, our hypothesis can also explain why dynamic contrast sensitivity field defects were commonly located eccentrically (Regan and Neima 1984; Neima, LeBlanc, and Regan 1984). Following this line of thought, and taking into account evidence that the magnocellular stream is important for visual sensitivity to motion (Shapley and Perry 1986), preferential damage to large ganglion cells could explain why some patients had elevated contrast threshold for motion/flicker perception while retaining normal contrast threshold for pattern perception. In the context of selective damage to motion-sensitive neurons, the recent report of Silverman, Trick, and Hart (1990) that thresholds for coherent motion within an extended (60 × 60 deg) centrally viewed display was elevated in some patients with OHT is of special interest.

The finding that contrast sensitivity fields for low spatial frequencies revealed damage that was far more diffuse than that revealed by clinical perimetry or by acuity perimetry may be relevant to the report of Quigley and his colleagues (Quigley, Addicks, and Green 1982; Quigley, Dunkelberger, and Green 1989) that a high proportion of ganglion cells can be lost before there is any field loss evident to clinical perimetry. Because ganglion cells with large dendritic fields have thick axons, our suggestion that the largest ganglion cells are most vulnerable to OHT and glaucoma may be related to the finding that axons of large diameter are preferentially affected in glaucoma (Quigley et al. 1987; Quigley, Dunkelberge, and Green 1988).

Multiple Sclerosis and Optic Neuritis

The Several Patterns of Contrast Sensitivity Loss in Multiple Sclerosis and Optic Neuritis   As noted above, patients with MS or optic neuritis who have normal visual acuity can show contrast sensitivity loss for grating stimuli. In some patients the contrast sensitivity loss depends on orientation, and when the loss is restricted to low and/or intermediate spatial frequencies it cannot be attributed to astigmatism (Regan et al. 1980; Kupersmith et al. 1984; Hess and Plant 1981; Regan and Maxner 1986). Orientation selectivity

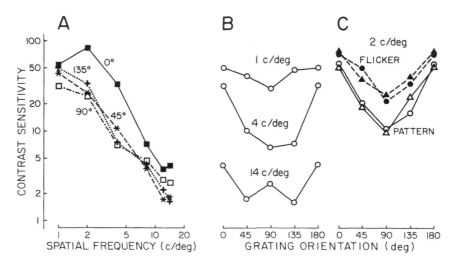

Figure 17.10 (A) Contrast sensitivity for pattern perception vs. grating spatial frequency. Filled square, 0 deg (vertical) grating orientation; open square, 90 deg (horizontal) orientation; asterisks; 45 deg orientation; plus, 135 deg orientation. (B) Contrast sensitivity for pattern perception vs. grating orientation for 8 Hz counterphase-modulated gratings of three spatial frequencies. (C) Contrast sensitivity for flicker perception (filled symbols) and pattern perception (open symbols) vs. grating orientation for a 2 c/deg, 8 Hz grating. Two sets of data obtained on two different days were plotted to indicate reproducibility. (From Regan and Maxner 1986. Reprinted with permission)

can be considerable. Figure 17.10B shows a 5:1 sensitivity ratio between horizontal and vertical thresholds at 4 c/deg. Ratios as large as 20:1 have been reported (Regan et al., 1980). On the grounds that strong orientation selectivity is not seen in neurons peripheral to striate cortex in nonhuman primates, we suggested that, in patients whose low-frequency loss is tuned to orientation, the damage responsible is at least in part sited at or central to striate cortex (Regan et al. 1980).

In this context it is interesting that, in some patients with MS and optic neuritis, the orientation selectivity of contrast sensitivity loss can be different at corresponding points in the left and right eyes (Regan et al. 1980; Kupersmith et al. 1983, 1984; Regan and Maxner 1986). Figure 17.11 illustrates this point. If the orientation-selective loss is caused by damage at or central to the striate cortex, this finding suggests that monocularly driven neurons are involved. Involvement of monocularly driven neurons is also consistent with the finding that the distribution of contrast sensitivity loss within the visual field can be patchy, with different distributions in the left and right eyes. Figure 17.12 illustrates this point.

Now we turn to the finding that pattern and motion-flicker thresholds can be differentially affected by MS. Some authors have claimed that the difference between pattern threshold and flicker/motion threshold (discussed above) is due merely to a criterion difference and that only one sensory mechanism is involved (Burbeck 1981; Derrington and Henning 1981). However, observa-

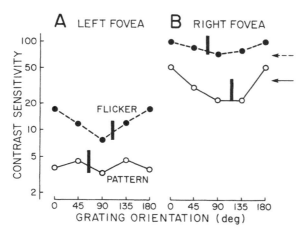

Figure 17.11 An example of completely selective orientation tuning for flicker in the fovea of one eye (A), while the fovea of the other eye showed alomost the converse: the effect of orientation was considerably stronger for pattern than for flicker (B). Horizontal arrows, lower normal 99 percent limits for contrast sensitivity for flicker (dashed line) and pattem (continuous line); vertical bars, if the distance between the highest and lowest points in the graph exceeds the length of the bar, then the effect of orientation is greater than norrnal at the 99 percent level. From Regan and Maxner 1986. Reprinted with permission)

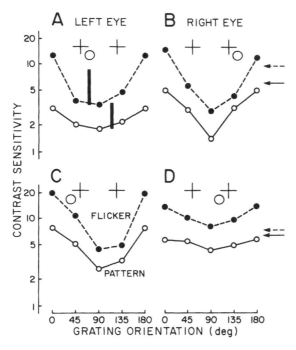

Figure 17.12 Contrast sensitivity for flicker (filled symbols) and pattern (open symbols) at 8 deg eccentricity at two corresponding sites in the left and right eyes. Inserts indicate stimulus location (circles) relative to the fovea (plusses). The pattem of loss could be quite different between different retinal sites and between corresponding points in the two eyes. Other details as for figure 17.11. (From Regan and Maxner 1986. Reprinted with permission)

tions on patients with MS conflict with this idea, and they indicate that the different contrast thresholds for pattern perception and for motion/flicker perception observed in control subjects reflect the existence of two neural mechanisms. Multiple sclerosis can alter the balance between thresholds for flicker and pattern in both foveal and peripheral visual fields (MacCana et al. 1983; Regan and Neima 1984). For example, in 10 patients the balance between pattern and flicker thresholds was upset in six, two of whom had a relative loss of flicker sensitivity while four of whom had a relative loss of pattern sensitivity (Regan and Neima 1984). In a series of 18 patients, foveal pattern sensitivity in six patients depended on orientation, but flicker/motion sensitivity did not; in three patients, flicker/motion sensitivity depended on orientation, but pattern sensitivity did not; and in seven patients both flicker/motion and orientation sensitivity depended on orientation (Regan and Maxner 1986). Figure 17.11 illustrates a case in which the left fovea showed orientation-tuned selectivity for flicker while the right fovea showed orientation-tuned selectivity for pattern. This finding indicates that (1) both motion/flicker and pattern thresholds are determined by orientation-tuned mechanisms, and (2) motion/flicker and pattern thresholds are determined by different mechanisms.

Possible Physiological Causes of Contrast Sensitivity Loss in Multiple Sclerosis and Optic Neuritis   Five candidate explanations for the findings listed above have been suggested, bearing in mind that different mechanisms of loss may occur in different patients and that in any given patient more than one of the proposed pathphysiological mechanisms may be effective at the same time.

1. One possible mechanism is that the spatial frequency specificity of loss is due to the well-known progressive increase of neural receptive field size with increasing eccentricity (K. Ruddock, personal communication 1978; W. Richards personal communication 1978; Hess and Plant 1986). The argument goes as follows. Suppose that a patient fixated the center of a circular stimulus field whose radius was, for example, 3 deg. Because the central fovea has the highest acuity, a small scotoma of, say, 0.5 deg radius would produce a loss of sensitivity to high spatial frequency gratings, but sensitivity to low spatial frequency gratings would be relatively unaffected because the area of the visual field between 0.5 and 3.0 deg radius was intact. Conversely, the effect of a circular annular scotoma extending from, say, 0.5 to 3.0 deg radius would have little effect on sensitivity to the highest spatial frequencies because the central fovea area is left intact, but sensitivity to low spatial frequencies would be relatively depressed. Because neural receptive field sizes are intermediate at intermediate eccentricities, a circular annular scotoma extending for, say, 0.5 to 1.0 deg radius would preferentially reduce sensitivity to gratings of intermediate spatial frequency.

It is difficult to see how this hypothesis could account for the finding that patients with normal Snellen acuity who were able to read high-contrast letters subtending 6.25 min arc or better were unable to read low-contrast letters subtending 25 min arc; in these patients, low-contrast visual loss existed within visual field areas less than 0.5 deg in diameter (Regan and Maxner 1986). Secondly, spatial frequency—specific visual loss is shown by patients with visual fields that are either intact or do not have the visual field loss required by hypothesis 1 (figure 17.4 and Regan and Maxner, 1986). Further objections to hypothesis 1 are that it does not explain low-frequency selective loss at peripheral sites; it does not explain orientation selectivity; and in itself it does not account for the different elevations of pattern versus flicker thresholds.

2. The second possible mechanism does not depend on the progressive increase of neural receptive field size with eccentricity. Contrast sensitivity loss is regarded as an aspect of visual field loss; contrast thresholds for a horizontal low-frequency grating will be higher than contrast thresholds for a vertical grating in regions of the visual field where the field loss reduces the effective area to a horizontal slit.

Although this mechanism may be effective in some patients, it seems unlikely that it is universally applicable. For example, even though the high-contrast and low-contrast isopters for the patient of figure 17.10 showed some vertical compression, this was far less than is required to explain 500 percent orientational tuning at 2 c/deg The ratio of horizontal to vertical sensitivities was changed by no more than about 50 percent when the visual field was restricted to a 1.0-deg slit in control subjects (Regan and Maxner, 1986).

3. The third possible mechanism is that orientational-selective visual loss is due to a directionally selective abnormality of eye movements. This is plausible because eye movement abnormalities are common in patients with MS. In particular, one might expect some patients with nystagmus to experience an orientation-selective loss of visual acuity and contrast sensitivity that is greatest for grating orientations perpendicular to the direction of eye movement. However, as noted earlier (Regan et al. 1980), it is difficult to understand how this mechanism could explain the presence of orientation tuning at low and/or intermediate spatial frequencies in cases in which high spatial frequencies are spared and grating acuity does not depend on orientation (e.g., figure 17.10B Regan et al. 1980), and in patients with no evident nystagmus.

4. As already mentioned, the fourth possible mechanism is monocular diplopia. However, although this mechanism may be involved in some cases of contrast sensitivity loss where acuity is relatively spared, it is easy to segregate patients and control subjects with chronic or transient diplopia by means of a preliminary screening. In any case, monocular diplopia cannot account for contrast sensitivity loss that is different in different parts of the field (Regan and Maxner 1986; Hess and Plant 1986), loss that extends over a broad range of low and intermediate frequencies (figures 17.4 and 17.5), nor does it explain cases in which flicker and pattern sensitivities are differentially affected (Regan and Neima 1984; Brussel et al. 1984) or in which contrast sensitivity loss is temporally as well as spatially tuned (Regan and Maxner 1986; Bodis-Wollner et al. 1984).

5. The fifth possible mechanism requires that several neural elements are driven from a single location in the visual field and that different elements respond best to different spatial frequencies and orientations (Braddick et al. 1978; Wilson and Bergen 1984; Wilson and Gelb 1984; De Valois and De Valois 1980). It has been suggested that MS can selectively reduce the sensitivity of such low, intermediate, or high-frequency elements (Regan et al. 1977) Recent findings in monkeys are relevant to this suggestion. Merigan and Eskin (1986) showed that, although the parvocellular stream plays a role in detecting static gratings of low spatial frequency, the magnocellular stream alone determines the detection of such gratings when they are temporally modulated. Accordingly, we suggested that an elevation of *motion/flicker threshold* for a temporally modulated grating of low spatial frequency (e.g., figures 17.10C, 17.11A, and 17.12A,B,C) is caused by damage to magnocellular-stream Y cells, while elevation of pattern threshold for the same temporally modulated grating (e.g., figures 17.10C, 17.11B, and 17.12B,C) is caused by damage to magnocellular-stream X cells (Regan and Maxner 1986).

Parkinson's Disease

Contrast Sensitivity Loss in Parkinson's Disease   Some patients with PD who have normal visual acuity for high-contrast letters show visual acuity loss for static low-contrast letters (Regan and Neima 1984) or contrast sensitivity loss for static gratings of low spatial frequency (Kupersmith et al 1982; Bulens et al 1986). However, the number of patients with reduced sensitivity to low-contrast targets is higher when temporally modulated rather than static test gratings are used. The severity of loss is also increased (Bodis-Wollner et al. 1987; Regan and Maxner 1987).

Bodis-Wollner documented this finding by measuring contrast sensitivity at many spatial frequencies for patients with PD. Figure 17.13 shows the mean contrast sensitivity curve for a control group (open triangles) with the characteristic peak at 2 to 5 c/deg obtained with counterphase-modulated gratings and compares it with corresponding data from two patients with PD. Bodis-Wollner described this finding as a narrowing of the bandwidth of the curve combined with a disappearance of low-frequency inhibition (Bodis-Wollner et al. 1987).

Contrast sensitivity loss is tuned to orientation in many patients with PD (Regan and Maxner 1987; Bulens et al. 1988) much as is described above for patients with MS. A second point of similarity with MS is that contrast sensitivity loss can be different at corresponding points in left and right eyes. A third point of similarity is that thresholds for pattern and for flicker/motion can be differentially affected. No explanation has been offered for this similarity in the visual manifestations of two diseases with such different etiologies.

Figure 17.14 details the effect of temporal frequency on orientation tuning in two patients with PD (Regan and Maxner 1987). Contrast sensitivity loss was greatest at about 4 to 8 Hz for the 2 c/deg grating used, and it fell off

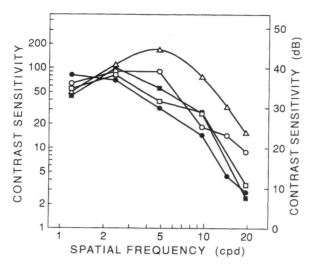

Figure 17.13   Spatial contrast sensitivity (1/contrast threshold) to a 4 deg, field is presented as a function of spatial frequency for the mean normal curve (open triangles) for each eye of a 60-year-old PD patient (right eye as open circle, left eye as filled circle), and for each eye of a 51-year-old PD patient (right eye as open square, left eye as filled square). Spatial contrast sensitivity is also shown in terms of decibels (dB) on the right vertical axis. (From Bodis-Wollner and Regan 1991. Reprinted with permission)

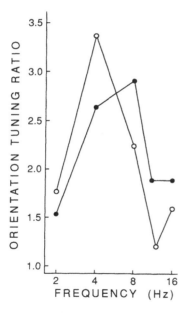

Figure 17.14   The effect of counterphase modulation frequency on the orientation selectivity of contrast sensitivity loss. The orientation tuning ratio is defined as the ratio of the highest to the lowest contrast sensitivity among four grating orientations (horizontal, vertical, and the two obliques). Data are shown for two patients with Parkinson's disease. The grating had a spatial frequency of 2 c/deg, subtended 3.5 deg, and was viewed foveally with one eye. (From Regan and Maxner 1987. Reprinted with permission.)

steeply at lower and higher frequencies. For the two patients shown, contrast sensitivity loss was highest for horizontal gratings. The quantity plotted as ordinate in figure 17.14 is the ratio between the lowest and highest contrast sensitivity among four grating orientations. (Note that the oblique effect is observed only for gratings of much higher spatial frequency than the 2 c/deg used here.)

Returning to figure 17.13, we note that control subJects, increasing the counterphase-modulation frequency of the test grating enhances contrast sensitivity in the 2 to 5 c/deg range, and the average increase is a little less than 2:1 (Robson 1966). Bodis-Wollner et al. (1987) found that for 8 out of 17 patients with PD this enhancement was abnormally low.

In normal human volunteers, the administration of dopaminergic drugs can improve contrast sensitivity, while the administration of dopaminergic blockers produces a similar loss of contrast sensitivity and change in the shape of the CSF as is shown in figure 17.13 (Domenici et al. 1985). This finding was the logical basis for a recent study on a single patient with PD. Contrast threshold for a 3.5 c/deg grating was tested when the grating was static and when it was counterphase-modulated at 8 Hz (Giaschi et al. 1992). After overnight withdrawal of medication, contrast sensitivity was markedly elevated when the grating was temporally modulated, but not when it was static. Within 90 minutes of restarting medication, dynamic contrast sensitivity was back to normal. This finding implies that the selective loss of contrast sensitivity for the temporally modulated grating was not caused by long-term damage to contrast-sensitive neurons, but rather directly by the absence of dopamine. Bodis-Wollner et al. (1987) studied patients with the on/off syndrome, and came to a similar conclusion. However, in spite of the selective loss of dynamic contrast sensitivity just described, a test of motion processing (recognition of motion-defined letters) showed no change during withdrawal of medication (Giaschi et al. 1992). A possible explanation is that, because the motion-defined letters were rendered visible by the relative motion of small dots, the initial encoding of motion was restricted to high spatial frequency mechanisms, while PD preferentially affects low spatial frequency mechanisms.

Possible Physiological Causes of Contrast Sensitivity Loss in Patients with Parkinson's Disease   We suggested that magnocellular stream Y-type neurons are preferentially damaged in patients who show contrast sensitivity loss for temporally modulated gratings of low spatial frequency (Regan and Maxner 1987). Our reasoning was the same as in the case of multiple sclerosis (see above). It was earlier suggested that the changes in spatiotemporal contrast sensitivity observed in PD are due to increased spatial summation caused by decreased surround inhibition that is caused, in turn, by a reduced level of retinal dopamine (Bodis-Wollner 1990). However, the finding that contrast sensitivity loss depends markedly on orientation in some patients implies that retinal dysfunction is not the whole story because, as noted earlier, precortical neurons are not strongly tuned to orientation.

ACKNOWLEDGMENTS

This chapter was partly based on research sponsored by the U.S. Air Force Office of Scientific Research (grant AFOSR-91-0080) and supported by the National Eye Institute; National Institutes of Health, Bethesda, MD; the Medical Research Council of Canada; the Multiple Sclerosis Society of Canada; and the Natural Sciences and Engineering Research Council of Canada.

NOTES

1. In practice, the pattern of loss observed may depend on grating orientation (Regan et al. 1980; Camisa, Mylin, and Bodis-Wollner 1981), grating temporal frequency (Bodis-Wollner et al. 1987; Regan and Maxner 1986, 1987), and location in the visual field (Regan and Maxner 1986, 1987; Regan and Neima 1984; Neima, LeBlanc, and Regan 1984; Hess and Plant 1986; Plant and Hess 1987).

2. The idea was even more obvious than I thought. According to Professor L. Frisen (personal communication, 1983), low-contrast letter charts were first described by a Swedish ophthalmologist in 1889. But, although the idea is literally antique, what is new is the possibility of understanding the results of a low-contrast letter test in terms of modern psychophysics and primate neurophysiology. Among modern letter charts, the Pelli-Robson chart provides a convenient means of measuring contrast sensitivity for letter recognition. Although the currently available Pelli-Robson chart offers only one letter size, there is no reason in principle why the same procedure should not be used for several letter sizes. The Regan letter charts measure visual acuity for letters of a given contrast, as does the chart described by Bailey (1982). The Regan charts provide eleven letter sizes, eight letters per line, and five contrasts (96, 50, 25, 11, and 4 percent). Different letter sequences are available for the purpose of repeat testing. There has been some discussion as to whether the Pelli-Robson and Regan charts provide the same data. It is possible that, if the patients' criterion was not adequately controlled by a forced-choice procedure, then the two kinds of charts might give different results. It is also possible that, because the number of letters per line on the two charts is different, the test-retest variability might be a little different. But, these minor points apart, there is no reason to suppose that the two kinds of charts do not provide essentially the same kind of data.

REFERENCES

Apkarian P, Tijssen R, Spekreijse H, Regan D (1987) Origin of notches in CSF: optical or neural? Invest Ophthalmol Vis Sci 28:607–612.

Atkin A, Wolkstein M, Bodis-Wollner I, Anders M, Kels B, Podos SM (1980) Interocular companson of contrast sensitivities in glaucoma patients and suspects. Brit J Ophthalmol 64: 858–862.

Bailey I. Simplifying contrast sensitivity testing (1982) Amer J Optom Physiol Opt 59:12P.

Bailey IL, Bullimore M (1992) A new test for the evaluation of disability glare. Optom Vis Sci 68:911–917.

Bergen JR (1991) Theories of visual texture perception. In: Spatial vision (Regan D, ed), pp 114–134. London: Macmillan.

Beverley KI, Regan D (1980) Device for measuring the precision of eye-hand coordination while tracking changing size. Aviat Space Environ Med 51:688– 693.

Blakemore C, Campbell FW (1969) On the existence of neurons within the human visual system selectively sensitive to the onentation and size of retinal images. J Physiol 15:439–440.

Blakemore C, Nachmias J (1971) The orientational specificity of two visual aftereffects. J Physiol 213, 157–174.

Bodis-Wollner I (1972) Visual acuity and contrast sensitivity in patients with cerebral lesions. Science 178:769–771.

Bodis-Wollner I (1987) The role of dopamine in vision and its impairment in Parkinson's disease. Arch Neurol 44:1209.

Bodis-Wollner I (1990) Visual deficits related to dopamine deficiency in experimental animals and Parkinson's disease patients. Trends in Neurosci 13:296–302.

Bodis-Wollner I, Hendley CD, Mylin LH, Thornton J (1979) Visual evoked potentials and the visuogram in multiple sclerosis. Ann Neurol 5:40–7.

Bodis-Wollner I, Marx MS, Mitra S, Bobak P, Mylin L, Yahr M (1987) Visual dysfunction in Parkinson's disease—loss in spatiotemporal contrast sensitivity. Brain 110:1675–1698.

Bodis-Wollner I, Mitra S, Bobak P, Guillory S, Mylin L (1984) Low frequency distortion in spatio-temporal surface in Parkinson's disease. Invest Ophthalmol Vis Sci (Suppl 25):313.

Bodis-Wollner I, Regan D (1991) Spatiotemporal contrast vision in Parkinson's disease and MPTP-treated monkeys: the role of dopamine. In: Vision and visual function (Regan D, ed), pp 250–260. London: Macmillan.

Braddick OJ, Campbell FW, Atkinson J (1978) Channels in vision: Basic aspects. In: Handbook of sensory physiology (Vol VIII, Perception) (Held R, Leiowitz H, Teuber HL, eds). Berlin: Spnnger.

Brussel EM, White CW, Mustillo P, Overbury O (1984) Inferences about mechanisms that mediate pattern and flicker sensitivity. Percept Psychophys 35:301–304.

Bulens C, Meerwaldt JD, van der Wildt GJ (1988) Effect of stimulus orientation on contrast sensitivity in Parkinson's disease. Neurology 38:76–81.

Bulens C, Meerwaldt JD, van der Wildt GJ, Keemink CK (1986) Contrast sensitivity in Parkinson's disease. Neurology 36:1121–1125.

Bulens C, Meerwaldt JD, van der Wildt GJ, Van Deursen JBP (1987) Effect of levodopa treatment on contrast sensitivity in Parkinson's disease. Ann Neurol 22:365–369.

Burbeck CA (1981) Criterion-free pattern and flicker thresholds. J Opt Soc Am 71:1343–1350.

Campbell FW, Green DG (1965) Optical and retinal factors affecting visual resolution. J Physiol 18:576–93.

De Valois RL, De Valois K (1980) Spatial vision. Ann Rev Psychol 31:309–341.

Camisa J, Mylin LH, Bodis-Wollner I (1981) The effect of stimulus orientation on the visual evoked potential in multiple sclerosis. Ann Neurol 10:532–9.

Derrington AM, Henning CB (1981) Pattern discrimination with flickering stimuli. Vision Res 21, 597–602.

Domenici L, Trimarchi C, Piccolino M, Fiorentini A, Maffei L (1985) Dopaminergic drugs improve human visual contrast sensitivity. Hum Neurobiol 4:195–197.

Drance SM, Lakowski R, Schulzer M (1981) Acquired color vision changes in glaucoma. Arch Ophthalmol 99:829–31.

Drucker MD, Savino PJ, Sergott RC, Bosley TM, Schatz NJ, Kubilis PS (1988) Low-contrast letter test to detect subtle neuropathies. Amer J Ophthalmol 105:141–145.

Fresco B, Giaschi D, Regan D (1991) Sensitive measurement of glare susceptibility in cataract patients. Invest Ophthalmol Vis Sci (Suppl. 32):1084.

Frisen L, Sjostrand J (1978) Contrast sensitivity in optic neuritis: a preliminary report. Documenta Ophthalmol Proc Ser 17:165-74.

Giaschi D, Regan D, Kothe A, Hong XH, Sharpe J (1991) Multiple sclerosis can degrade detection and/or discrimination of motion-defined form while sparing motion sensitivity. Invest Ophthalmol Vis Sci (Suppl. 32):1282.

Giaschi D, Regan D, Kothe A, Hong XH, Sharpe J (1992) Motion-defined letter detection and recognition in patients with multiple sclerosis. Ann-Neurol, in press.

Giaschi D, Lang A, Reed B, Duff J, Hong XH, Regan D (1992) Motion and contrast processing in the ON and OFF periods in Parkinson's disease. Ann Neurol, submitted.

Harnois C, Deziel A, Marcotte G (1986) Contrast sensitivity of diabetic patients on contrast letter charts. Invest Ophthalmol Vis Sci 27(Suppl):307.

Henkind P (1978) Retina. In: Glaucoma (Heilmann K, Richardson KT, eds), pp 73-77. Philadelphia: Saunders.

Hess RF, Plant GT (1986) The psychophysical loss in optic neuritis: spatial and temporal aspects. In: Optic neuritis (Hess RF, Plant GT, eds), pp 109- 151. Cambridge: Cambridge University Press.

Holladay JT, Prager TC, Irajillo J et al (1987) Brightness acuity tester and outdoor visual acuity in cataract patients. J Cataract Refract Surg 13:67-69.

Kleiner RC, Enger C, Alexander MF, Fine SL (1988) Contrast sensitivity in age-related macular degeneration. Arch Ophthalmol 106:55-57.

Kulikowski JJ, Tolhurst DJ (1973) Psychophysical evidence for sustained and transient detectors in human vision. J Physiol 232:149-162.

Kulikowski JJ, Tolhurst DJ (1979) Psychophysical evidence for sustained and transient detectors in human vision. J Physiol (London) 232:149-162.

Kupersrnith MJ, Nelson JI, Seiple WH, Carr RE, Weiss PA (1983) The 20/20 eye in multiple sclerosis. Neurology 33:1015-1020.

Kupersmith MJ, Nelson JI, Seiple WH, Carr RE, Weiss PA (1984) Contrast sensitivity loss in multiple sclerosis. Invest Ophthalmol Vis Sci 25:632-639.

Kupersmith MJ, Shakin E, Siegel IM, Lieberman A (1982) Visual system abnormalities in patients with Parkinson's disease. Arch Neurol 39:284-286.

Lerner B, Ehger C, Alexander M, Fine SL (1986) Macular dysfunction after resolution of central serous chorioretinopathy. Invest Ophthalmol Vis Sci 27(Suppl):21.

MacCana F, Kulikowski JJ, Bhargava SK (1983) Changes in spatial resolution for pattern and movement detection in clinical cases. Ophthal Physiol Optom 3:47-54.

Medjbeur S, Tulunay-Keesey U (1985) Spatiotemporal responses of the visual system in demyelinating diseases. Brain 108:123-138.

Medijbeur S, Tulunay-Keesey U (1986) Suprathreshold responses of the visual system in normals and in demyelinating diseases. Invest Ophthalmol Vis Sci 27:1368-1378.

Merigan WH, Eskin TA (1986) Spatio-temporal vision of macaques with severe loss of P_β retinal ganglion cells. Vision Res 26:1751-1761.

Miller D, Benedek GB (1985) Intraocular light scattling. Illinois: Springfield.

Moskowitz A, Sokol S, Bardenstein D, Schwartz B (1985) Perforrnance of ocular hypertension and glaucoma patients on high and low contrast letter charts. Invest Ophthalmol Vis Sci (Suppl. 26):225.

Nadler MP, Miller D, Nadler DJ (1990) Glare and contrast sensitivity for clinicians. New York: Springer.

Neima D, LeBlanc R, Regan D (1984) Visual field defects in ocular hypertension and glaucoma. Arch Ophthalmol 102:1042–1045.

Paragon Services (1985) Handbook to Regan low contrast acuity charts. P.O. Box 113, Lower Sackville, Nova Scotia, Canada B4C 2S8.

Plant G, Hess RF (1987) Regional threshold contrast sensitivity within the central visual field in optic neuritis. Brain 110:489–515.

Quigley HA, Addicks EM, Green WR (1982) Optic nerve damage in human glaucoma: III qualitative correlation of nerve fibre loss and visual defect in glaucoma, ischemic neuropathy, disc edema and toxic neuropathy. Arch Ophthalmol 100:100–106.

Quigley HA, Addicks EM, Green WR (1982) Optic nerve damage in human glaucoma. Arch Ophthalmol 100:135–146.

Quigley HA, Dunkelberger GR, Green WR (1988) Chronic human glaucoma causes selectively greater loss of large optic nerve fibres. Ophthalmology 95:357–361.

Quigley HA, Dunkelberger GR, Green WR (1989) Retinal ganglion cell atrophy correlated with automated perimetry in human eyes with glaucoma. Am J Ophthalmol 107:453–459.

Quigley HA, Sanchez RM, Dunkelberger GR, L'Hemault NL, Baginski TA (1987) Chronic glaucoma selectivity damages large optic nerve fibres. Invest Ophthalmol Vis Sci 28:913–918.

Regan D (1981) Psychophysical tests of vision and hearing in patients with multiple sclerosis. In: Demyelinating disease: basic and clinical electrophysiology (Waxman SG, Ritchie JM, eds), pp 217–237. New York: Raven.

Regan D (1982) Visual information channeling in normal and disordered vision. Psych Rev 89:407–444.

Regan D (1991) Detection and spatial discriminations for objects defined by colour contrast, binoculardisparity and motion parallax. In: Spatial vision (Regan D, ed), pp. 135–178. London: Macmillan.

Regan D, Bartol S, Murray TJ, Beverley K (1982) Spatial frequency discrimination in normal vision and in patients with multiple sclerosis. Brain 105:735–754.

Regan D, Beverley K (1983) Visual fields described by contrast sensitivity, by acuity, and by relative sensitivity to different orientations. Invest Ophthalmol Vis Sci 24:754–759.

Regan D, Beverley KI (1985) Postadaptation orientation discrimination. J Opt Soc Am A2: 147–155.

Regan D, Giaschi D, Sharpe JA, Hong XH (1992) Visual processing of motion-defined form: selective failure in patients with parieto-temporal lesions. J Neurosci, in press.

Regan D, Hong HX (1992) Recognition and detection of texture-defined letters. Vision Res, submitted.

Regan D, Kothe AC, Sharpe JA (1991) Recognition of motion-defined shapes in patients with multiple sclerosis and optic neuritis. Brain 114:1179–1155.

Regan D, Maxner C (1986) Orientation-dependent loss of contrast sensitivity for pattern and flicker in multiple sclerosis. Clin Vis Sci 1:1–23.

Regan D, Maxner C (1987) Orientation-selective visual loss in patients with Parkinson's disease. Brain 110:239–271.

Regan D, Neima D (1983) Low contrast letter charts as a test of visual function. Ophthalmology 90:1192–1200.

Regan D, Neima D (1984) Balance between pattern and flicker sensitivities in the visual fields of ophthalmological patients. Br J Ophthalmol 68:310–315.

Regan D, Neima D (1984) Low-contrast letter charts in early diabetic retinopathy, ocular hypertension, glaucoma, and Parkinson's disease. Br J Ophthalmol 68:885–889.

Regan D, Neima D (1984) Visual fatigue and visual evoked potentials in multiple sclerosis, glaucoma, ocular hypertension and Parkinson's diseasee. J Neurol Neurosurg Psychiat 47:673–678.

Regan D, Raymond J, Ginsburg A, Murray TJ (1981) Contrast sensitivity, visual acuity and the discrimination of Snellen letters in multiple sclerosis. Brain 104:333–350.

Regan D, Silver R, Murray TJ (1977) Visual acuity and contrast sensitivity in multiple sclerosis—hidden visual loss. Brain 100:563–579.

Regan D, Whitlock J, Murray TJ, Beverley KI (1980) Orientation-specific losses of contrast sensitivity in multiple sclerosis. Invest Ophthalmol Vis Sci 19:324–328.

Robson JG (1966) Spatial and temporal contrast-sensitivity functions of the visual system. J Opt Soc A m 56:1141–1142.

Robson JG, Graham N (1982) Probability summation and regional variation in contrast sensitivity across the visual field. Vis Res 21:409–418.

Rock WJ, Drance SM, Morgan RW (1972) A modification of the Armaly visual field screening technique for glaucoma. Can J Ophthalmol 7:283–292.

Schwartz B, Rieser JC, Fishbein SL (1977) Fluorescein angiographic defects of the optic disc in glaucoma. Arch Ophthalmol 95:1961–1974.

Shapley R, Perry VH (1986) Cat and monkey retinal ganglion cells and their functional roles. Trends Neurosci 9:229–235.

Silverman SE, Trick GL, Hart WM Jr (1990) Motion perception is abnormal in primary open-angle glaucoma and ocular hypertension. Invest Ophthalmol Vis Sci 31:722–729.

Talhurst DJ (1973) Separate channels for the analysis of shape and movement of a moving visual stimulus. J Physiol (London) 231:384–402.

Travis D, Thompson P, Gilchrist J (1987) Monocular diplopia in multiple sclerosis. Clin Vis Sci 2:103–110.

Tulunay-Keesey U (1972) Flicker and pattem detection: a comparison of thresholds. J Opt Soc Am 62:466–468.

Tyler CW (1981) Specific defects of flicker sensitivity in glaucoma and ocular hypertension. Invest Ophthalmol Vis Sci 20:204–212.

Tytla ME, Trope GE, Buncic JR (1990) Flicker sensitivity in treated ocular hypertension. Ophthalmology 97:36–43.

Wilson HR, Gelb DJ (1984) Modified line-element theory for spatial-frequency and width discrimination. J Opt Soc Am Al:124–131.

Wilson HR, Regan D (1984) Spatial frequency adaptation and grating discrimination: predictions of a line element model. J Opt Soc Am A1:1091–1096.

Wyszecki G, Stiles WS (1967) Colour science, concepts and methods: Quantitative data and formulas. New York: Wiley.

Zimmern RL, Campbell FW, Wilkinson IMS (1979) Subtle disturbances of vision after optic neuritis elicited by studying contrast sensitivity. J Neurol Neurosurg Psychiat 42:507–512.

Retina Research Foundation

The Retina Research Foundation is a publicly supported, tax-exempt charitable organization headquartered in Houston, Texas. Since 1973 the Foundation has sustained a multifaceted basic science and clinical research program to find the causes of and cures for the many retinal diseases that annually threaten millions of citizens worldwide with the prospect of blindness or serious visual impairment. It is dedicated to the prospect that blindness is a foe that can be fought successfully through research.

The Retina Research Foundation offices are located at 6560 Fannin, Suite 2200, Houston, Texas 77030

Index

Printed in the United States
by Baker & Taylor Publisher Services